DISEASE AND DEATH
IN EARLY COLONIAL MEXICO

Dellplain Latin American Studies

Dellplain Latin American Studies

PUBLISHED IN COOPERATION WITH
THE DEPARTMENT OF GEOGRAPHY
SYRACUSE UNIVERSITY

Editor

David J. Robinson

Editorial Advisory Committee

John K. Chance
Arizona State University

William M. Denevan
University of Wisconsin

John E. Kicza
Washington State University

Asunción Lavrin
Howard University

W. George Lovell
Queen's University

Publication Design and Cartography

Marcia J. Harrington
Syracuse University

DISEASE AND DEATH IN EARLY COLONIAL MEXICO

SIMULATING AMERINDIAN DEPOPULATION

Thomas M. Whitmore

Dellplain Latin American Studies, No. 28

Westview Press

BOULDER • SAN FRANCISCO • OXFORD

Dellplain Latin American Studies

This Westview softcover edition is printed on acid-free paper and bound in library-quality, coated covers that carry the highest rating of the National Association of State Textbook Administrators, in consultation with the Association of American Publishers and the Book Manufacturers' Institute.

Copyright © 1992 by the Department of Geography, Syracuse University

Published in 1992 in the United States of America by Westview Press, Inc., 5500 Central Avenue, Boulder, Colorado 80301-2847, and in the United Kingdom by Westview Press, 36 Lonsdale Road, Summertown, Oxford OX2 7EW

Library of Congress Cataloging-in-Publication Data
Whitmore, Thomas M.
  Disease and death in early colonial Mexico : simulating
Amerindian depopulation / by Thomas M. Whitmore
    p. cm.—(Dellplain Latin American studies ; no. 28)
  Includes bibliographical references and index.
  ISBN 0-8133-8188-6
  1. Indians of Mexico—Population. 2. Indians of Mexico—
Mortality. 3. Demographic anthropology—Computer simulation.
I. Title. II. Series.
F1219.3.P73W47   1991
305.897′072—dc20

91-18346
CIP

Printed and bound in the United States of America

The paper used in this publication meets the requirements
of the American National Standard for Permanence of Paper
for Printed Library Materials Z39.48-1984.

10   9   8   7   6   5   4   3   2   1

To Andrea

Contents

List of Tables

List of Figures

Acknowledgments

Since in one sense a book is the result of all of one's life work up to the present, a truly comprehensive acknowledgment would approach the already considerable bulk of this document. For that reason, if for no other, this acknowledgement must be circumscribed. I entreat those who do not appear here not to judge me harshly for omission, for even if not publicly acknowledged, your help is sincerely appreciated.

This book is based on my doctoral dissertation at Clark University. I am in debt to my dissertation committee, for they are as congenial and helpful a group of scholars as is imaginable. Without their help this document would probably never have been attempted or completed and certainly would have been much the poorer; thank you all. Specifically, I would like to express my appreciation to my chairman, Bill Turner. Friend and critical reader, Bill's good humor, enthusiasm, and confidence in my ability inspired me. I hope his sterling example of productivity and professionalism somehow rubbed off on me. Many thanks are also due to my good friend Doug Johnson. Doug is at least partly responsible for my interest in systems and first interested me in systems dynamics. Doug's gift for competent, beautifully written expression is a benchmark to which I aspire. In large measure this work is an outgrowth of an earlier project of Robert Kates' that I had the good fortune to participate in. Bob's generous and inspirational support, especially over the rocky patches, made this labor bearable, even exciting. Thank you, Bob. I am grateful to David Robinson, whose suggestion of using population simulation to overcome some of the problems of the early colonial historical demography of the New World was the immediate inspiration for this work and whose helpful, careful reading of this manuscript is much appreciated. Acknowledgment is also needed to Sam Ratick, whose timely help with some of the difficult modeling problems is greatly appreciated. Several conversations with Bill Denevan about the issues surrounding this study were also stimulating.

I must also acknowledge the help and support of several fellow graduate students who through their example and support made this project a bit less lonely and intimidating. Thanks to Lee Dillard, Tom Downing, Dominic Golding, Abe Goldman, and Dick Perritt. Especial thanks to Mark Johnson.

In addition to my Clark "family," I owe a debt of gratitude to my family. Thank you dear Andrea; only you know how much I needed your help during this long process. To Karen, Jim, and Alan, thanks much for the encouragement, cheerful support, love, and understanding; it really helped. My mother and brother have tolerated vague reports of my progress through graduate school with equanimity; thank you for your understanding.

Many thanks to those in the Graduate School of Geography office, especially Madeleine Grinkis, whose unselfish help made coping with the University bureaucracy almost a pleasure, and Jean Heffernan for keeping the place running so smoothly. Thanks also to Joan McGrath in Clark's Research office for help in keeping my grant accounts straight.

No acknowledgment would be complete if I failed to mention the help rendered by numerous librarians, especially those at Clark's Goddard Library, particularly Mary Hartman and Kokab Arif. Thanks also to the staff at the University of California, Berkeley libraries.

Ann Gibson of Clark Cartographic competently rendered the map from my vague suggestions.

Thanks are also due to the people at High Performance Systems, especially Steve Peterson, who were helpful in sorting out some problems in STELLA.

Thanks also to Marcia Harrington of Syracuse University, whose competent and patient work on this manuscript is greatly appreciated.

This research was partially supported by a National Science Foundation doctoral dissertation improvement grant (No. SES-87116764). An article length version of this research first appeared in the *Annals of the Association of American Geographers*.

Thomas Whitmore

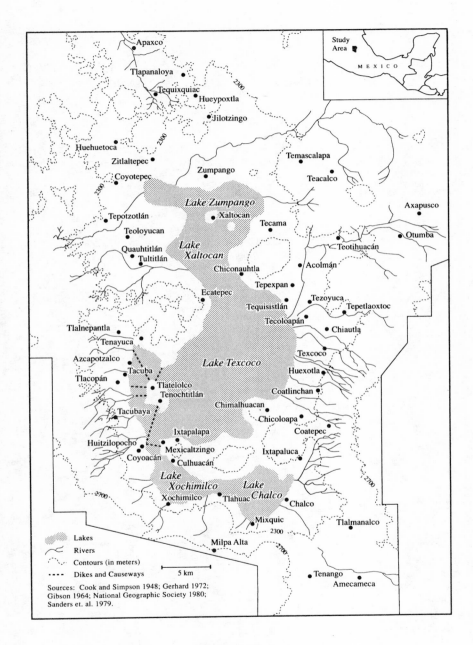

Apaxco

Tlapanaloya

Tequixquiac
Hueypoxtla

Jilotzingo

2300

Huehuetoca

Zitlaltepec

Coyotepec

Temascalapa

Zumpango

Teacalco

Axapusco

Lake Zumpango

Tepotzotlán

Xaltocan

Tecama

Teoloyucan

Lake
Xaltocan

Otumba

Quauhtitlán

Tultitlán

Teotihuacán

Chiconauhtla

Acolmán

Tepexpan

Ecatepec

Tequisistlán

Tezoyuca

Tepetlaoxtoc

Tecoloapán

Chiautla

Tlalnepantla

Tenayuca

Texcoco

Azcapotzalco

Tacuba

Lake Texcoco

Huexotla

Tlacopán

Tlatelolco

Tenochtitlán

Coatlinchan

Tacubaya

Chimalhuacan

Chicoloapa

Coatepec

Ixtapalapa

Huitzilopocho

Mexicaltzingo

Coyoacán

Culhuacán

Ixtapaluca

Lake
Xochimilco

Lake
Chalco

Xochimilco

Tlahuac

Chalco

2700

Mixquic

Tlalmanalco

2300

Milpa Alta

2700

Tenango

Amecameca

Legend:
- Lakes
- Rivers
- Contours (in meters)
- Dikes and Causeways

5 km

Sources: Cook and Simpson 1948; Gerhard 1972;
Gibson 1964; National Geographic Society 1980;
Sanders et. al. 1979.

Study
Area

MEXICO

1.1 The Study Area

Chapter 1

HOLOCAUST OR NOT? THE DEBATE ON AMERINDIAN DEPOPULATION IN THE SIXTEENTH CENTURY

Comparison with other parts of the world at comparable levels of culture leads us to throw in our lot with Rosenblat [for low pre-conquest Amerindian populations]. This saves us from having to face the second improbability ... a fall of 90 percent in the course of the sixteenth century. History knows of no population of comparable magnitude suffering such catastrophic decline.[1]

In its extent this phenomenon [the Amerindian population collapse] is without parallel in the modern history of the world's population.[2]

✛ ✛ ✛

The eve of the sixteenth-century Spanish conquest of the New World found an abundantly populated hemisphere, particularly within the regions of "high civilization" in Mesoamerica and Andean South America. But within 100 years, the Amerindian population was reduced to a struggling remnant of its former size. This Amerindian depopulation is not seriously disputed. Virtually everything else about this tragedy is: the size of the immediate pre-Colombian Amerindian populations, the magnitude of their sixteenth- and seventeenth-century declines, and the purported causes of the collapse.

While the estimates of Amerindian populations have been subject to an impressive volume of able and intense scrutiny, there remain significant

---

[1] C. McEvedy, and R. Jones, *Atlas of World Population History*, London: Penguin Books, 1978, p. 292.

[2] N. Sánchez-Albornoz, "The Population of Colonial Spanish America," in Leslie Bethell (ed.), *The Cambridge History of Latin America, Volume II: Colonial Latin America*, Cambridge: Cambridge University Press, 1984, p. 7.

differences in the reconstructions of population size, and these differences are exemplified by the "eve-of-the-conquest" hemispheric estimates. They range from greater than 100 million[3] to only 8-15 million.[4] The high estimate is substantially greater than the 60-80 million estimated for the entire European population of the time,[5] and the low estimates barely double that of the sixteenth-century Iberian population.[6] The post-conquest (ca. A.D. 1650) hemispheric population minimum is subject to less debate, with estimates ranging from approximately 4.5 million[7] to 10 million.[8]

As a consequence of these divergent estimates, the relative collapse of the sixteenth-century Amerindian populations ranges from the 18 percent loss calculated by McEvedy and Jones[9] to the 95 percent loss derived by Dobyns.[10] By comparison, the range of estimates for the fourteenth-century population holocaust due to the Black Death is less diverse. For England, McEvedy and Jones and Slack argue for a conservative figure,[11] a loss of one-third from A.D. 1300-1400, while Russell and Hatcher argue for more liberal estimates ranging from 40-50 percent loss for the same period.[12]

While the range of estimates in the debate about the scale of collapse is large, there is more agreement about its causes. Virtually all scholars recognize the primacy of epidemic disease mortality as the major cause of the Amerindian population collapse. The *conquistadores* introduced European epidemic diseases such as measles, smallpox, and typhus to an Amerindian population with no previous exposure to them, causing widespread epidemics and very high loss of life. While epidemics may have been foremost, some scholars implicate the deliberate Spanish cruelty,

---

3   H. F. Dobyns, "Estimating Aboriginal American Population: An Appraisal of Techniques with A New Hemisphere Estimate," *Current Anthropology* 7 (1966), p. 415.

4   A. L. Kroeber, *Cultural and Natural Areas of North America*, University of California Publications in American Archaeology and Ethnology Vol. 38, Berkeley: University of California Press, 1939, 81; and McEvedy and Jones, *Atlas*, p. 270.

5   Murdo J. MacLeod, *Spanish Central America A Socioeconomic History, 1520-1720*, Berkley: University of California Press, 1973, p. 18; and McEvedy and Jones, *Atlas*, p. 18.

6   McEvedy and Jones *Atlas*, p. 105.

7   Dobyns "Estimating," p. 415.

8   A. Rosenblat, *La población y el mestizaje en America*, Vol. 1. Buenos Aires: Editorial Nova, 1954, pp. 9, 102, 105, 122-4.

9   McEvedy and Jones, *Atlas*, p. 270.

10   Dobyns "Estimating," p. 415.

11   McEvedy and Jones, *Atlas*, 42; and Paul Slack, *The Impact of Plague in Tudor and Stuart England*, London: Routledge & Kegan Paul, 1985, p. 15.

12   Josiah Cox Russell, *British Medieval Population*, Albuquerque, NM, 1948, pp. 260-281; and John Hatcher, *Plague, Population and the English Economy 1348-1530*, London and Basingstoke: The Macmillan Press Ltd., 1977, p. 68.

homicide, mistreatment, and slavery in the holocaust as well.[13] Changes in the economic and social systems are claimed by others to have aided in the collapse, perhaps by leading to a loss of the "will to survive."[14]

These controversies serve as the general problematics for this study, which uses a system dynamics computer simulation methodology to examine the magnitude and causes of the immediate post-conquest population decline in one key area: the Basin of Mexico.

The Basin of Mexico: A Microcosm of the Debate

Situated in the central Mexican highlands, the Basin of Mexico is an elevated plain surrounded by high mountains on all but its northern side and there by low hills (Figure 1.1). Its morphology resembles a large, shallow, flat-bottomed bowl. This analogy is apt, since for most of its inhabited history, the Basin's most distinguishing feature was an interconnected series of large, shallow lakes that occupied much of the southern and central areas. It was a closed hydrological unit until the largest lake, Texcoco, was drained in the eighteenth century.[15]

At the beginning of the sixteenth century, the Basin possessed an agricultural complex of diversity, sophistication, and high productivity. This complex was harnessed to provide for the needs of a large urban population, centered in the island capital of Tenochtitlán-Tlateloco, and for a number of other large settlements girding the lakes. This water-bound metropolis was one of the great cities in the world on the eve of the Spanish conquest, and its population may have totaled 150-200,000.[16] The total population in the Basin at that time was undoubtedly larger than it had ever been in the past .[17]

---

13 For example, See N. Sánchez-Albornoz, *The Population of Latin America: A History*, Berkeley: University of California Press, 1974, p. 52.

14 Sherburne F. Cook and Woodrow Borah, *Essays in Population History*, Vol. 1. Berkeley: University of California Press, 1971, p. 409; and Sánchez-Albornoz, *The Population of Latin America*, p. 55.

15 Ross Hassig, *Trade, Tribute, and Transportation, The Sixteenth-Century Political Economy of the Valley of Mexico*, Norman: The University of Oklahoma Press, 1985, p. 209; and W. T. Sanders, J. R. Parsons, and R. S. Santley, *The Basin of Mexico: Ecological Processes in the Evolution of a Civilization*, New York: Academic Press, 1979, p. 81.

16 Charles Gibson, *The Aztecs Under Spanish Rule*, Stanford, California: Stanford University Press, 1964, p. 5; and Edward E. Calneck, "The Internal Structure of Tenochtitlan," in E. R. Wolf (ed.), *The Valley of Mexico, Studies in Pre-Hispanic Ecology and Society*, Albuquerque: The University of New Mexico Press, 1976, p. 288.

17 Thomas M. Whitmore, and B. L. Turner II, *Population Reconstruction of the Basin of Mexico: 1150 B.C. to Present*, Millennial Longwaves of Human Occupance Project: Technical Paper #1, Clark University, 1986, p. 3.

Because the mountain barriers served to differentiate and separate Amerindian peoples in the Basin from those without, even as the Basin's lakes served to attract and hold them, the Basin may be thought of as a "naturally" demarcated region.[18] While this region has been continuously settled since at least 1500 B.C.,[19] the pattern of settlement and population size was anything but uniform and there have been at least two long periods of population growth followed by significant decline.[20] The decline that truncated the second of these population growth "waves" (the immediate pre-Hispanic population florescence), is the subject of this study.

Because of its importance in pre-Hispanic and colonial history, the population history of the Basin of Mexico has received substantial attention. Further, because of the quantity and quality of population and other data available for the Basin is unexcelled, it has long been the focus for population study. For the period of interest here (the sixteenth and early seventeenth centuries) Gibson and Sanders derive Basin-specific population estimates.[21] Other estimates for the Basin in this period may be extracted from Cook and Simpson, Cook and Borah, Borah and Cook, Rosenblat, Gerhard, and Slicher van Bath.[22] Despite this attention, or perhaps because of it, the estimated population values vary widely, however.

Without dwelling on these estimates (which will be detailed in Chapter 3), it is important to note that there is a wide diversity in both the eve-of-the-conquest values and the subsequent nadir values. The lowest estimate for 1519 is that of Sanders, at 1.16 million, while the highest is that derived from Borah and Cook, 2.96 million.[23] Thus, the largest estimate for this

[18] Gibson, *The Aztecs*, p. 2.

[19] Sanders, *et al.*, *The Basin of Mexico*, p. 93.

[20] Whitmore and Turner, *Population Reconstruction of the Basin of Mexico*, pp. 2-3.

[21] Gibson, *The Aztecs*; and W. T. Sanders, "The Population of the Central Mexican Symbiotic Region, the Basin of Mexico, and the Teotihuacán Valley in the Sixteenth Century," in W. M. Denevan (ed.), *The Native Population of the Americas in 1492*, Madison, WI: University of Wisconsin Press, 1976.

[22] Sherburne F. Cook and Lesley Bird Simpson, *The Population of Central Mexico in the Sixteenth Century*, Ibero-Americana 31, Berkeley: University of California Press, 1948; Sherburne F. Cook and Woodrow Borah, *The Indian Population of Central Mexico, 1531-1610*, Ibero-Americana 44, Berkeley: University of California Press, 1960; Woodrow Borah and Sherburne F. Cook, *The Population of Central Mexico in 1548*, Ibero-America 43, Berkeley: University of California Press, 1960; A. Rosenblat, *La Población de América en 1492, Viejos y Nuevós Cálculos*, México City: El Colegio de México, 1967; Peter Gerhard, *A Guide to the Historical Geography of New Spain*, Cambridge: Cambridge University Press, 1972; B. H. Slicher van Bath, "The Calculation of the Population of New Spain, Especially for the Period Before 1570," *Boletín de Estudios Latinoamericanos y del Caribe*, 24, (1978; and Sherburn F. Cook, and Woodrow Borah. *Essays in Population History*, Vol. 3. Berkeley: University of California Press, 1979.

[23] Sanders, "The Population of the Central Mexican Symbiotic Region"; and Woodrow Borah and Sherburne F. Cook, *The Aboriginal Population of Central*

date is over 2.5 times as large as the lowest. An even larger spread obtains
for the nadir populations. The largest of these, 0.346 million (in 1597), is
derived from Cook and Simpson, while the lowest is obtained from Cook
and Borah, 0.073 million (in 1620).[24] The spread here is even larger, since
the larger value is over 4.5 times as large as the smaller.

Thus, depending on one's choice, an argument may be made that the
sixteenth-century depopulation of the Basin was catastrophic, falling from
2.96 to 0.073 million (a fall to scarcely 3 percent of the initial figure). An
alternative argument may be made that the fall was much less severe, from
1.16 to 0.346 million (a decline to about 30 percent of the initial value). It is
this diversity of estimates (and the differing interpretations of history that
result) that frames the specific problem to be examined here. Because its
diversity in population estimates mirrors those on larger scales and because
the issues surrounding this question are similar in the Basin case and
elsewhere, the Basin of Mexico constitutes a microcosmic study for all
sixteenth-century Amerindian depopulation controversies.

The central question is: could a large and healthy population suffer the
catastrophic collapses implied by the larger pre-conquest population
estimates? While the method employed in this study is novel, its topic of
study, the initial Amerindian population decline, has its roots in the
sixteenth century. To place this study in perspective, it is useful to review
briefly the general issues and debate on the broad topic of Amerindian
population change.

Background to the Amerindian Depopulation

The Debate and Evidence

The initial basis of the debate on Amerindian population numbers lies
in the conflicting European eyewitness reports. Borah points to Las Casas'
three million estimate for Hispaniola and to Gonzalo Fernández de Oviedo's
reckoning of 2 million for Central America and Panama as examples of
early high figures for places that were not seats of high cultures, therefore
implying potentially higher populations for Central Mexico and Peru.[25]

Mexico on the Eve of the Spanish Conquest, Ibero-America 45. Berkeley:
University of California Press, 1963.

24 Cook and Simpson, *The Population of Central Mexico in the Sixteenth Century*;
and Cook and Borah *Essays in Population History*, Vol. 3, p. 1.

25 Woodrow, Borah, "Historical demography of aboriginal and colonial America: An
attempt at perspective," in W. M. Denevan (ed.), *The Native Population of the
Americas in 1492*, Madison, WI: University of Wisconsin Press, 1976, p. 14;
Bartolomé de Las Casas, *Obras Escogidas de Fray Bartolomé de las Casas*, J. Pérez
de Tudela (ed.). Madrid: Ediciones Atlas, 1957-1958, pp. 51-52; and Gonzalo
Fernández de Oviedo y Valdés, *Historial general y natural de las Indias*, Vol. 4. Juan
Pérez de Tudela (ed.). Madrid: Ediciones Atlas, 1959, p. 353.

Rosenblat, Kroeber, Steward, and others argue that such estimates were much too large, and even Borah notes Díaz del Castillo's objection to what he viewed as inflated numbers, especially of warriors, reported to Spain.[26] Nevertheless, MacLeod, Sauer, Dobyns, Cook and Borah, and others argue for the essential credibility of contemporary testimony for Central Mexico, most of which supports large estimates.[27]

One of the present extremes of the debate was set by the late eighteenth century.[28] Historians examined the recorded testimony and other evidence and compared it with what was known or assumed to be known about pre-Colombian societies to determine the veracity of particular documents and other lines of evidence. The extremes of this debate are exemplified by Clavijero who estimated a 30 million pre-contact Central Mexican population and Robertson who argued that the Spanish found only sparse settlements of barbarians and were led to exaggerate in official reports back to Spain.[29]

The twentieth-century debate revolves about the same issues, and much of the early work reflects different interpretations of history and different assumptions about the nature of pre-Colombian societies. Among the better known early twentieth-century estimates, Spinden, influenced perhaps by his Maya expertise, argued for a large pre-contact hemispheric total of 40-50 million.[30] Similarly, Means, another expert on a high culture, the Inca, used social structure to estimate 16-32 million for the Inca alone.[31] Sapper, using what might be described as a resource potential argument, estimated the late fifteenth-century hemispheric population as between 37 million and

26 Rosenblat, *La Población y el mestizaje*, p. 101; Kroeber, "Cultural Areas"; Borah, "Historical Demography," p. 14; and B. Díaz del Castillo, *Historia verdadera de la conquista de la Nueva España*. Vol. 1, Mexico City: Porrúa, 1960, p. 79; and J. H. Steward, "The Native Population of South America," in J.H. Steward (ed.), *Handbook of South American Indians*, Vol. 5. Smithsonian Institution, Bureau of American Ethnology Bulletin No. 143, Washington DC: U.S. Government Printing Office, 1949, p. 656.

27 MacLeod, *Spanish Central America*, p. 18; Dobyns "Estimating"; Sherburn F. Cook, and Woodrow Borah, "On the Credibility of Contemporary Testimony on the Population of Mexico in the Sixteenth Century," *Suma Antropología en Homenaje a Roberto J. Weitlaner*, Mexico City: Instituto Nacional de Antropología e Historia, 1966; and C. O. Sauer, *The Early Spanish Main*, Berkeley: University of California Press, 1966.

28 Borah, "Historical demography," p. 14.

29 F. J. Clavijero, *Historia Antigua de México*, Mexico City: Editorial Porrúa, 1964, II: pp. 561-70; W. Robertson, *The History of America*, Vol. 2. London, 1777, pp. 293-302, 409-450, pp. 459-461, 483-486; and Borah, "Historical Demography," p. 14.

30 H. J. Spinden,"The Population of Ancient America," *Geographical Review*, 18 (1928), p. 660.

31 P. A. Means, *Ancient Civilizations of the Andes*, New York: Charles Scribner's Sons, 1931, p. 296.

48.5 million.[32] In contrast to the association of scholars of "high culture" to high population estimates,[33] a single high estimate, Rivet's 40-50 million population for the hemisphere, was derived using North American depopulation data.[34]

By comparison with the "high" Amerindian cultures, some experts on North and South American Amerindian societies produced notably lower estimates.[35] Mooney totaled the aboriginal population of North America at 1.15 million.[36] Kroeber lowered Mooney's figure for North America to 0.9 million and estimated only 8.4 million for the entire hemisphere.[37] Steward estimated the aboriginal population of South America as 9.129 million and projected an hemispheric total of 15.59 million.[38]

The challenge of this diversity of estimates highlights the contribution of the detailed work that is the hallmark of the so called "Berkeley School." This impressive body of scholarship begins with and draws inspiration from Sauer's Ibero-Americana monograph, *The Aboriginal Population of Northwestern Mexico*.[39] For over 30 years this group of productive scholars—S.F. Cook, L.B. Simpson, W.W. Borah, H. Ashmann, and later, W.M. Denevan—has explored pre-conquest and early colonial Amerindian population dynamics in the Ibero-Americana series. This body of work includes monographs detailing ecology and demography on a small scale in Mexico, Baja California, South America, and California.[40] An

---

32 K. Sapper, "Die Zahl und die Volkdichte der Indianischen Bevolkerung in Amerika von der Conquista und in der Gegenwart," In *Proceedings of the Twenty-first International Congress of Americanists, First part*, Leiden: E. J. Brill, 1924, pp. 95-104.

33 Borah, "Historical Demography," p. 15.

34 P. Rivet, "Langues américaines," in A. Meillet and M. Cohen (eds.), *Les Langues des Monde*, Vol. 12. Paris: Collection Linguistique, Société du Linguistique, 1924, p. 601.

35 Borah, "Historical Demography," p. 15.

36 J. Mooney, *The Aboriginal Population of America North of Mexico*, Miscellaneous Collections 80, No. 7. Washington, DC: Smithsonian Institution, 1928, p. 33.

37 Kroeber, "Cultural Areas," pp. 131-181.

38 Steward, "The Native Population of South America," pp. 655-668.

39 C. O. Sauer, *Aboriginal Population of Northwestern Mexico*, Ibero-Americana 10, Berkeley: The University of California Press, 1935; and William M. Denevan, "Carl Sauer and Native Population Size in the New World, "Paper presented at the annual meeting of the Association of American Geographers, Baltimore, MD. 1989.

40 See H. Aschmann, *The Central Desert of Baja California: Demography and Ecology*, Ibero-Americana 42, Berkeley: University of California Press, 1959; Sherburne F. Cook, *Population Trends Among the California Mission Indians*, Ibero-Americana 17, Berkeley: University of California Press, 1940; Sherburne F. Cook, *The Historical Demography and Ecology of the Teotlapan*, Ibero-Americana 33, Berkeley: University of California Press, 1949a; Sherburne F. Cook, *Santa Mariá Ixcatlán: Habitat, Population, Subsistance*, Ibero-Americana 41, Berkeley:

8

influential group of monographs in this series exploits methodological advances that allow the use of various Hispanic documents and transcriptions of pre-Hispanic Aztec codices to produce relatively well supported population estimates for dates in the early and mid-sixteenth century.[41]

In addition to their demographic focus, the "Berkeley" scholars explored aspects of the economic, environmental, and epidemiological history of the immediate pre-Hispanic and Colonial period.[42]

These monographs and a variety of local studies[43] and journal articles[44] are characterized by their methodological sophistication, including

University of California Press, 1958; Sherburne F. Cook and Woodrow Borah, *The Population of the Mixteca Alta*, Ibero-Americana 50, Berkeley: University of California Press, 1968.; and W.M. Denevan, *The Aboriginal Cultural Ecology of the Llanos de Mojos of Bolivia*, Ibero-Americana 48, Berkeley: University of California Press, 1966.

[41] For example, see Borah and Cook, *The Population of Central Mexico in 1548*; Borah and Cook, *Aboriginal Population of Central Mexico*; Cook and Borah, *The Indian Population of Central Mexico*; and Cook and Simpson, *The Population of Central Mexico in the Sixteenth Century*.

[42] See Woodrow Borah *New Spain's Century of Depression*, Ibero-Americana 35, Berkeley: University of California Press, 1951; Woodrow Borah, *Early Colonial Trade and Navigation between Mexico and Peru*, Ibero-Americana 38, Berkeley: University of California Press, 1954; Woodrow Borah and Sherburne F. Cook, *Price Trends of Some Basic Commodities in Central Mexico, 1531-1570*, Ibero-Americana 40, Berkeley: University of California Press, 1958; Sherburne F. Cook, *The Extent and Significance of Disease Among the Indians of Baja California, 1697-1773*, Ibero-Americana 12, Berkeley: University of California Press, 1937; Sherburne F. Cook, "Smallpox in Spanish and Mexican California, 1770-1845," *Bulletin of the History of Medicine* 7 (1939), pp. 153-191; Sherburne F. Cook, "The Incidence and Significance of Disease Among the Aztecs and Related Tribes," *Hispanic American Historical Review* 26 (1946), pp. 320-335; and Sherburne F. Cook, *Soil Erosion and Population in Central Mexico*, Ibero-Americana 34, Berkeley: University of California Press, 1949.

[43] See Sherburne F. Cook, "The Aboriginal Population of the San Joaquin Valley, California," *Anthropological Records*, Berkeley: University of California Press, 1955, Vol. 16: pp. 31-78; Sherburne F. Cook, "The Aboriginal Population of the North Coast of California," *Anthropological Records*, Berkeley: University of California Press, 1956, Vol. 16: pp. 81-129; Sherburne F. Cook, "The Aboriginal Population of Alemeda and Contra Costa Counties, California," *Anthropological Records*, Berkeley: University of California Press, 1957, Vol. 16, pp. 131-154.

[44] See Woodrow Borah, "América Como Modelo? El Impacto Demográfico de La Expansión Europea Sobre el Mundo no Europeo," *Cuadernos Americanos* 6 (1962), pp. 176-185; Woodrow Borah, "The Historical Demography of Latin America: Sources, Techniques, Controversies, Yields," in Paul Deprez (ed.), *Population and Economics: Procedings of Section V of the Fourth Congress of the International Economic History Association*, Winnipeg: University of Manitoba Press, 1970; Borah and Cook, "La Despoblación del México Central en El Siglo XVI," *Historia*

the explicit identification and careful assembly of sources and the cross-checking of their validity.[45] In addition to the care exhibited in treating the sources, the manipulation and interpretation of these massive data assemblies are carried out with an eye for statistical validity. The population figures that result are subject to statistically competent treatment as well.

Different assumptions about the nature of Amerindian societies and about the interpretation of history color these population estimates.[46] The most lively debates, however, concern the nature of the evidence used to compile the estimates and its treatment. Central to this debate are: criticisms of the veracity of colonial documents used to estimate populations;[47] criticisms of the choice of documents, their interpretation, and the assumptions necessary to use them;[48] and criticisms of the methodology used to produce the estimates.[49]

DATA SOURCES

As is evident in the brief chronology noted above, a wide variety of data sources is employed in investigating the sixteenth-century population history of the New World. Among the most widely used class of data are Hispanic eyewitness accounts, including letters and diaries containing the initial estimates of the conquistadors. Military estimates of the number of warriors in allied armies and opposing forces have been creatively utilized by Cook and Simpson and Cook and Borah to generate population estimates.[50] Similarly, early clerical estimates of the numbers of baptisms, conversions, and of initial populations have been used by Cook and Cook and Simpson.[51] These sources are not without their critics, however. Rosenblat, Sanders, and Henige object to them, arguing that they were

---

Mexicana 12 (1962), pp. 1-12; and Sherburne F. Cook and Woodrow Borah, "The Rate of Population Change in Central Mexico," *Hispanic American Historical Review* 37 (1957), pp. 463-470.

[45] Dobyns, "Estimating," p. 403.

[46] Borah, "Historical Ddemography," pp. 18-19.

[47] See Sanders, "The Population of the Central Mexican Symbiotic Region."

[48] See D. Henige, "On the Contact Population of Hispañola: History as Higher Mathematics," *Hispanic American Historical Review* 58 (1978), pp. 217-237; and Slicher van Bath, "The Calculation of the Population of New Spain."

[49] R. A. Zambardino, "Mexico's Population in the Sixteenth Century: Demographic Anomaly or Mathematical Illusion?" *Journal of Interdisciplinary History*, 11 (1980).

[50] Cook and Simpson, *The Population of Central Mexico in the Sixteenth Century*, pp. 22-30; and Cook and Borah, *Essays in Population History*, Vol. 1, pp. 8-9, 376-401.

[51] Cook, *The Extent and Significance of Disease*, 7; and Cook and Simpson, *The Population of Central Mexico in the Sixteenth Century*, pp. 19-21.

biased to impress the Spanish Crown and the Church.[52] Further, the sources are often incongruent, and for that reason the choice of particular accounts is important and to some degree subjective.

By far the most statistically compelling data sources are the civil records of the Spanish colonial government. Documents such as the *Suma de visitas* and the *Matrícula de Tributarios*, which record counts of tribute paying Indians (among other useful economic and demographic facts), were produced as early as the mid-1500's to assess the numbers of *tributarios*, and hence to assess the taxation rates. These documents form the backbone of much of the historical demographic research in the Americas. Cook and Simpson, Cook and Borah, Borah and Cook, Cook, Friede, Sanders, and Gibson among others all used or relied on such documents.[53] Similar demographic and economic surveys, the *Relaciones Geográficas*, have been used by Gerhard and Cook and Simpson.[54] Counts used for resettlements have also been used by Cook and Borah.[55] Ecclesiastical sources of similar utility, such as parish registers of births and deaths, have been utilized by Sauer, Cook, and Aschmann.[56]

Sanders and Henige have criticized over-reliance on these sources, especially the tribute assessment documents.[57] They cite several reasons: possibilities of fraud that may bias the counts; the inconsistency of the data from place to place and among different sources; the physical problems that may have precluded the careful coverage and detail that is implied in the

---

[52] Rosenblat, *La Población y el mestizaje* pp. 96-102; A. Rosenbladt, "The Population of Hispanola at the time of Columbus," in W. M. Denevan (ed.), *The Native Population of the Americas in 1492*, Madison, WI: University of Wisconsin Press, 1976, pp. 47-66; Sanders, "The Population of the Central Mexican Symbiotic Region, p. 103; and Henige, "On the Contact Population of Hispañola," pp. 221-222.

[53] Cook and Simpson, *The Population of Central Mexico in the Sixteenth Century*; Cook and Borah, "The Rate of Population Change in Central Mexico"; Cook and Borah, *The Indian Population of Central Mexico*; Cook and Borah, *The Population of the Mixteca Alta*; Cook and Borah, *Essays in Population History*, Vol. 1.; Borah and Cook, *The Population of Central Mexico in 1548*; Nobel David Cook, *Demographic Collapse: Indian Peru, 1520-1620*, New York: Cambridge University Press, 1981; Juan Friede, "Demographic Changes in the Mining Community of Muzo after the Plague of 1629," *Hispanic American Historical Review*, 47 (1967), pp. 338-343; Sanders, "The Population of the Central Mexican Symbiotic Region"; and Gibson, *The Aztecs*.

[54] Gerhard, *Historical Geography of New Spain*; Peter Gerhard, *The Southeast Frontier of New Spain*, Princeton: Princeton University Press, and 1979; Cook and Simpson, *The Population of Central Mexico in the Sixteenth Century*, pp. 3-9.

[55] Cook and Borah, *The Indian Population of Central Mexico*, pp. 10-11.

[56] Sauer, *Aboriginal Population*, 2; Cook, *The Extent and Significance of Disease*, 7; and Aschmann, *Baja California*, pp. 152-4.

[57] Sanders, "The Population of the Central Mexican Symbiotic Region," pp. 94-98; and Henige, "On the Contact Population of Hispañola," p. 232.

documents (hence the recorded figures may be partially imaginary); and their incomplete survival that makes complete coverage an impossibility. Nevertheless, their availability and their relatively extensive coverage make these documents the most important single source of early colonial demographic data.

In addition to the early Spanish eyewitness and bureaucratic data, the Spanish transcribed a number of pre-Columbian documents. Borah and Cook use transcribed Aztec records, such as the *Codex Mendoza*, which record quantities of tribute paid to Aztec emperors, to produce an estimate of the A.D. 1492 central Mexican population.[58] The pitfalls inherent in such complex transformations are cogently pointed out by Sanders and Cook.[59]

Other indigenous sources of data, such as informers and direct observation of contemporary Indians, have been used by Cook, Vellard, and others.[60] The psychology of human memory and other problems in using these data sources are explored by Cook.[61]

In addition to these documentary surrogates, a variety of "physical" surrogates, drawn largely from archaeology, have been creatively employed to generate population estimates. For example, Sanders and colleagues used surface shards and other settlement remains to estimate the immediate pre-contact population of the Basin of Mexico.[62] This method, and that of using relic settlement structures (e.g., house mounds), have been widely employed to estimate population throughout Mesoamerica, but especially in the Maya area.[63] In addition, Adams has produced estimates based on the remains of monumental architecture.[64] These surrogates, all occupational

---

[58] Borah and Cook, *Aboriginal Population of Central Mexico*.

[59] Sanders, "The population of the Central Mexican Symbiotic Region," pp. 112-114; and Cook, *Demographic Collapse*, p. 58.

[60] Cook, "Aboriginal Population of the North Coast of California"; and J. Vellard, "Causas Biológicas de la Desaparición de los Indios Americanos," *Boletín del Instituto Riva Agüero* 2 (1956).

[61] Cook, "Aboriginal Population of the North Coast of California," pp. 81-82.

[62] Sanders, *et al.*, *The Basin of Mexico*, Chapter 2, p. 184.

[63] See R. E. Blanton, *Monte Albán: Settlement Patterns at the Ancient Zapotec Capital*, New York: Academic Press, 1978; K. V. Flannery, *The Early Mesoamerican Village*, New York: Academic Press, 1976; and B. L. Turner II, "Comparisons of Agrotechnologies in The Basin of Mexico and Central Maya Lowlands: Formative to the Classic Maya Collapse," in A. G. Miller (ed.), *Highland-Lowland Interaction in Mesoamerica, Interdisciplinary Approaches*, Washington, DC: Dunbarton Oaks Research Library and Collection, 1983.

[64] R. E. W. Adams, "Settlement Patterns of the Central Yucatan and Southern Campeche Regions," in W. Ashmore (ed.), *Lowland Maya Settlement Patterns*, Albuquerque: University of New Mexico Press, 1981.

remains, and the populations derived from them, have been critically examined by Tolstoy and Fish, Turner, and Whitmore and Turner.[65]

Potential population, judged by agroecosystem/resource system potential has been explored for small, homogenous regions by Cook and Sanders for central Mexican valleys.[66] Sapper expanded the horizon and estimated the entire Mexican and hemispheric population using resource potential.[67] The complexity of these methods, the fact that they can only estimate the possible, the problems of evidence, and the problems in defining the potential itself have been cited by Cook and Turner among other investigators of pre-Hispanic and colonial cultural ecologies.[68]

Disease mortality models, using historical evidence of the timing, frequency, and mortality of epidemics, have also been used to estimate the scale of the post-contact Amerindian population decline. Dobyns, Crosby, Gerhard, and Ashburn have led the way in outlining the descriptive history of epidemic disease in Spanish colonial America.[69]

METHODOLOGY

The ingenuity and sophistication evident in the choice of data sources used to estimate populations are matched by that employed in the interpretation of the source data, its extension to wider spatial scales, and its temporal expansion. Since virtually all of the source data are only surrogates for the desired population data, the interpretation, choice, and conversion of these

---

[65] P. Tolstoy, and S. K. Fish, "Surface and Subsurface Evidence for Community Size at Coapexco, Mexico," *Journal of Field Archaeology* 2 (1975); B. L. Turner II, *Population Reconstruction of the Central Maya Lowlands: 1000 B.C. to Present*, Millennial Long Waves of Human Occupance Project, Technical Paper # 2, Clark University, 1986; and Whitmore and Turner, *Population Reconstruction of the Basin of Mexico*.

[66] Cook, *Teotlapan*, pp. 39-41; and W. T. Sanders, "The Agricultural History of the Basin of Mexico," in E. R. Wolf (ed.), *The Valley of Mexico*, Albuquerque: The University of New Mexico Press, 1976, pp. 139.

[67] Sapper, "Die Zahl und die Volkdichte," p. 100.

[68] Cook, *Demographic Collapse*, pp. 28-29; Turner, "Comparisons of Agrotechnologies," p. 15; and Turner, *Population Reconstruction of the Central Maya Lowlands*.

[69] P. M. Ashburn, *The Ranks of Death: A Medical History of the Conquest of America*, Frank D. Ashburn (ed.). New York: Coward-McCann, Inc., 1947; Alfred W. Crosby, "Conquistador y Pestiliencia: The First New World Pandemic and the Fall of the Great Indian Empires," *Hispanic American Historical Review* 47, (1967), pp. 321-337; Alfred W. Crosby, *The Colombian Exchange: Biological and Cultural Consequences of 1492*, Westport, CN: Greenwood Press, 1972, p. 44; Alfred W. Crosby, "Virgin Soil Epidemics as a Factor in the Aboriginal Depopulation in America," *William and Mary Quarterly* 33, (1976), pp. 289-299; H. F. Dobyns, "An Outline of Andean Epidemic History to 1720," *Bulletin of the History of Medicine*, 37 (1963), pp. 493-515; and Gerhard, *Historical Geography of New Spain*, p. 23.

surrogate data remain the most intensely debated aspect of New World historical demography. In addition to the full discussions that accompany many estimates, especially those of the "Berkeley School," there is a considerable volume of scholarship that critiques other estimates in addition to producing new ones.

Befitting their pre-eminence as data sources, the conversion of tribute and other colonial demographic/economic survey data into population figures has attracted the most critical review. Discussions of the documentary survey evidence include various aspects of the data and conversion methodology such as: (i) the interpretation of the inconsistent terminology in the sources; (ii) the numbers of Amerinds exempt from tribute and labor service; (iii) the reliability and accuracy of the documents; and (iv) the assumptions of family size that define the multiplier which converts the number of *tributarios* to a total population count.[70] The aptness of choice among documents is discussed by Sanders and Henige.[71] Dobyns points to the importance of knowing the timing (date) of the counts.[72] Uncertainty in the definition of an Amerindian and charges of bias on the part of scholars are pointed to by Petersen and Henige.[73]

To extend population estimates that are derived using local-scale data to larger spatial entities, three general techniques have been used. In the first of these, estimates for larger areas have been calculated by multiplying sample densities times the desired regional area.[74] Similarly, sample depopulation ratios have been applied to hemispheric nadir population figures to generate pre-conquest hemispheric totals.[75] Denevan and Kehoe and Kehoe have objected to the assumptions of societal consistency inherent

[70] Cook, *Demographic Collapse*, pp. 75-90; Henige, "On the Contact Population of Hispañola," p. 232; George Kubler, "Population Movements in Mexico 1520-1600," *Hispanic American Historical Review*, 22 (1942), pp. 606-643; Rosenblat, "The Population of Hispañola," pp. 45-54, 59-64; Rosenblat, *La Población*, pp. 32-81; Rosenblat, *La población y el mestizaje*, p. 101; Sanders, "The Population of the Central Mexican Symbiotic Region," pp. 94-101; and Slicher van Bath, "The Calculation of the Population of New Spain."

[71] Sanders, "The Population of the Central Mexican Symbiotic Region," pp. 114-115; and Henige, "On the Contact Population of Hispañola," pp. 221-222.

[72] Dobyns, "Estimating," p. 402.

[73] W. Petersen, "A Demographers View of Prehistoric Demography," *Current Anthropology* 16 (1975), p. 386; W. Petersen, *Population*. Third ed. New York: MacMillan Publishing Inc., 1975, p. 236; and Henige, "On the Contact Population of Hispañola," pp. 221-222.

[74] See O. G. Ricketson, Jr., and E. Bayles. *Uaxactun Guatemala, Group E - 1926-1931, Part 1: The Excavations; Part 2: The Artifacts*, Carnegie Institutions of Washington Publication No. 477, 1937.

[75] See Rivet "Langues Américaines," 601; and Dobyns, "Estimating," p. 415.

in hemispheric projections.[76] The general problem of aggregation bias for spatially dependent correlations (i.e., the differing correlations obtained when identical data are correlated at different scales of aggregation) has not been specifically addressed for Spanish American historical demography, but Clark and Avery, Curry, Robinson, Neprash, Thomas and Anderson, and others have addressed the theoretical issues.[77]

The second method, the "filling in" of missing data for particular locales at particular times has been widely accomplished by calculating a mean (or median) ratio of population for sites with data at two dates and using the resulting figure to "fill in" data for sites with data for only one of the dates in question. This technique is widely used by the "Berkeley School" scholars, Cook, Simpson, and Borah. In theory, this technique suffers from the same "aggregation" bias problems as the spatial projection technique.

The third spatial extension methodology involves the summation of local values to produce estimates for larger regions. Summation has been done on all scales; Denevan summed sub-hemispheric regions to produce a hemisphere-wide estimate; Mooney summed individual tribal populations to produce a North American estimate; and Sanders and Gibson summed estimates for individual communities to produce a Basin of Mexico figure.[78]

Much of the most reliable sixteenth-century data was not compiled until the last half of the century. For that reason, estimates for immediate pre-contact populations commonly rely on temporal extension techniques to generate values for earlier dates. The most rudimentary of these methodologies involves the use of simple ratios. A ratio of known initial to subsequent populations for a community or region is calculated and divided by the number of years between the dates in question. The resulting value

76 W. M. Denevan, *The Native Population of the Americas in 1492*, Madison, WI: University of Wisconsin Press, 1976, p. 429; and T. F. Kehoe, and A. B. Kehoe, "Comments on H. F. Dobyns, 'Estimating Aboriginal American Population: An Appraisal of Techniques with a New Hemisphere Estimate'," *Current Anthropology* 7 (1966), p. 434.

77 W. A. V. Clark, and K. L. Avery. "The Effects of Data Aggregation in Statistical Analysis," *Geographical Analysis* 8 (1976), pp. 428-438; L. Curry, "A Note on Spatial Association," *The Professional Geographer* 18 (1966), pp. 97-99; A. H. Robinson, "The Necessity of Weighing Values in Correlation Analysis of Areal Data," *Annals of the Association of American Geographers*, 46 (1956), pp. 233-236; J. A. Neprash, "Some Problems in the Correlation of Spatially Distributed Variables," *American Statistical Association Supplement* 29, (1934), pp. 167-168; and E. N. Thomas, and D. L. Anderson. "Additional Comments on Weighting Values in Correlation Analysis of Areal Data," *Annals of the Association of American Geographers* 55, (1965), pp. 492-505.

78 Denevan, *The Native Population of the Americas in 1492*, p. 291; Mooney, *Aboriginal Population*, p. 882; Sanders, "The Population of the Central Mexican Symbiotic Region," p. 130-131; and Gibson, *The Aztecs*, p. 142-143.

of population change per year may be used to extend estimates to dates before and after the initial pair by multiplying the ratio times the number of years in the desired interval and adding (or subtracting) the resultant to the initial figure. This is equivalent to the linear graphical extension used by Sanders.[79] It assumes, however, that the absolute amount of population change per year is invariant, and for that reason this method is reasonably accurate only for very short extension intervals.

Cook and Borah derive a different technique that assumes equal rates of change per year.[80] Their "coefficient of population movement, ω," is the geometric mean rate of change derived from known initial and subsequent populations figures for a community. The population at another desired date can be estimated by multiplying either the initial or subsequent population times the "coefficient of population movement" and multiplying this product times the number of years the desired date is distant from the starting date.

Yet another method that relies on rates of change is used by Cook and Shea.[81] Here, the rate of change of population between two dates is figured assuming that the change follows an exponential function in 'e.' By solving the equation,

$$P_2 = P_1 \times e^{rt}$$

(where 'P_1' is the initial population, 'P_2' is the subsequent population, 't' is the time interval in years, 'r' is the annual rate of change, and 'e' is the base of the natural logarithms),

for 'r' from two known populations at known dates, the average annual rate of change is obtained. The population at a desired date can be estimated by multiplying the initial population by e^{rt}, where t is the number of years the desired date is distant from the initial date. This method is similar to the graphical technique using semi-log paper employed by Cook and Borah and Zambardino.[82] A common fault shared by all temporal extension techniques is that the accuracy of the projected estimates is likely to decrease proportionally the further away in time the desired date is from the initial one.[83]

Innovative additive/subtractive techniques have been used to recreate populations at different dates. For example, Aschmann and Cook have used parish records and other data on disease mortalities to reconstruct previous

---

79 Sanders, "The Population of the Central Mexican Symbiotic Region," 114-115, 123, 124.

80 Cook and Borah, *Essays in Population History.* Vol. 1, Chapter 2.

81 Cook, *Demographic Collapse*, 90-95; and D. E. Shea, "A Defense of Small Population Estimates for the Colonial Andes in 1520," in W. M. Denevan (ed.), *The Native Population of the Americas in 1492*, Madison, WI: University of Wisconsin Press, 1976, pp. 158-80.

82 Cook and Borah, *Essays in Population History*, Vol. 1, Chapter 2; and Zambardino, "Mexico's Population," pp. 21-22.

83 Zambardino, "Mexico's Population," pp. 21-22.

populations.[84] Using a method that does not require population data for two dates, Cook uses a computer simulation of disease mortalities to derive relative depopulation figures, and uses these to estimate earlier populations by the addition of the numbers shown to have perished in epidemics to the remaining population.[85] Using another innovative method, Cook employs stable population theory to derive an expected population size and structure for a date subsequent to an initial figure and compares this expected value with the historically recorded value.[86] In this way he can deduce the probable degree of "excess" mortality due to epidemic disease in the interval. This "excess" mortality represents the population change between intervals, so he can estimate populations at earlier dates.

Zambardino cogently notes that all techniques that are based on surrogates or that must be extended spatially or temporally are liable to unacceptably high levels of uncertainty due to the multiplication of the uncertainty inherent in each step of the conversion.[87] In general, the more steps such a factorial method has, the greater the possible uncertainty. Further, few of these studies specifically addresses the problems that migration would produce in the archival data.[88]

CAUSES

With only a few exceptions, the determination of the scale of Amerindian population collapse has been methodologically divorced from considerations of the causes of the collapse. Nevertheless, the probable causes of the Indian population decline have been vigorously debated. Indeed, Dobyns notes that failure to consider adequately the effects of Spanish induced epidemics was a factor contributing to Kroeber's and others' low estimates of pre-Hispanic Indian populations.[89]

Sánchez-Albornoz recognizes four interrelated causes.[90] The first of these is the so-called "homicide theory."[91] In their letters and accounts, Las Casas, Motolinéa, Zorita, and others argued that the Spanish conquerors resorted to systematic killing as a terror weapon to compensate for their

---

84 Aschmann, *Baja California*; Cook, "Smallpox in California"; and Cook, *Population Trends.*

85 Cook, *Demographic Collapse*, pp. 100-106.

86 Ibid.

87 Zambardino, "Mexico's Population," pp. 6-8; and R. A. Zambardino, "Critique of David Henige; 'On the Contact Population of Hispanola: History as Higher Mathematics'," *Hispanic American Historical Review* 58 (1978), p. 706.

88 David J. Robinson, "Introduction: Towards a Typology of Migration in Colonial Spanish America," in D. J. Robinson (ed.), *Migration in Spanish Colonial America*, CAmbridge: Cambridge University Press, 1990, p. 12.

89 Dobyns, "Estimating," p. 411.

90 Sánchez-Albornoz, *The Population of Latin America*, pp. 51-66.

91 Kubler "Population Movements," pp. 606-643.

numerical disadvantage.[92] Forced movement, slavery, and famine resulting from Spanish seizure of food reserves, and routine military encounters are also cited by Sánchez-Albornoz as contributing to Indian population decline.[93] Sauer and others also note the massacre of submissive Indian groups by rebellious ones as being indirectly caused by the Spanish presence.[94] Friede argues that hundreds of archival documents refer to excessive work (especially in the mines), general cruelty and ill-treatment, and conscription for expeditions as factors in the Indian population decline.[95]

The loss of the "will to survive" is also implicated in the Amerindian collapse. The aloofness and laziness attributed to Indians in Hispanic colonial documents is interpreted as a general state of depression and the loss of the will to live by Sánchez-Albornoz.[96] Citing Jaramillo Uribe, Sauer, Gonzáles and Mellafe, Sánchez-Albornoz argues that pre-conquest families were larger than those in early colonial times and that there were also many unmarried adults after the conquest.[97] He attributes this reduced total fertility to psychological and socioeconomic situations brought about by the disruptions of the conquest.[98] For example, women avoided conception since child bearing only added to their overwork or provided the Spanish with slaves.[99] They sought to induce abortion for the same reasons, and committed infanticide to spare their children the hardships of Spanish colonial servitude. Similarly, Kubler argues that overwork and ill-treatment led Indians to suicide.[100]

The economic and social readjustment engendered by Spanish domination is also cited as a contributing factor to indigenous population decline by Cook and Borah.[101] Sánchez-Albornoz cites Chevalier, Simpson, and Friede who argue that the widespread conversion of *tierra caliente* to Spanish export crops, such as sugar, dyes, and cacao, led to the

---

[92] Sánchez-Albornoz, *The Population of Latin America*, p. 51.

[93] Sánchez-Albornoz, *The Population of Latin America*, p. 52.

[94] Sauer, *Aboriginal Population*.

[95] Friede, "Demographic changes," p. 339.

[96] Sánchez-Albornoz, *The Population of Latin America*, p. 55.

[97] J. Jaramillo Uribe,"La Población Indígena de Colombia en el Momento de la Conquista y sus Transformaciones Posteriores," *Anuario Colombiano de Historia Social y de la Cultura*, 1 (1964), pp. 239-293; Sauer, *The Early Spanish Main*; E. R. Gonzáles, and R. Mellafe, "La Función de la Famila en la Historia Social Hispanoamericana Colonial," *Anuario del Instituto Investigaciones Históricas*, 8 (1965), pp. 57-81; and Sánchez-Albornoz, *The Population of Latin America*, p. 54.

[98] Sánchez-Albornoz, *The Population of Latin America*, pp. 54, 56.

[99] T. T. Veblen, "Native Population Decline in Totonicapan Guatemala," *Annals of the Association of American Geographers*, 67, (1977), p. 493.

[100] Kubler, "Population Movements," pp. 633-639.

[101] Cook and Borah, *Essays in Population History*, Vol. 1, p. 409.

expropriation of Indian lands in that realm and forced them to a more marginal existence with higher death rates and lower fertility rates.[102] The rapid population expansion of Spanish domesticated animals also contributed to the marginalization of the indigenous economy by displacing Indians to less desirable locales, altering the local ecosystems, and damaging the existing crops.[103] Kubler and Lipschutz point to the role the forced relocation and collectivization of the Indian populace had in elevating death rates.[104]

These circumstances notwithstanding, a great many scholars of the early colonial period believe that the primary cause of Indian population decline was excessive mortality caused by the introduction of Old World diseases into a non-immune population.[105]

The controversy about the magnitude of the population decline and the critiques of the methods used to estimate it indicate that analyses of documentary sources of tributary numbers (population surrogates), when coupled with a deficient set of cultural ecological, geographic, and demographic assumptions, are inadequate to produce unambiguous estimates. The heat, if not the light, generated by these debates has attracted demographers who have taken an interest in the Amerindian collapse and other collapses of indigenous peoples in the face of culture conflicts. They have raised serious questions about the validity of all such estimates. McArthur argues that the paucity of demographic structure data so degrades

---

102   Sánchez-Albornoz, *The Population of Latin America*, p. 57; F. Chevalier, *Land and Society in Colonial America*, L. B. Simpson (ed.). Berkeley: University of California Press, 1963; L. B. Simpson, *Exploitation of Land in Central Mexico in the Sixteenth Century*, Ibero-Americana 36, Berkeley: University of California Press, 1952; and Juan Friede, "De la Encomienda Indiana a la Propiedad Territorial y su Influencia Sobre el Mestizaje," *Anuario Colombiano de Historia Social y de la Cultura* 4, (1969), pp. 35-62.

103   Simpson, *Exploitation*; and Sánchez-Albornoz, *The Population of Latin America*, pp. 58-59.

104   Kubler, "Population Movements," pp. 633-639; and A. Lipschutz, "La despoblación de las Indias después de la Conquésta," *América Indígena*, 26 (1966), pp. 227-247.

105   See Sánchez-Albornoz 1974: p. 65; J. H. Elliott, "The Spanish Conquest and Settlement of America," in Leslie Bethell (ed.), *The Cambridge History of Latin America*, Vol. 1. Cambridge: Cambridge University Press, 1984, p. 202; N. Wachtel, "The Indian and the Spanish Conquest," in L. Bethell (ed.), *The Cambridge History of Latin America*, Vol. 1. Cambridge: Cambridge University Press, 1984, p. 213; Dobyns, "An Outline of Andean Epidemic History"; Ashburn, *Ranks of Death*; Cook, "Disease Among the Aztecs"; Cook, *The Extent and Significance of Disease*; Crosby, "Conquistador y Pestiliencia"; Crosby, "Virgin Soil Epidemics"; Denevan, *The Native Population of the Americas in 1492*, pp. 4-5; Gerhard, *Historical Geography of New Spain*, p. 23; Gerhard, *The Southeast Frontier of New Spain*, p. 25; William H. McNeill, *Plagues and Peoples*, Garden City, NY: Anchor Books, 1976, pp. 180-185; Gibson, *The Aztecs*, p. 136; and MacLeod, *Spanish Central America*, p. 19.

many studies that even those efforts that are acceptable may raise more questions than they answer.[106] Petersen argues that the scarcity of quality data diminishes the believability of population collapse figures, and that systematic bias on the part of scholars leads to unrealistically large depopulation figures.[107] Further, Petersen notes that documents used to estimate populations and the analyses that flow from them, no matter how historically accurate, cannot correctly answer questions about population dynamics if the data important to understanding of the dynamics are not recorded.[108] McArthur agrees, and points to the importance of data on demographic structure (both before contact and during the population decline) and migration as key to helping explain the course of a population decline.[109]

Much, if not most, of the effort expended in analysis of the Amerindian collapse has consisted of detailed description and classification. This approach, however, fails to link proposed causes for the collapse to the statistics gathered on the magnitude of the collapse, impeding the exploration of explanation. Potentially important causal factors in the collapse may have been ignored because they did not surface in the descriptive accounts of the holocaust. Further, without a model of the causal interactions, the assumptions used to construct the depopulation estimates may not be valid. Thus, a model of explanation is necessary to have confidence in the statistical collapse figures as well as to have a better understanding of its causes.

While historically-based estimates may be faithful to their sources, they may fail to reproduce the actual population dynamics of the times. Specialists in Latin American population history are cognizant of these problems. Borah advocates using the best historical verification techniques to investigate documentary sources, but also calls for comparative study and integration of demographic, social structural, resource, settlement structural, and technological variables into historical population studies.[110] Robinson notes that weaknesses in the evidence of settlement structure, subsistence systems, and local ecologies diminish understanding of post-contact Amerindian population dynamics.[111] To overcome the many problems of data shortfall and inadequate analysis, Robinson advocates simplifying the necessary assumptions in a controlled way. He suggests

---

106 N. McArthur,"The Demography of Primitive Populations," *Science,* 167 (1970), 1098-1099, p. 1101.

107 Petersen, "A Demographers View," pp. 384-386; and Petersen, *Population,* pp. 235-236.

108 Petersen, "A Demographers View," p. 396.

109 McArthur, "Demography of Primitive Populations," pp. 1098-1099.

110 Borah, "Historical Demography," pp. 22-24, 29.

111 David J. Robinson "Introduction," in D. J. Robinson (ed.), *Studies in Spanish American Population History.* Boulder, CO: Westview Press, 1981, pp. 2-3.

using simulation models of change, such as computer models of disease diffusion.[112]

This study explores such a modelling approach by means of system dynamics computer simulations applied to the sixteenth-century population collapse in the Basin of Mexico.[113] This location was selected because it was diverse and well populated before the Spanish intrusion, and continued to be distinctive after the conquest. The Basin was the Aztec imperial homeland with a large and probably growing population. The Spanish subjugation of the Basin was rapid and sustained by occupation and "Hispanicization" of the landscape. In addition, this case was selected because it has been the subject of extensive historical examination from which considerable data can be drawn.[114]

The preceding discussion of the background, general methodological problems, and controversy inherent in the various historical estimates of the Basin's population suggest that by addressing three broad questions about the sixteenth-century population history of the Basin, a significant advance in scholarship about these issues may be achieved. These questions, then, serve as the *raison d'être* for this study.

1. Was the severe depopulation implied by most of the historical analyses possible? That is to say, is it reasonable to believe that the purported causes of the population decline could drive a large and healthy population to suffer such a collapse in the span of 100 years?

2. What was the scale of the decline? In particular, are the relatively extreme estimates of Cook and Borah supportable, is the less profound depopulation implied by Cook and Simpson more likely, or is some other reconstruction better? These questions embody several others:

   a. What is the most reasonable 1519 population estimate for the Basin?
   b. Despite the poor data used to estimate the populations for the first half-century of Hispanic occupancy, historical reconstructions point to a severe collapse in this period. Was this likely, and what was its scale?
   c. What was the overall rate of depopulation in the Basin and when was the nadir of population?

---

[112] Robinson, "Introduction," p. 7.

[113] J. W. Forrester, *Principles of Systems*, Cambridge, MA: Wright-Allen Press, Inc., 1968.

[114] See Cook and Borah, *The Indian Population of Central Mexico*; Cook and Simpson, *The Population of Central Mexico in the Sixteenth Century*; Gibson, *The Aztecs*; Sanders, "The Population of the Central Mexican Symbiotic Region"; and others.

    d. What is the nature of the "fine-structure" of the population trajectory? That is to say, how did the collapse proceed, in phases or more-or-less uniformly?

3. What was the major cause of the depopulation? Again, this question implies more detailed ones:

    a. Besides increased mortality, how significant were the other demographic causes of population decline, decreased fertility and/or emigration?

    b. Is it possible that introduced epidemic diseases were mostly responsible for the population loss?

    c. What other causal factors (e.g., homicide or famine) were important and how significant were they?

Resolving fundamental questions such as these is required if the general debate around the Amerindian depopulation is to approach resolution. The simulation methodology developed here provides one of the most rigorous means of resolving these questions (assuming, of course that new historical documentation that is above challenge is not found).

Simulation as Methodology

Unlike most of the previous work, the modeling approach used here does not address the population collapse by way of historical arguments (i.e., arguments based on textual choice, veracity, or interpretation of population counts). Instead, the scale of collapse is examined indirectly through the operation of a causal model of population change. The model's structure is based on law-like generalities of the "middle range," combined with data derived for the Amerindian situation. This model is used to simulate the dynamic behavior of the system in response to the known perturbations of disease, conflict, famine, and so on. In essence, this model consists of a set of hypotheses. These relate the structure of the system, the rates which control change in the state variables, and assumptions as to the initial values of state variables. These hypotheses are calibrated by examining the dynamic behavior of the system to ascertain if it operates in a manner consistent with the values of known historical variables, or "reasonable" values if specific values are unknown. In this case, the results from the calibrated simulations will be compared to the historically derived population estimates.

Hypotheses that seek to explain dynamic behavior must be developed by reference to process laws.[115] In the historical demography of Western Europe, process laws were determined from data extracted from the

---

[115] G. Bergmann, *Philosophy of Science*, Madison, WI: University of Wisconsin Press, 1966, p. 93; and D. Harvey, *Explanation in Geography*, New York: St. Martin's Press, 1969, pp. 418-419.

historical record.[116] These process laws may be described as structural frameworks that show how a variety of variables affected, and were affected by, the basic elements of population change (i.e., mortality, fertility, and migration rates). Detailed data on such basic elements are not available for the early collapse period in the New World, and may never be.[117]

These problems notwithstanding, potential explanation can be attempted for this period by applying the process laws developed elsewhere to create a hypothetical population system. Similarly, values for state variables and rates can be estimated from data for analogous situations elsewhere. This approach assumes that human populations behave according to culturally invariant process laws and that human population dynamics can be thought of as a system of interrelated parts. This assumption is implicit in virtually all conceptions of population dynamics.[118] The dynamic behavior exhibited by such a construction can be compared with the historically derived empirical record, and, to the extent to which it agrees, the structure can be tentatively accepted as a potential explanation. It is important to note, however, that all such models contain simplifying assumptions. For that reason, close fit with the empirical data is not proof of the validity of the structure or rate

---

116   See Confrees Bellagio Conference, "The Relationship of Nutrition, Disease, and Social Conditions: a Graphical Presentation," in R. I. Rotberg and T. K. Rabb (eds.), *Hunger and History, The Impact of Changing Food Production and Consumption Patterns on Society*, Cambridge: Cambridge University Press, 1983, pp. 305-308; D. E. C. Eversley, "Population, Economy, and Society," in D.V. Glass and D.E.C. Eversley (eds.), *Population in History*, Chicago: Aldine Publishing Co., 1965, pp. 23-69; H. J. Habakkuk, *Population Growth and Economic Development Since 1750*, Leicester, U.K: Leicester University Press, 1971, Chapter 1; Hatcher, *Plague, Population and the English Economy*, pp. 55-62; T. McKeown, "Food, Infection, and Population," in R. I. Rotberg and T. K. Rabb (eds.), *Hunger and History, The Impact of Changing Food Production and Consumption Patterns on Society*, Cambridge: Cambridge University Press, 1983, pp. 29-50; J. D. Post, *Food Shortage, Climatic Variability, and Epidemic Disease in Preindustrial Europe*, Ithaca, NY: Cornell University Press, 1985, pp. 17-29; N. S. Scrimshaw, "Functional Consequences of Malnutrition for Human Populations: A Comment," in R. I. Rotberg and T. K. Rabb (eds.), *Hunger and History*, pp. 211-214; S. C. Watkins, and E. van der Walle. "Nutrition, Mortality, and Population size: Malthus' court of last resort," in R.T. Rotberg and T.K. Rabb (ed.), *Hunger and History*, pp. 7-28; and E.A. Wrigley, and R.S. Schofield, *The Population History of England 1541-1871: A Reconstruction*, London: Edward Arnold, 1981, Chapter 11.

117   But see Robinson's edited volume *Studies in Spanish American Population History*, Boulder, CO: Westview Press, 1981) for examples of the application of the "European method" to later periods in the New World.

118   See M.W. Flinn, *The European Demographic System, 1500-1820*, Brighton, UK: Harvester Press, 1981.

assumptions in such models.[119] Further, a close fit with historical data does not completely clarify the situation, since the empirical record is incomplete and untrustworthy.

In general, models are formalized expressions of theory, in this situation, theories of process. Since no general theory of population change is universally agreed upon, it is impossible to demonstrate that such a model is formally derived from theory. A model in this case is a temporary device: representing what we believe the structure to be; suggesting theory; and allowing manipulations and conclusions to be drawn without a formal, general theory.[120] To increase the chance that such a model reflects a valid theory, it is critical that the model be as isomorphic as possible with the "real world." This requirement is equivalent to Bergmann's: that all the influences acting upon the relevant variables (in this case the variables of the demographic equation) are encompassed by the explanatory system.[121] To that end, each element and relationship in the model must have real world meaning and exhibit the quantitative behavior of the real world variable. In addition, the model structure must reflect relationships demonstrated elsewhere (i.e., reflect generally agreed-upon partial theory).[122]

A Forrester system dynamics simulation is an appropriate type of methodology to be applied to this modeling problem.[123] It asserts causal relationships, thereby proposing explanation. It assumes that dynamic tendencies of the system arise from the interaction of the systemic causal structure and external perturbations, thereby incorporating theories of the middle range.[124] Nevertheless, it does not assert perfect predictability, only aggregate or average system behavior.[125] By providing precise and explicit exposition of the values and structures within the model, it enhances falsifiability.[126] By allowing the state of the system to alter the strength of relationships, it accommodates changing conditions. Further, it explicitly deals with time lags in responses, an important facet for population dynamics. Lastly, it is not particularly sensitive to parameter changes—only

119   Harvey, *Explanation*, p. 404.

120   Harvey, *Explanation*, p. 146.

121   Bergmann, *Philosophy of Science*, 94.

122   D. H. Meadows, "The Unavoidable A Priori," in J. Randers (ed.), *Elements of the System Dynamics Method*, Cambridge, MA: The M.I.T. Press, 1980, p. 36.

123   Forrester, *Principles of Systems*.

124   Meadows, "The Unavoidable A Priori," 25-27; and R. Woods, *Theoretical Population Geography*, Burnt Mill, UK: Longman Group Ltd., 1982, pp. 5, 7-8.

125   Meadows, "The Unavoidable A Priori," pp. 25-27

126   J. A. Bell, and J. F. Bell, "System Dynamics and Scientific Method," in J. Randers (ed.), *Elements of the System Dynamics Method*, Cambridge, MA: M.I.T. Press., 1980, 16, 19; and Meadows, "The Unavoidable A Priori," pp. 25-27.

to structural changes, therefore incomplete or imprecise data are less of a problem.[127]

Foremost, this simulation methodology increases the level of confidence in the descriptive statistics of the collapse—that is, it identifies which population reconstructions are most plausible. It also offers a means of detailing the scenarios of the causes of depopulation so that the most likely scenarios and their operations can be determined. In sum, this study produces a structured, dynamic cultural ecology of population change in this region.

This method is advantageous in a number of ways. It explicitly couples population change to those causal factors believed responsible for it, thereby enhancing the believability of the results. Further, it illuminates the relative importance of different elements. A number of important variables (some noted above) that are not incorporated in previous studies are explicitly linked in a model of change. A third advantage is that the approach makes explicit the assumptions and purported mechanisms of change and is, for that reason, falsifiable on grounds other than the controversial ones of the selective choice of sources, their assumed veracity, or the methodologies used in their interpretation.

While the preceding justifies the use of simulation to explore historical population change, it does not address the larger problem of examining existing historically-derived estimates. To apply a simulation methodology to this type of problem, it is necessary to *compare* simulation results with historical reconstructions. In such comparisons, the fundamental assumption is that historical population reconstructions that "match" simulation population reconstructions also draw on the same causal structures. Thus, doubt is cast on the validity of an historical reconstruction that requires the simulation model to use extreme or historically inaccurate data values in order to produce a run that mimics the historical reconstruction trajectory.

The general method necessary to realize these comparisons involves a multi-step process. The first step is to identify and quantify historically-derived Basin population estimates. The second step is to arrange the individual historical estimates into groups that reflect a similar set of assumptions about the sixteenth-century depopulation. The population trajectory created by the simulation will be matched against these historical possibilities.

The third step is to create the simulation itself. Since the simulation is created without input from the historically-derived population estimates, it is necessary to calibrate the simulation so that its "nominal" population output closely "matches" the population dynamics of each of the grouped historical reconstructions. Once a simulation run is created that matches an historical reconstruction, interpretations about the validity or probability of this family of historical estimates may be made by referencing the assumptions needed to produce the matching simulation. Simulations that necessitate extreme or

---

[127] Meadows, "The Unavoidable A Priori," pp. 25-27.

impossible assumptions in order to match an historical group or those that generate data that is contradicted by other historical data are rejected. By inference, the historical group that matches the rejected simulation is discarded as well. This complex method is more fully described in Chapters 3 and 4. Aspects of the construction of the simulation model are discussed below and more fully in Chapter 2.

Model Description

To understand population dynamics, it is necessary to understand the dynamics of the elements of the demographic equation (i.e., the dynamics of fertility, mortality, and migration). Each of these elements is, in turn, related to a set of intermediate factors, which determine the resulting dynamic. These intermediate factors do not operate singly or in isolation but are interconnected in a system. Hence, to understand the operation of the immediate factors, and thus the dynamic of the demographic elements, it is necessary to consider the web of "geographical" influences, the physical environment, human society, and biology, or as Sinnecker has put it for epidemiology: the environmental system, the host system, and the causative agent.[128]

Since data do not exist to measure directly the dynamics of the demographic elements for the early collapse period, it is necessary to consider the intermediate and secondary influences on these elements. The fundamental assertion of this simulation methodology is that data do exist to estimate the influence of these elements, and simulation can generate the demographic equation dynamics from the dynamics of these other variables.

Turning first to the intermediate factors associated with mortality, four stand out. The first two, endemic diseases and famines are clearly related facets of the indigenous system. Tuberculosis, pneumonia, other respiratory diseases, dysentery, diarrheas, other intestinal infections, parasitic worms, nutritional deficiency diseases, suppuration, fevers, and syphilis are widely recognized as endemic in the pre-conquest New World.[129] Famine is also reported in Aztec codices.[130] Violent death, the third factor, was clearly an aspect of Amerindian mortality before the conquest. Spanish homicide in the form of forced labor, military action, and

---

[128] J. M. May, "Medical Geography: Its Methods and Objectives," *Geographical Review* 40, (1950), 11; and H. Sinnecker, *General Epidemiology*, Translated by N. Walker, London: Wiley, 1976, p. 24.

[129] Ashburn, *Ranks of Death*, Chapters 10 and 11; Cook, *Teotlapan*; and Crosby, *The Colombian Exchange*, Chapter 4.

[130] Cook, *Soil Erosion*, 332-333; and Ross Hassig, "The Famine of One Rabbit: Ecological Causes and Social Consequences of a Pre-Colombian Calamity," *Journal of Anthropological Research* 37 (1981), pp. 171-182.

wanton cruelty is also widely documented.[131] The fourth, but clearly the most prominent mortality factor in the immediate post-conquest period, is epidemic disease.[132]

On the fertility side, three sets of intermediate variables are pertinent.[133] The first of these are factors affecting exposure to intercourse (i.e., factors governing the formation of unions and those governing exposure to intercourse within unions). The second variables are the factors that affect exposure to conception, that is to say variables that affect fecundity. Lastly, variables that influence gestation and successful partition are counted among the intermediate fertility-affecting variables.

For the purposes of this model, net migration in pre-Hispanic times is assumed to be zero. Its exclusion will do no violence to the model since the factors influencing migration were radically different in post-contact times. Migration in post-contact times was, very generally, of two types. Petersen argues that the first of these, spontaneous migration in the face of local epidemics, social disruption and/or economic deprivation, famines, natural hazards, or war, was perhaps the most typical response to troubled times.[134] Other voluntary migration types included migration to more attractive places; from the services-rich cities and the potentially rich mining camps, to the shift in the labor force that accompanied the shift to colonial agricultural estates.[135] The Spanish tribute counts in the later periods recognized this and included a category for non-locals, *forasteros*, and their numbers were often significant.[136] The second type of migration in colonial times was forced migration in the form of human movements associated with forced labor and relocations or regroupings *(congregaciones)* of entire Indian communities.[137]

---

[131] Kubler, "Population Movements," pp. 606-643; Friede, "Demographic changes," pp. 339; and Sánchez-Albornoz, *The Population of Latin America,* pp. 52.

[132] Ashburn, *Ranks of Death*; Cook, *The Extent and Significance of Disease*; Cook, "Disease Among the Aztecs"; Crosby, "Conquistador y Pestiliencia"; Crosby, "Virgin Soil Epidemics"; Denevan, *The Native Population of the Americas in 1492*, pp. 4-5; Dobyns, "An Outline of Andean Epidemic History"; Elliott, "The Spanish Conquest and Settlement of America," p. 202; Gerhard, *Historical Geography of New Spain*, p. 23; Gerhard, *The Southeast Frontier of New Spain*, p. 25; Gibson, *The Aztecs*, p. 136; MacLeod, *Spanish Central America*, p. 19; McNeill, *Plagues and Peoples*, p. 176; and Sánchez-Albornoz, *The Population of Latin America*, p. 65; and Wachtel, "The Indian and the Spanish Conquest," p. 213.

[133] United Nations Department of Economic and Social Affairs, *The Determinants and Consequences of Population Trends*, Vol. 1. New York: The United Nations, 1973, pp. 77-78.

[134] Petersen, *Population*, p. 386.

[135] Robinson, "Typology of Migration," pp. 14-15.

[136] For example, see Cook, *Demographic Collapse*, p. 86.

[137] Robinson, "Typology of Migration," p. 13.

Each of the intermediate factors listed above for fertility, mortality, and migration are influenced by a variety of secondary factors. For simplicity, these may be described in five general classes; historical, demographic, epidemiological, cultural, and agroecological. These classes capture the essence of Woods' six "factors controlling population growth [and decline];" biological, environmental, economic, social, political, and technological.[138] It is from consideration of these secondary factors that level, rate, and lag data are derived in the simulation. The following is a general discussion of how secondary factors are used to derive model parameters. Each determination of a model parameter reflects a synthesis, utilizing theoretical arguments and Old and New World empirical data.

Historical factors include the dating and identification of epidemic disease outbreaks. These data exist in the secondary literature of the history of the post-conquest period.[139] Data for war casualties and figures for forced labor migrations are less obvious in the interpretative literature. Estimates may have to be made from general arguments about the size of armies and their rate of casualty, and general estimates of the number of forced laborers in the mines and on plantations. These historical data are used in estimating several model constituents, including: epidemic disease, migration rate, and total mortality.

Assumptions as to the pre-conquest demographic structure are obtained by utilizing stable population tables.[140] These are chosen based on informed scholarly interpretations as to the mortality and fertility schedules for pre-conquest Amerindians as well as using theoretical arguments.[141] Fertility rates for post-conquest populations are determined in the model by the modification of an assumed "natural fertility" by secondary factors.[142] Similarly, non-crisis mortality is calculated from an assumed "natural" benchmark. Demographic structure data also influences endemic and epidemic mortality rates.

Arguments as to the innate susceptibility of the indigenous population to the epidemic diseases of the period are derived from the epidemiological

---

138 Woods, *Theoretical Population Geography*, pp. 9-15.

139 Outstanding examples are found in Dobyns, "Andean Epidemic History"; Wachtel, "The Indian and the Spanish Conquest," p. 213; Cook, *Demographic Collapse*, pp. 60-61; Gerhard, *Historical Geography of New Spain*, p. 23, and Gibson, *The Aztecs*, Appendix IV.

140 A. J. Coale, and P. Demeny, *Regional Model Life Tables and Stable Populations*, Princeton: Princeton University Press, 1966.

141 See Cook, "Disease among the Aztecs"; Cook, *Demographic Collapse*, pp. 100-106; and United Nations, *The Determinants and Consequences of Population Trends*, p. 78.

142 United Nations, *The Determinants and Consequences of Population Trends*, p. 78.

literature dealing with each disease.[143] Similarly, the virulence of the several diseases are estimated by recourse to the medical literature and the literature of the disease impacts in America.[144] The social, environmental, and demographic factors influencing transmission of epidemic infections are also found in the epidemiological literature related to each disease.

Inferences as to the effects of particular cultural practices, such as the reported post-conquest practices of abortion, voluntary celibacy, and infanticide, on demographic variables are made from an analysis of the primary Hispanic accounts as well as their interpretation by scholars exemplified by Sánchez-Albornoz, Jaramillo Uribe, and Sauer.[145] Similarly, cultural factors important to the epidemiological variables, such as settlement structure, density, and the reported lack of a concept of contagion, are obtained from primary accounts and their interpretation.

Consideration of the agroecosystem in this population dynamics model is important because of the role that famine played in communities besieged by epidemic and other deaths. Food production variables, including the timing and level of labor inputs to agriculture, are clearly influenced by the rate of epidemic mortality, the quantity of labor withdrawn by Spanish *encomenderos*, and other labor withdrawal factors. Other production variables (e.g., adoption of new cultigens, reduction of subsistence crop area, cultivation methods, amount of normal surplus generated, and vulnerability to drought) are affected by these labor changes. The diminished production resulting from these changes is partially responsible for famine. In addition to the obvious link of malnutrition to susceptibility, famine is implicated in epidemic spread through an acceleration process of the epidemic's diffusion, as demonstrated by Post for Europe.[146] Estimates and descriptions of the indigenous production systems such as Turner's and Sanders and colleagues' are the sources for these data.[147]

This study is a dynamic and comparative cultural ecology of a structured subset of environment-society relationships, an outgrowth of traditional geographical "human-nature" studies. It attempts to link the factors directly governing human population change to elements in the broader environmental, sociocultural, technical, and historical *milieux*. As such it invokes primarily the "vertical" geographical syntheses identified by

---

143 See A. S. Evans, "Epidemiological Concepts and Methods," in A. S. Evans (ed.), *Viral Infections of Humans*, New York and London: Plenum Medical Book Company, 1976, pp. 1-32, for viral diseases.

144 See Ashburn, *Ranks of Death*; and Cook, *Demographic Collapse*; Chapter 5.

145 Sánchez-Albornoz, *The Population of Latin America*, p. 55; Jaramillo Uribe, "La Población Indígena de Colombia"; and Sauer, *The Early Spanish Main*.

146 Post, *Food Shortage*.

147 Turner, "Comparisons of Agrotechnologies"; and Sanders, et al., *The Basin of Mexico*.

Turner.[148] Topically it lies along a well-worn path of geographical exploration in Amerindian population studies blazed by Carl Sauer and his "Berkeley School" legacy and the more recent efforts of Robinson. Seen in another light, the subject and goals of this study lie within the general definition of population geography put forth by Ogden and Zelinsky.[149]

The findings of this study are significant to and will extend research on the Amerindian collapse in several ways. First, this simulation modelling approach represents an alternative to the historical-accounting approach which dominates the literature, and, significantly, serves as a relatively independent "test" of the conclusions implicit in that literature. Second, it postulates an explicit set of causes and interactions within a modelled population system. For that reason, the conclusions reached are, in principle, falsifiable—and this is an aid to reaching a theory of the collapse. Further, testing of the explicit set of causal relationships within the simulations sheds light on the interaction of causal factors and their relative importance. Lastly, while the conclusions reached for this case study are applicable strictly to the single area examined, the implications of this method and findings are important for research in the Amerindian collapse in general. Indeed, any study of population collapse, historic or prehistoric, may benefit from the insights generated in this study. In sum, the study weds a method little-developed by geographers and historical demographers to a subject and sub-field that has a long tradition in geography and that, by its very "complexity," should benefit from such a method.

This work is organized in five chapters. The long second chapter describes the construction of simulation models in general, and of MEXIPOP in particular. This simulation model is the heart of the methodology developed here, and its three major sub-systems are described and justified in detail.

The shorter third chapter has three parts that provide the bridge between the simulations and the historical estimates. The first details the historical population estimates for the Basin and groups them to facilitate analysis. The second part calibrates the MEXIPOP simulation runs and produces a group of standardized simulation runs. The third part "mates" the standardized simulation runs with historical reconstruction groups.

The fourth chapter has a dual function. First, it serves to interpret the population dynamics, the causal linkages, the longer-term demographic trends, and some of the implications suggested by the simulations. Second,

---

[148] B. L. Turner, II. "The Specialist-Synthesis Approach to the Revival of Geography: The Case of Cultural Ecology," *Annals of the Association of American Geographers,* 79 (1989).

[149] P. E. Ogden, "Population Geography," in R. J. Johnston (ed.), *The Dictionary of Human Geography,* Oxford: Basin Blackwell Ltd., 1981; and W. Zelinski, *A Prologue to Population Geography,* Englewood Cliffs, NJ: Prentice-Hall, 1966, p. 5.

using the data developed in the first section, it describes the rationale for the choice among the potential simulations and describes the choice.

The last chapter is a forum to discuss the major findings of this work and their significance. To that end, it details the "answers" to the basic questions that drive this work and describes their significance. Further, it speculates on the wider methodological significance of the techniques developed here and suggests other potential uses for the methods developed here.

Chapter 2

SIMULATION METHOD AND JUSTIFICATION

The General Model

This chapter describes and explains the elements and interconnections of the STELLA system dynamics population model developed for this study: MEXIPOP. To clarify how this complex and abstract model was constructed and how it relates to the issues of interest here, it is useful to show the work from a "thought model," through a causal loop diagram, to a quantifiable dynamic model. Since this is tedious for the large MEXIPOP model, an example is used to highlight the general technique. Here, an example "thought model" of the interactions of a simple population system, and the resulting causal model and STELLA diagram are explained. The full MEXIPOP model is discussed in subsequent sections.

The Thought Model

The behavior of a human population may be modeled as an interacting system of causal variables whose behavior determines the dynamics of the population. These types of interrelationships may be simply illustrated by use of a causal diagram that displays the underlying logic of these connections and suggests the nature of each relationship.

In this example (Figure 2.1), the size of a population is determined by the three basic demographic variables, fertility, mortality, and migration. This relationship is symbolized in the diagram by the arrows connecting these variables to the *population size* variable. The "+" sign near the arrowhead connecting *fertility* to *population size* indicates that these variables are related positively so that an increase in *fertility* results in an increase in *population size*. Similarly, a decrease in *fertility* brings about a decrease in *population size*. The "-" sign near the arrows connecting *mortality* and out-migration to *population size* indicates a negative or inverse relationship so that a decrease in *mortality* or out-migration results in an

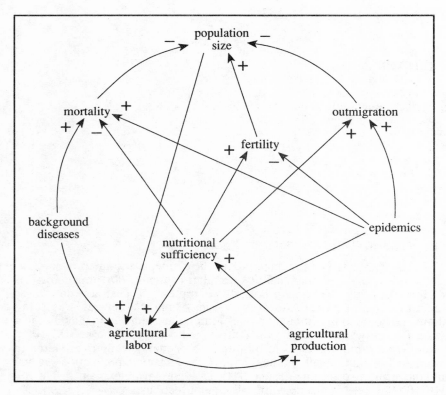

Figure 2.1 Interactive Thought Model

increase in *population size*. As would be expected, *mortality* is shown to vary positively with the incidence of *epidemics, background diseases*, and negatively with *nutritional sufficiency* (Figure 2.1). Similarly, *out-migration* varies positively with *epidemics* and negatively with *nutritional sufficiency*. By contrast, *fertility* varies negatively with *epidemics* and positively with *nutritional sufficiency*. The variable, *epidemics*, is shown without any "incoming" arrows, indicating that it is independent of the other variables in this model. *Nutritional sufficiency* is dependent on *agricultural production*, which is, in turn, dependent on *agricultural labor*. The model's connections are completed by the dependence of *agricultural labor* with *population size, background diseases, famines*, and *epidemics*. Circular connections such as those that link *famines* to *agricultural labor, agricultural labor* to *agricultural production*, and *agricultural production* finally back to *famines* again are termed feedback loops. This small loop is a "positive feedback loop" since an increase in *agricultural labor* will increase *agricultural production* which will decrease *famine*, which will, ultimately, further increase *agricultural labor*.

The Stella "Causal Model"

The presence of many, complex, and reciprocal causal relationships (i.e., nested feedback loops) in any system provides the justification for using system analysis since they highlight the complexity and counter-intuitive nature of the behavior of even a simple system. To exploit the advantages of this systemic description, however, it is necessary to go beyond these simple mental models and to define the relationships between the variables numerically. In essence, this consists of constructing a system of equations that define these relationships. The simulation of the dynamics of the system is accomplished by having a computer solve these equations iteratively (i.e., to use the values obtained for one time increment to solve for the next). In this case, STELLA, a microcomputer system dynamics program, is used to accomplish this. In STELLA simulations, the state of the model (i.e., the values of the variables) at the beginning of the temporal simulation is set by the initial assumptions. Subsequently, the model's structure determines the values of variables.

There are several symbols used to denote variables and the logical connections between them in STELLA model diagrams. The variables are italicized in the text and labeled with identifying names in which the "_" character replaces the "blank space" between words. These variable names may be complete, descriptive words or phrases or simple abbreviation-like notations. A quick tour of the STELLA diagram representing the example model above will make the diagrams more comprehensible (see Figure 2.2). The rectangular STOCK symbol (e.g., *population_size* and *agricultural_labor*) symbolizes anything that accumulates. A common example of a STOCK is the amount of water in a bathtub at any moment; this quantity is the value of that STOCK at that moment. Associated with STOCKS are pipe and valve-like FLOW icons (e.g., *deaths*, *births*, and *increment* in Figure 2.2). These are conduits for carrying (into or out of) the things that accumulate in the stocks. Using the bathtub analogy, the drains and taps are FLOW variables. They can link STOCKS or connect STOCKS with CLOUDS (e.g., *deaths*, *births*, and *increment* in Figure 2.2). The CLOUDS are the sources or sinks of the FLOWS and represent things that lie outside the model. The FLOW icons have valve-like regulators that show that they determine the rate of the flow. Round icons without flow pipes are CONVERTORS (e.g., *mortality, fertility, background_diseases, famines, epidemics*, and *agricultural_production* in Figure 2.2). These may act to convert one variable into a form usable by another or may be independent variables or constants that affect other elements in the model. The logic of the connections between the model elements is symbolized by the connection ARROWS (e.g., between *epidemics* and *mortality* in Figure 2.2). The nature of the connection between elements is definable by equation or graphically. For example, *population_size* (at time 2) = *population_size* (at time 1) + *births - deaths -out-migration* (during the interval). The nature of these connections is numerically specified and may be simple or complex depending on the specific situation. The MEXIPOP

34

model developed in this study uses the same logic and symbolization as in the example. For clarity, it is discussed in three parts (or sub-systems), the demographic, the health/interaction, and the production. For all the simulations in this study, the data are reported and interpreted using a standard one-year time interval. The STELLA simulation actually recalculates in shorter intervals, of 0.25 year, to enhance simulation accuracy. [1]

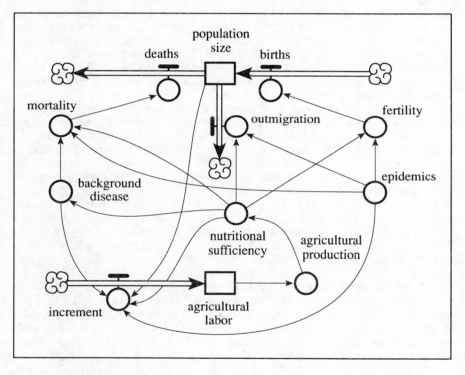

Figure 2.2 Stella Structural Diagram

---

[1] Throughout this and subsequent chapters some specific values and detailed logic of the numerical calculations of model variables are not detailed. They appear, instead, in Appendix 1. The general logic and justification of the model is detailed within the text of this chapter. Throughout the text, reference to the illustrative figures will amplify and clarify the arguments.

Demographic Sub-system

DEMOGRAPHIC MODELS

The population sub-system (Fig 2.3) is modeled using six age-class groups. Each of these groups has an associated mortality and migration function. In addition, there is a natality component that augments the population. Such age division is necessary to model adequately the effects of disease and famine on a population since the age of the affected individual is among the most important considerations in assessing the epidemiological impact of an epidemic or famine event.[2] Further, modeling the demographic dynamics, in particular the number of "able-bodied" adults, is important in understanding the ability of a population to support its dependents (both the youth and the aged as well as those external to the population, such as Spanish landlords).[3]

Since detailed demographic data for the pre-conquest population of the Basin are lacking, the initial numeric values for mortality, natality, and the age structure of the model populations are derived from life tables found in *Regional Model Life Tables and Stable Populations.*[4] In this work, the authors abstract (from 326 contemporary and historical national censuses world-wide) four general patterns ("families") of mortality, which they label "north," "south," "east," and "west".[5] These are distinguished by their different age-class mortality structure. Within each "family" of mortality there are 24 levels of mortality and fertility and corresponding age-structure (e.g., level 1 corresponds to high mortality, high fertility conditions, while level 24 represents the opposite conditions of low mortality and low fertility). Additionally, within each "level" there are separate calculations for different rates of growth or decline. Hence, the tables make it possible to model slowly growing populations of high fertility and mortality as well as rapidly growing populations of high fertility and mortality. The tables are calculated for "stable" populations (i.e., those with unchanging mortality patterns and uniform rates of growth or decline) and as such have stable age structures (i.e., for a given rate of growth the relative proportions of people at different ages are constant over time). It is from Coale and Demeny's detailed individual tables that the initial mortality, fertility, and age structure values for the models are calculated.

The specific "family" of mortalities for the immediate pre-contact Basin is not known. For that reason, we agree with Coale and Demeny who

---

2   Evans, "Epidemiological Concepts," p. 1; S. H. Preston, *Mortality Patterns in National populations, With Special Reference to Recorded Cause of Death*, New York: Academic Press, 1976, p. 91; Sinnecker, *General Epidemiology*, pp. 89-90; and S. C. Watkins and J. Menken, "Famines in Historical Perspective," *Population and Development Review*, 11 (1985), p. 655.

3   Hassig, *Trade, Tribute, and Transportation*, pp. 181-182.

4   Coale and Demeny, *Model Life Tables.*

5   Coale and Demeny, *Model Life Tables*, [7].

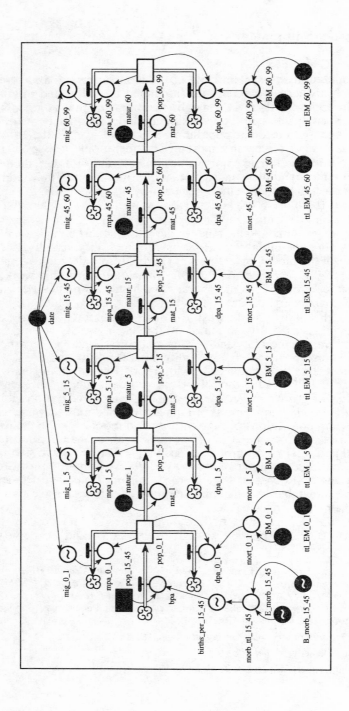

Figure 2.3 Demographic Sub-system

suggest "...utilizing the "West" family in the usual circumstances of underdeveloped [primarily agrarian?] countries where there is no reliable guide to the age pattern of mortality".[6] A less specific argument also supports the choice of the "west" family of mortalities. Since the "north", "south," and "east" patterns are specific to populations outside of Latin America, they are not appropriate choices for Amerindian populations. We are left with the "west" family, which represents a composite of non-regionally specific mortality patterns.[7] While the values in this family are not derived from pre-Hispanic Amerindian population data, there is little reason to believe that the general mortality patterns of the pre-Colombian New World were significantly different than those exhibited by other pre-industrial populations. The "west" pattern has high infant mortality, lower childhood and young adult mortalities, and relatively high mortalities for the aged.

N. D. Cook used the "West" model, level 3, to simulate the immediate pre-contact Peruvian population, and Hassig argues that this model population is also a good fit to the Basin in terms of social organization, population density, medical expertise, and epidemiological vulnerability.[8] Since such population assumptions are important in the simulations, both level 3 "West" and the lower mortality-lower fertility level 8 "West" population assumptions are used here. Augmenting these differing population models, two assumptions for the rate of population growth for each are used. The first presumes a virtually zero growth situation, and the other assumes a relatively rapid (for a paleolithic technology based civilization) growth rate of a little over 0.5 percent. This latter roughly corresponds to the growth rate implicit in Sanders and colleagues' archaeological reconstruction for the immediate pre-contact era Basin population.[9]

MEXIPOP SIMULATION LOGIC[10]

Age Structure

In STELLA modeling terms, the population is represented by population stocks (levels) for the 6 age-classes (e.g., *pop_0_1*) with birth

---

6   Coale and Demeny, *Model Life Tables*, p. 29. Also see below for more detailed argument about the choice of the "West" family.

7   Coale and Demeny, *Model Life Tables*, [14].

8   Cook, *Demographic Collapse*, p. 100; and Hassig, *Trade, Tribute, and Transportation*, p. 179, note 61.

9   Sanders, *et al.*, *The Basin of Mexico*; and Whitmore and Turner, *Population Reconstruction of the Basin of Mexico*, p. 34.

10   Throughout this chapter, reference is made to the MEXIPOP model diagram. Figures 2.3, 2.4, 2.5, 2.9, and 2.10 display the most relevant sections of this large model. The remaining parts are displayed in Figures A.1, A.2, and A.3 in the Appendix. A complete list of defining equations and graphical relationships for each relationship in MEXIPOP is found in the Appendix.

in-flows (e.g., *bpa*) augmenting the age 0-1 class stock and death (e.g., *dpa_0_1*), maturation (e.g., *mat_1*), and migration (e.g., *mpa_1_15*) out-flows depleting the age-class numbers (Figure 2.3). The following paragraphs will describe this structure and each variable, discuss the assumptions underlying them, and justify the values assumed for each.

The choice of these age-class divisions (i.e., 0-1, 2-5, 6-15, 16-45, 46-60, and 61-99) is based on Coale and Demeny's 5-year age-classes.[11] Coale and Demeny use separate tables for each sex, but since these sex-related mortality differences are relatively small and the proportions of each sex are quite similar, I have averaged them to produce male-plus-female age-class totals (Table 2.1). I have left unchanged the important infant and

TABLE 2.1 MODEL POPULATION PROPORTIONS

	Population model			
AGE-CLASS	3W ZPG (%)	3W + (%)	8 W ZPG (%)	8 W + (%)
	(a)	(a)	(b)	(b)
0-1	3.28	3.72	2.38	2.75
2-5	9.64	10.81	7.97	9.09
6-15	20.86	22.60	18.30	20.17
16-45	47.04	46.44	45.72	45.83
46-60	12.99	11.42	15.57	13.90
61-99	6.21	5.04	10.06	8.28

("ZPG" => no growth; "+" => 0.5% growth)
Calculated from:
(a) Coale & Demeny, 1966: 31, 127
(b) Coale & Demeny, 1966: 41, 137

young child groups, ages 0-1 and 2-5, but I have grouped some five-year age-classes to produce a "childhood" age-class of ages 6-15, a "young adult" age-class of ages 16-45, a "mature adult" age-class of ages 46-60, and an "elderly" age-class of ages 61-99, producing the 6 in the model (Figure 2.4 and Table 2.1). This alteration greatly simplifies the model. Any such accumulation of different ages necessarily introduces errors greater than those obtained from using finer divisions, however, since the entire age-group is assigned a mortality rate that is a population-proportion-adjusted average of the mortality rates of the constituent 5-year age-class. Yet, because the differences in age-group mortalities differ most strongly in the early ages (and these are not altered), this "age clumping" does not detract from the ability of the model to simulate the population dynamics to a degree of precision adequate in this type of study.

---

[11]   Coale and Demeny, *Model Life Tables*, [41].

39

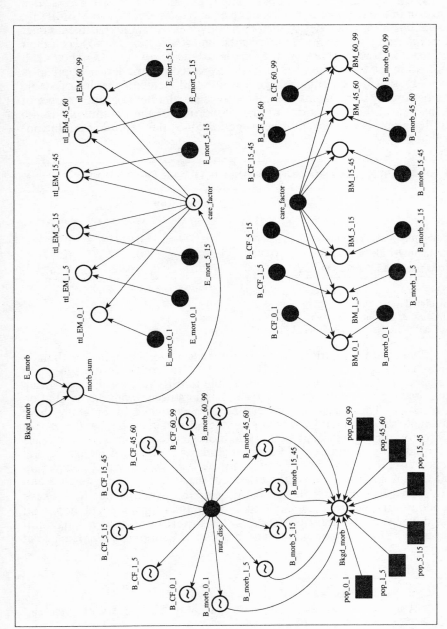

Figure 2.4 Health—Interaction Sub-system

Births

The first "flow" into the population, the number of live births, is a function of the number of mating couples and their fertility. In MEXIPOP, annual births (*bpa*) are determined by a converter that multiplies the number of births expected per the fertile population (*births_per_15_45*) (i.e., their fertility) by the number of the fertile adults (*pop_15_45*). For each population model the number of births expected per the fertile population (aged 15 to 45) are computed from Coale and Demeny's tables of stable populations by dividing the community-wide birth rates (i.e., the number of births per 1,000 population) by the proportion of the community in the fertile ages (i.e., the number aged 15-45 per 1,000 population) (Table 2.2).[12]

TABLE 2.2 COMMUNITY-WIDE BIRTH AND DEATH RATES

	Population model			
	3W ZPG (A)	3W +(A)*	8 W ZPG (B)	8 W + (B)
Community-wide death rates	0.0419	0.0427	0.0277	0.0261
Community-wide birth rates	0.0419	0.0477	0.0277	0.0311
Births per 15-45 population	0.0890	0.1026	0.0605	0.0679

("ZPG" => no growth; "+" => 0.5% growth)
Calculated from:
(a) Coale & Demeny, 1966: 31, 127
(b) Coale & Demeny, 1966: 41, 137

These simplifications may encompass more complexity than is immediately apparent, however. Both the definition of the fertile age-group (i.e., *pop_15_45*) and the calculation of the fertility rate for this age-group (i.e., *births_per_15_45*) draw on several assumptions about the population in question. These assumptions can best be examined by breaking them down into the behavioral and biological factors that contribute to the pattern of fertility for a given population. The biological component of fertility is determined by a complex of factors including: the ages of menarche and menopause, the prevalence of permanent sterility, the effects of postpartum and lactational amenorrhea, the effects of crisis induced amenorrhea and low sperm quality, and the probability of inter-uterine death.[13] These fecundity variables set the upper limit on fertility in a given population. That this upper limit is rarely achieved is due to fertility-limiting behavioral factors. The most important of these behavioral factors include: late age at

---

[12] Coale and Demeny, *Model Life Tables*, pp. 31, 41, 127, 137.

[13] J. Bongaarts, "Does Malnutrition Affect Fertility? A Summary of Evidence," *Science*, 208 (1980), p. 565.

marriage, marital disruption, deliberate birth control, and the pattern of breast feeding.[14]

Dealing first with the mating age-group variable, the model defines the 15-45 population age-class (i.e., *pop_15_45*) as the fertile age-group. Examining the length of the female fertile period will show that this is not an unreasonable assumption. Considerable research in this topic has shown that the ages of menarche and menopause are primarily functions of nutrition.[15] [16] The range of published ages of menarche varies from 13-16 years for low income, rural, modern populations[17] to from 14-16.5 years in nineteenth-century English working-class populations.[18] While most of the data are for first-world or South Asian populations, there do not seem to be geographic or racial-cultural differences aside from those of nutrition since Huss-Ashmore found contemporary, rural, highland Mexican populations to have similar ages of menarche, ranging from 14-17 years.[19] These data suggest that the age of menarche may be assumed here to be at or below 15 years of age. Similarly, the age of menopause also varies, and through a wider range. Frish found ages of menopause for nineteenth-century English working-class populations to range from 45-50, and Huss-Ashmore found a mean age of 47.5 years for Europeans in the same century.[20] Contemporary data from highland Mexico indicate an even lower age range of 38-43 years.[21] A menopausal age of 45 years thus seems to be an appropriate choice based on these data.

The other determinant of the ages of the breeding age-group is behavioral, the age of marriage or cohabitation. Here, the evidence is slim, but what little data there are suggest that the assumed average age of

---

14 Bongaarts, "Does Malnutrition Affect Fertility?" p. 564.

15 R. E. Frish, "Some Further Notes on Population, Food Intake, and Natural Fertility," in H. Levidon and Menken (eds.), *Natural Fertility*, Liege, Belgium: Ordina Editions, no date, p. 139; and W. H. Mosley, "The Effects of Nutrition on Natural Fertility," in H. Levidon and Menken (eds.), *Natural Fertility*, p. 88.

16 Further, the age of menarche does not mark the beginning of full potential fecundity because there is a period of several years of so-called "adolescent sterility" in which fecundity is below potential. There is also a period of "tapering-off" fecundity before menopause. These complex effects are incorporated in the *births_per_5_45* variable.

17 Frish, "Some Further Notes," p. 139; R. Huss-Ashmore, "Fat and Fertility: Demographic Implications of Differential Fat Storage," in K. A. Bennett (ed.), *Yearbook of Physical Anthropology*, New York: Alan R. Liss, Inc., 1980, p. 73; and Mosley, "The Effects of Nutrition," p. 88.

18 R. E. Frish, "Demographic Implications of the Biological Determinants of Female Fecundity," *Social Biology*, 22 (1975), p. 19.

19 Huss-Ashmore, "Fat and Fertility," p. 71.

20 Frish, "Some Further Notes," p. 139; and Huss-Ashmore, "Fat and Fertility," p. 71.

21 Huss-Ashmore, "Fat and Fertility," p. 71.

marriage, at 15, is not unreasonable. Cook and Borah unearthed late seventeenth-century church record data from Oaxaca that recorded early ages of marriage.[22] Of marriages in which the participants were younger than 25 years (a group apparently chosen to minimize the averaging problems when second and other late marriages skew the data), the mean age for men was 18.41 years and for women 15.49 years.[23] The median age for women in the entire sample was 16.2 years and for men, 20.51 years.[24] Further, they found that 48.2 percent of brides in their sample were younger than 16.0 years old, and 60.3 percent were younger than 18.0 years.[25] Cook and Borah's data, even though it is for 200 years later, echo Soustelle's assertion that Aztec men married at age 20-22. Alas, Soustelle gives no estimate about the marriage age of Aztec women.[26]

Gibson points to the difficulty in analyzing this topic by citing a 1579 document that argues that the age of marriage (presumably Christian marriage) in colonial times was 25 for women and 30 for men, and had risen from pre-conquest values, estimated at 12 in another document.[27] On the face of it, neither of these extreme values seem all that likely, since age 12 was likely to be pre-menarcheal and 25-30 is a late (but certainly not unknown) age of marriage in a traditional society. These extremes may be put down to exaggeration on the part of the sixteenth-century writers, were there not evidence that marriage, in the sense of a Christian, church wedding, may have been postponed in order to avoid tribute.[28] Acting against this was the practice of *encomenderos* forcing early marriage on the part of their potential *tributarios* to raise tribute amounts.[29] It may well be that marriage in the demographic sense of union with the possibility of procreation, may have occurred well before "legal," ecclesiastical marriage.

The mating age-group fertility variable, *births_per_15_45*, reflects assumptions about both biological and behavioral aspects of fertility. Foremost of these is an assumption of "natural fertility" for historical and non-Western populations. Natural fertility describes a population with no usual conscious effort to control the number of offspring.[30] The other behavioral variables (marital disruption, age of marriage, and pattern of breast feeding) and the biological variables (ages of menarche and

---

22   Cook and Borah, *Essays in Population History*, Vol. 2. p. 278.

23   Ibid.

24   Ibid.

25   Ibid.

26   Cook and Borah, *Essays in Population History*, Vol. 2, p. 278; and J. Soustelle, *The Daily Life of the Aztecs on the Eve of the Spanish Conquest*, London: Weidenfield and Nicholson, 1961, p. 173.

27   Gibson, *The Aztecs*, p. 151, note 72.

28   Ibid.

29   Ibid.

30   Mosley, "The Effects of Nutrition," p. 88.

menopause, prevalence of sterility, probability of inter-uterine death, and effects of postpartum and lactational amenorrhea) are incorporated in the fertility schedules that underlie the calculation of the "model life tables," since they are generalizations of the fertility and mortality experience of actual populations.[31] The value for the *births_per_15_45* variable is calculated from the crude fertility rate for the model population (i.e., that one chosen from Coale and Demeny) of the assumed mortality and age structure.

In compiling the model life tables, Coale and Demeny deliberately excluded population statistics from countries undergoing crises such as warfare or epidemics since a population's fertility and mortality are affected by such crises.[32] Since a goal of this study is to model the consequences of such crises for a population, the effect of crises on fertility is modeled by using the *morb_ttl_15_45* variable to modify the age-group fertility variable, *births_per_15_45*, in times of epidemic and famine (Figure 2.3). Figure 2.5 demonstrates the relationship between the morbidities of the fertile populations and the resulting birth rates. In general, the minimum birth rate, achieved when the morbidity levels approach 1.0 (i.e., everyone in the age-class is sick), is roughly 1/3 that obtaining in "normal" conditions.[33] The relationships are not modeled as linear ones since an increase in morbidity for a population with morbidity near zero will affect the resultant fertility less than the same increase in morbidity in a population that is already quite ill (i.e., the morbidity is large).

These relationships reflect the general decline in fertility due to changes in both biological and behavioral components of fertility during a subsistence or epidemic crisis. Behavioral changes such as postponement of marriage are widely reported in famines and a similar reaction is likely during epidemics as well.[34] Similarly, sexual abstinence and reduced frequency of intercourse due to the absence of spouses in search for food are also commonly reported in famines.[35] Epidemics are also likely to

---

31 Coale and Demeny, *Model Life Tables*, [6].

32 Coale and Demeny, *Model Life Tables*, [7].

33 Sara Millman, personal communication, 1988.

34 Watkins and Menken, "Famines in Historical Perspective," p. 656; and Emmanuel Le Roy Ladurie, "Famine Amenorrhea (Seventeenth-Twentieth Centuries)," in Robert Forster and Orest Ranum (eds.), *Biology of Man in History: Selections from the Annales Economies, Sociétés, Civilisations*, Trans. Elborg Forster and Patricia M. Ranum, Baltimore and London: The Johns Hopkins University Press, 1975, p. 164.

35 Le Roy Ladurie, "Famine Amenorrhea," p. 164; and Watkins and Menken, "Famines in Historical Perspective," p. 656.

44

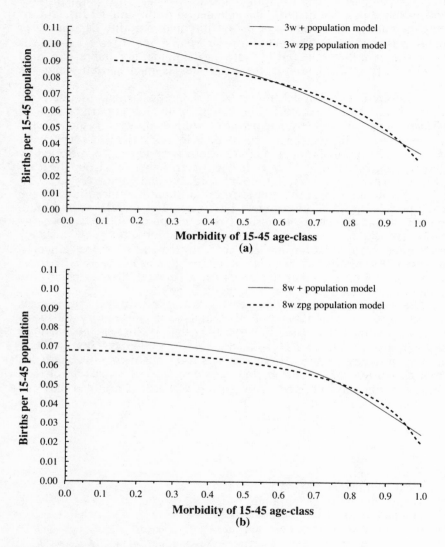

Figure 2.5 Birth Rate—Morbidity Interaction

reduce the frequency of intercourse due to illness. Watkins and Menken and Le Roy Ladurie also report crisis fecundity modifications such as famine amenorrhea and increased spontaneous abortion.[36] The loss of libido is also commonly noted and may have a basis in physiological or behavioral modifications due to crises.[37]

TABLE 2.3 MODEL POPULATION MORTALITY RATES

	Population model			
AGE-CLASS	3W ZPG (A)	3W + (A)	8 W ZPG (B)	8 W + (B)
0-1	0.2571	0.3192	0.2454	0.2629
1-5	0.0628	0.0628	0.0360	0.0348
5-15	0.0106	0.0106	0.0065	0.0063
15-45	0.0187	0.0185	0.0120	0.0115
45-60	0.0374	0.0372	0.0255	0.0274
60-99	0.1003	0.0993	0.0826	0.0784

("ZPG" => no growth; "+" => 0.5% growth)
Calculated from:
(a) Coale & Demeny 1966: 31, 127
(b) Coale & Demeny 1966: 41, 137

Deaths

The second set of "flows" out of the population, the yearly death totals for each age-class (e.g., *dpa_0_1*), are a product of the number of individuals within each age-group by the mortality rate for that age-class (e.g., *mort_0_1*) (Figure 2.3). In a situation without crises, the age-class mortalities, while different from one to another (and different between population models), are unchanging over time. In MEXIPOP, the period immediately before Spanish contact in 1519 is considered to be crisis free so the initial values of these mortalities are the same as the values in later, crisis-free, periods. These initial values for the age-class mortalities are calculated from the *Regional Model Life Tables and Stable Populations* by multiplying the proportions of total deaths accruing to the age-class by the community-wide death rate, and dividing by the age-class population proportion (results of these calculations are displayed in Table 2.3).[38] It is in this calculation and that of the maturation from one age-class to another (below) that the effect of "lumping" different age groups is felt. A life table with single year age-classes would assign a different mortality to each age. Any consolidation of ages, such as that in Demeny and Coale's tables or in

---

36 Watkins and Menken, "Famines in Historical Perspective," p. 656; and Le Roy Ladurie, "Famine Amenorrhoea," p. 164.

37 Le Roy Ladurie, "Famine Amenorrhoea," p. 164; and Watkins and Menken, "Famines in Historical Perspective," p. 656.

38 Coale and Demeny, *Model Life Tables*, pp. 30-31, 40-41, 126-127, 136-137.

this model, "averages" the mortalities for the different ages and assigns a "weighted average" mortality to the summed age-class. The weighting is necessary since the numbers of individuals in each age-class is different. As a rule, the mortalities for children decline with increasing age and from middle-age onwards mortalities increase (Table 2.3). But these changes are not uniform since there is little difference in the mortalities of the middle years especially, while there are sharp differences of mortality between individual years in childhood and in late maturity. The 6 age-group divisions in the model take advantage of this property to consolidate ages with generally similar mortalities, thus minimizing the averaging error. A later section will detail the construction of these age-class mortalities from the "background" and "epidemic" mortalities (e.g., *ttl_EM_0_1* and *BM_0_1*) shown in Figure 2.3.

Maturation

The age-groups within the population are linked by a third set of flow variables. The maturation of surviving individuals from one age-class to the next are symbolized by the maturation flow variables (e.g., *mat_1*). Thus for the 0-1 age-group, the *mat_1* variable reduces the number within the age-class, while it increases the number in the 1-5 age-class. The number of graduates from an age-class 'n' years in width is a function of the number of entrants to the age-class 'n' years ago. Hence, the number of individuals maturing from an age-class 'n' years in width in any year 'z' is given by the general expression:

$$\text{grads}_{t=z} = \text{entrants}_{t=z-n} * \text{survival rate}_{t=z} * \text{survival rate}_{t=z-1} \ldots * \text{survival rate}_{t=z-n}$$

'Entrants$_{t=z-n}$' is the number entering the age-class at time 'z-n' (i.e., the number entering the 'n' year wide age-group 'n' years before the date in question). The 'survival rates' equal 1 minus the mortality rate obtaining for the age-class in the years noted. The Stella modeling of this simple relationship is rather tedious. Figure 2.6 shows the logic of the calculations to determine the number maturing from the 1-5 age-group. For any date, the upper group of convertors "remembers" the number of entrants to the 1-5 age-group 4 years previous (e.g., *mat_1_lag_4*). The lower group of convertors in Figure 2.6 calculates the survival rate (equal to 1 minus the mortality rate) for the age-class for each year (e.g., *surv_1_5*, *S_1_5_lag_1*, ... , *S_1_5_lag_3*) and multiplies these by the number of entrants of 4 years earlier, *mat_1_lag_4*, to produce the number of graduates from the age-class, *matur_5* (for convenience, this variable is set to equal the *mat_5* variable in Figure 2.3). The logic is identical for the other maturation variables, except that it is more involved for wider age-classes.

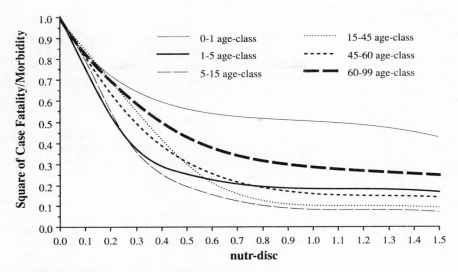

Figure 2.6 Background Case Fatality and Morbidity

Migration
The remaining flow determinant of the population is migration. Temporary or permanent movement is commonly cited as a major component of the demographic responses to famines and epidemics.[39] In the model (Figure 2.3), migration (e.g., *mig_0_1*) is simulated as a function of the calender date, using the *date* variable to regulate the out-flow of population.[40] This structure allows simulation of crisis or forced migration at specified times. The demographic sub-system is linked to the rest of the model primarily through the determination of the morbidity and mortality of the population in the health interaction sub-system.

---

[39] E. Colson, "In Good Years and in Bad: Food Strategies of Self-Reliant Societies," *Journal of Anthropological Research,* 35 (1979), pp. 25-26; G.J. Hugo, "The Demographic Impact of Famine: A Review," in B. Currey and G. J. Hugo (eds.), *Famine as a Geographical Phenomena*, Boston. D. Reidel Publishing Co., 1984, 13, p. 23; and Watkins and Menken, "Famines in Historical Perspective," p. 652.

[40] The convertor symbol for the date variable (Fig. 2.3) is shown in solid black rather than outline form. This symbolization shows that this variable is defined elsewhere in the model and only reproduced here. This convention obviates the need for long and possibly confusing logical connection lines from the variable *date* to all the other variables logically dependent on it. This convention is widely used in MEXIPOP wherever clarity is improved by its use, but it does not alter the logical relationships.

Health/Interaction Sub-system

This sub-system simulates the interconnections between the health experience of the population and its mortality and how these variables influence the production of food and vice versa. Before explaining this sub-system, it is helpful to sketch three of the general structural properties of the sub-system here. First, the overall mortality in the population is divided into two types, "background" and "epidemic" (see Figure 2.4) Background mortality represents the indigenous, endemic disease and nutritional problems common to pre-Hispanic Amerindian populations (see e.g., *BM_0_1* in Fig 2.4). Epidemic mortality is that additional mortality that obtains during an epidemic of an introduced fatal disease (see, for example, *ttl_EM_0_1* in Figure 2.4). Second, mortalities are modeled as a product of the standard epidemiological concepts, the morbidity and case fatality of each event. Morbidity is defined as the proportion of the total population (or of the age-class population if the age-class is the unit examined) that is affected by the mortality-causing famine, epidemic or endemic disease. Case fatality is the proportion of those affected who die. Thus, the product of the two yields the proportion of the population who die from the event (i.e., the mortality of the event). This division makes it possible to distinguish wide-spread, but relatively mild events from more lethal but less inclusive events. Lastly, it is sometimes necessary to convert age-class-specific morbidity values to community-level data. For that reason, there is a complex of converters that produce community-level data from age-class-specific values. These are symbolized in the STELLA modeling language by the variables, *Bkgd_morb* (i.e., the total background mortality for the whole community) and its corresponding set of 6 age-class background morbidities (such as *B_morb_0_1*), and *E_morb* and its corresponding age-class morbidities (such as *E_morb_0_1*) (Figures 2.4 and 2.7).[41]

BACKGROUND MORTALITY

It is clear that the initial, or pre-Hispanic, mortality configuration is dramatically changed by the entrance of Europeans and their diseases. As the discussion below elaborates, this simulation is based on the premise that periods of social disruption, epidemics, and famines will alter the demographic variables, but in periods of relative tranquility the pre-existing pattern continues. In essence, I argue that the general patterns of mortality and fertility are elements of the "deep structure" of Amerindian groups and were changed minimally, if at all, during the first century of Spanish colonialism.[42] Over time, fundamental changes in productive and health technology, ideology, and socioeconomic structures altered these basic

---

41 The ~ symbol within converters, such as *B_CF_0_1*, indicates that the latter are determined graphically from the values of the determining variables, in this case *nutr_disc*. These may be linear or curvilinear relationships.

42 See Watkins and Menken, "Famines in Historical Perspective," p. 659.

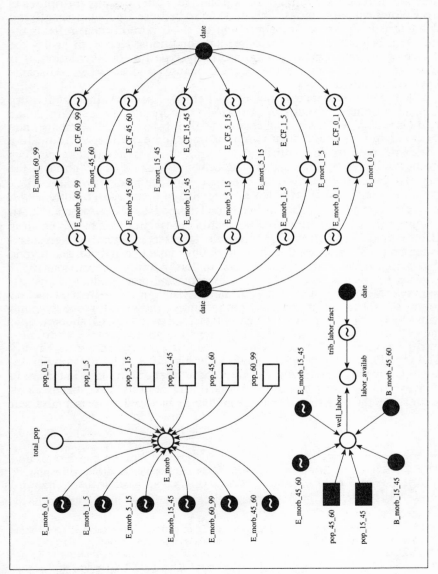

Figure 2.7 Epidemic Sub-system

demographic structures. Nevertheless, they only began to exert strong influence after the initial century of depopulation.

The population structure and mortality pattern used in these simulations reflect the types of background mortality-causing infirmities in pre-Colombian populations. This must be so because a population suffers a characteristic age-specific pattern and level of mortality that reflects the prevalent behavioral and environmental conditions. Hence, to justify the choice of an appropriate general mortality type for the simulation, it is necessary to examine the evidence for the causes of death for pre-Hispanic Amerindian populations.

While the evidence is not overwhelming, several lines of inquiry suggest a general pattern of Amerindian mortality. Discussing Aztec medicine, Rogers notes that catarrh (i.e., influenza-like ailments) and rheumatism must have been common since there were specific healing deities devoted to these illnesses.[43] Similarly, he notes that respiratory problems, including tuberculosis and bronchitis, had specific terms in the Nahuatl language.[44] Physical evidence for respiratory problems (i.e., pneumonia and tuberculosis) have been noted in Peruvian mummies, and it is likely that these problems were widespread in the Americas.[45] An extensive list of likely pre-Colombian ailments is provided by Newman.[46] These include: (1) bacillary and amoebic dysentery; (2) viral influenza and pneumonia; (3) various arthritides; (4) various insect born rickettsial fevers; (5) various viral fevers; (6) American leishmaniasis (protozoan); (7) American trypanosomiasis; (8) round worms and other endoparasites; (9) non-venereal syphilis and *pinta*; (10) nutritional deficiency diseases such as goiter; (11) a range of bacterial pathogens including streptococcus and staphylococcus; (12) salmonella and other food poisons; (13) tuberculosis; and (14) perhaps typhus. Several of these ailments such as the arthritides, nutritional deficiencies, and skin diseases (e.g., *pinta*) are not commonly fatal though they figure in the total morbidity suffered by the population. And while it may be unlikely that all of these were experienced in the Basin of Mexico, the most common killers must certainly have been. Cook summarizes the pattern of Amerindian disease as revealed in his analysis of

---

[43] S. L. Rogers, "A Comparison Between Sixteenth Century Medicine in Europe and Pre-Cortesian Mexico," *Actas XLI Congreso Internacional de Americanistas*, 1 (1974), p. 52.

[44] Rogers, "A Comparison," p. 55.

[45] M. J. Allison, A. Pezzia, and E. Gerszten. "Infectious Diseases in Precolombian Inhabitants of Peru," *American Journal of Physical Anthropology*, 41 (1974), p. 468.

[46] M. T. Newman,"Aboriginal New World Epidemiology and Medical Care, and the Impact of Old World Disease Imports," *American Journal of Physical Anthropology*, 45 (1978), p. 668.

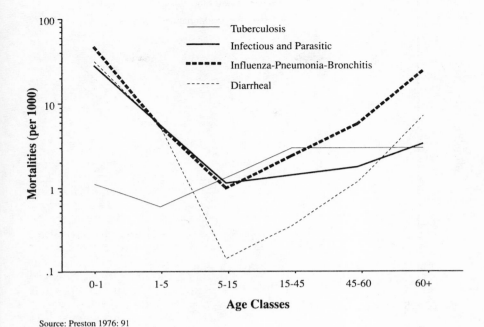

Source: Preston 1976: 91

Figure 2.8 Mortality by Cause

herbals, "... the aboriginal tribes in particular, suffered extensively from infections of the respiratory and gastrointestinal tracts."[47]

By distilling these diseases into Preston's generalizations of mortality by cause, "infectious and parasitic" (i.e., the rickettsial and viral fevers, American leishmaniasis, American trypanosomiasis, the endoparasites, and streptococcus and staphylococcus bacteria), "respiratory" (i.e., influenza, pneumonia, and bronchitis), "diarrheal" (i.e., the bacterial and amoebic dysenteries), and "tuberculosis," we can compare the general pattern of mortality suffered by a pre-conquest Amerindian population experiencing these problems with a model mortality pattern calculated from Coale and Demeny.[48] Comparison of Figure 2.8 (which shows Preston's cause-specific age-group mortalities) and Figure 2.9 (which compares the total [i.e., all causes] mortality in Preston's data with a similar curve derived from the "level 8 west" section of the *Regional Model Life Tables and*

---

47   Cook, "Disease among the Aztecs," p. 327.

48   Preston, *Mortality Patterns*, p. 91.

52

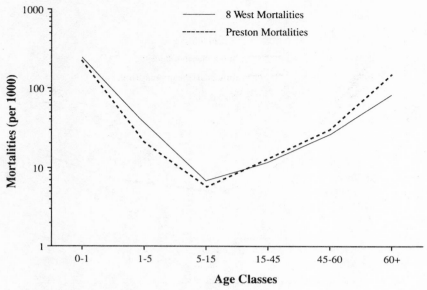

Sources: Preston 1976: 91; Coale & Demeny: 1966: 40-41, 136-137

Figure 2.9 8 West and Preston Mortalities Compared

Stable Populations) shows that the curves are similar enough to support the choice of the "west" family of mortalities.[49]

EPIDEMIC MORTALITY

It is fortunate that there are relatively detailed lists of the most notable periods of illness and disease in the Basin of Mexico. Unfortunately, it is not known if these surviving data are complete. It is likely, however, that the most severe events are recorded, and for that reason it is assumed that the temporal sequence of epidemics developed here is sufficient to simulate the most important demographic effects. Table 2.4 displays 19 epidemic episodes in the Basin from 1520 through 1625, compiled primarily from Gibson, Gerhard, and Hassig.[50]

In some cases, such as for the epidemic(s) in 1576-81, the original

---

49 The graph of Preston's composite mortality (Fig. 2.7) adds the mortality due to cardiovascular diseases, and other diseases of infancy. These were excluded in Figure 2.6 to simplify the presentation, but since the pattern of these mortalities generally parallels that of the general pattern (i.e., the other diseases of infancy raises the infant mortalities and the cardiovascular diseases generally raise the mortality of the aged), this exclusion does not affect the argument.

50 Gibson, *The Aztecs*, pp. 448-450; Gerhard, *Historical Geography of New Spain*, pp. 23-24; and Hassig, *Trade, Tribute, and Transportation*, pp. 155-156.

TABLE 2.4 EPIDEMIC SEQUENCE IN THE BASIN OF MEXICO

Year	Notes (after Gibson 1964: 448-450)
1520-21	Hueyzahuatl, viruelas, lepras, sarna [mange]; = Smallpox (Gerhard 1972: 24)
1531-32	Zahuatl, sarampión, viruelas, zahuatl tepiton; = measles (Zinnser 1934: 256)
1538	Viruelas, [minor variety of smallpox?]
1545-48	Great pestilence, cocoliztili, nose and eye bleeding; = typhus [tabardillo] (Humboldt 1822: 117; Zinsser 1934: 256; & Gerhard 1972: 24) or = pneumonic plague (MacLeod 1973: 19)
1550	Paperas [mumps]
1558	Death and famine
1559	Symptoms like 1545 and 1576 [typhus or pneumonic plague]
1563-64	Zahuatl, sarampión, matlaltotonqui [pleurisy]
1566	Cocoliztili
1576-81	Great pestilence, affects all Indians, few Spanish; nosebleeds common; = typhus (Zinsser 1934: 257 Gerhard 1972: 24)
1587-88	Cocoliztili
1590	Tlatlacistli with many deaths; = influenza (Gerhard 1972: 24)
1592-93	Tlatlasistli, sarampion, mostly children [probably measles]
1595-97	Sarampión, paperas, & tabardillo, high morbidity, low mortality
1601-02	Cocoliztili
1604-07	Sarampión, cocoliztili, diarrhea, high mortality
1613	Cocoliztili
1615-16	Sarampión, viruelas, minor epidemic

source materials record differing dates for the onset or termination of an Indeed, little is known about where in the Basin epidemics were initiated, hence their spatial diffusion patterns are also uncertain, although it is a reasonable guess that Tenochtitlán/Mexico City (or perhaps the Basin's eastern extremity through which most people, and infections, entered) was the Basin origin for many. This is an important point since the settlement pattern of the Basin was non-uniform.

Nevertheless, it is the total "at risk" population of the Basin that is of interest here rather than the micro-spatial epidemiology. In order to efficiently deal with the total population, it is necessary to simplify this simulation and it is assumed here that the effect of each epidemic was spatially uniform throughout the Basin and concentrated in the single year noted in Table 2.4 and the dates are those recorded by Gibson.[51] By concentrating epidemic affects in this way, the impact of any epidemic may be multiplied since the *care factor* variable will multiply the mortality more for a single high-morbidity event than for a series of lower morbidity events, even if the total morbidity is the same for both. This multiplying

---

51 Gibson, *The Aztecs*, pp. 448-450.

effect may more closely simulate actual events, however, since it is the local morbidity totals that really affect the ability to care for the ill, and while different scattered communities may not have been stricken simultaneously, individual households or whole communities likely were made victim more-or-less simultaneously and thus, suffered from increased mortality.

While the information as to the timing of epidemics seems reasonably satisfactory, the identity of the pathogens responsible for individual outbreaks is less certain. In many cases the identity of diseases must be established from the recorded symptoms, and this is a problem since the descriptions are often vague and in many cases the same symptom could result from several illnesses. Ramenofsky goes further to argue that there is a logical problem with using modern epidemiological data to infer the identity of historical epidemics since the microbes and hosts likely have changed over time, rendering the historical descriptions inaccurate as a mirror of contemporary symptoms.[52] While this point is well taken, it seems unlikely that the general symptomatology of particular infections has changed all that significantly even if the virulence of particular pathogens or the resistance of hosts has changed. A more difficult complication arises from the fact that there may have been multiple epidemics raging in a community at the same time, thus producing a confusing record of symptoms.[53] For many diseases, it is secondary infection that produces the most noticeable symptoms and, indeed, produce much of the mortality (an example of this point for measles is noted below). This complexity notwithstanding, simplicity argues for assigning each simulated epidemic event to a specific disease. The issue is no less clear when particular outbreaks are identified by name. There is disagreement both about the identity of diseases referred to by their Nahuatl names (e.g., *cocoliztli*) and those referred to in Spanish (e.g., *tabardillo*). These identity issues will be discussed in the sections below devoted to each disease.

As in the case of background mortality, epidemic mortality is modeled as the product of case fatality and morbidity. It is necessary to aggregate these by age-group since case fatality is age specific and the morbidity of different age-groups is a function of their previous experience with the particular pathogen. This is because most of the important introduced pathogens convey a lifetime immunity to survivors of earlier infections. For example, a smallpox epidemic that affects a large proportion of the population will render the infected survivors immune to further occurrences of the same virus, hence a re-occurrence of smallpox in the surviving population will only affect those who have been born since the last smallpox epidemic and those who avoided infection the first time. Its importance notwithstanding, there is significant uncertainty as to the age-

52 A. F. Ramenofsky, *Vectors of Death. The Archaeology of European Contact.* Albuquerque: University of New Mexico Press, 1987, p. 137.

53 Crosby, "Virgin Soil Epidemics," p. 294; and H. Zinsser, *Rats, Lice and History.* Boston: Little Brown and Company, 1934, p. 120.

specific case fatality and morbidity of individual pathogens. Such data are difficult to obtain even in contemporary situations since the population at risk, the numbers infected of this population, and the numbers succumbing to the particular disease must be recorded. Nevertheless, such data must be developed, so to explicate and justify the epidemic models developed here, the identity and virulence of each type of pathogen will be treated in turn, more-or-less in their historical order of occurrence.

The first post-contact epidemic in the Basin, in 1520-21, is usually identified as smallpox (*Variola major*) (Table 2.4).[54] Early chroniclers such as Díaz del Castillo, López de Gómara, Motolinia, Sahagún and Mendieta[55] note a disease that they identify as *viruelas* (Spanish for smallpox) or *hueyzahuatl* (Nahuatl, presumably same disease). The identification of *viruelas* also occurs for epidemics in 1531, 1538, and 1615.[56] It is not certain that smallpox was the major epidemic in 1531 or 1615, however, since Motolinía, Mendieta, Cisneros, and Chimpalpahin also record *sarampíon* (measles) and/or *zahuatal tepiton* for these dates. Hopkins argues that the Nahuatl term for smallpox was *hueyzahuatl*, while *tepitonzahuatl* (clearly the same term as *zahuatal tepiton*) referred to measles.[57] Since, even for contemporary observers, measles and smallpox are frequently confused, it seems reasonable to agree with Gibson that *zahuatal tepiton* referred to measles.[58] Adding to the complication in all this, however, is the fact that there are two major types of smallpox, *Variola major* and *Variola minor*, the latter having very low mortality in all its forms.[59] It is possible, therefore, that *zahuatal tepiton* referred to the less virulent form of smallpox. This possibility notwithstanding, it is not unreasonable to assume that smallpox was the major epidemic only in 1520-21 and 1538.

There are very little data on case fatalities for smallpox in virgin-soil populations, and for that reason, historical case fatality figures for non-virgin-soil populations such as those derived here, are used to model the case fatality of smallpox in the Amerindian population. Further, despite the commonality of smallpox in the past, mortality figures for non-virgin-soil unvaccinated communities are not widespread in the literature. Nevertheless, the general outlines of virgin-soil-like smallpox epidemics are given by Dixon who notes 35-36 percent community-wide mortalities in

---

54 Gerhard, *Historical Geography of New Spain*, 23; Gibson, *The Aztecs*, 488; MacLeod, *Spanish Central America* 19; and McNeill, *Plagues and Peoples*, p. 183.

55 All cited in Gibson, *The Aztecs*, p. 448.

56 Gibson, *The Aztecs*, pp. 448-449.

57 D. R. Hopkins, *Princes and Peasants, Smallpox in History*, Chicago: University of Chicago Press, 1983, p. 206.

58 C. W. Dixon, *Smallpox*, London: J. and A. Churchill, 1962, p. 120; and Gibson, *The Aztecs*, p. 448.

59 Dixon, *Smallpox*, pp. 6-7.

TABLE 2.5 SMALLPOX CASE FATALITY RATES

(all rates expressed as percentages)

Location and Date	Community Case Fatality	Reference
19th C. USA	38.50	Crosby (1976: 292)
19th C. Pueblo	74.00	Stearn & Stearn (1945: 15)
19th C. Hawaii	77.70	Judd (1977: 550)
20th C. Madras	37.80	Benenson (1976:444-445)
19th C. Boston	16.40	Mercer (1985: 293)
19th C. France	16.20	Mercer (1985: 302)
19th C. Verona	46.70	Mercer (1985: 302)
19th C. Milan	38.50	Mercer (1985: 302)
19th C. Bohemia	29.80	Mercer (1985: 302)
Average	41.73	

AGE SPECIFIC CASE FATALITY RATES

Age-class	Berlin (a)	London (a)	Dixon (low) (b)	Dixon (high) (b)	Average
0-1	40.00	60.00	42.00	60.00	50.50
1-5	40.00	60.00	42.00	60.00	50.50
5-10	40.00	—	—	—	40.00
10-15	27.00	23.00	—	—	25.00
15-20	27.00	40.00	—	—	33.50
20-25	27.00	40.00	—	—	33.50
25-30	27.00	40.00	—	—	33.50
30-35	27.00	40.00	—	—	33.50
35-40	27.00	40.00	—	—	33.50
40-45	39.00	40.00	—	—	39.50
45-50	39.00	40.00	—	—	39.50
50-55	39.00	40.00	42.00	60.00	45.25
55-60	39.00	40.00	42.00	60.00	45.25
60+	39.00	40.00	42.00	60.00	45.25

(a) Razzell (1977: 126-127)
(b) Dixon (1962: 326)

severe eighteenth-century epidemics in Iceland and South Africa.[60] Aggregate as these figures are, they do provide a basis to estimate age-class-specific figures. Assuming a 90 percent morbidity in these situations implies a community-wide case fatality of approximately 40 percent. This simple estimate is buttressed by examining the recorded or estimated smallpox case fatality figures for unvaccinated communities shown in Table 2.5. While these have ranged from about 15 percent to over 70 percent, the

---

[60] Dixon, *Smallpox*, pp. 207-208.

average is close to the 40 percent figure calculated above (Table 2.5).[61] The even-more-scarce age-specific case fatality data are summarized in Table 2.5 and are averaged to create age-class case fatality values. The community-wide case fatality implied in these age-class-specific figures will, of course, vary according to the age structure of the victim population, but these values do not seem inconsistent with the community-wide averages noted above.

The age-class case fatality values calculated in Table 2.5 (and for all the epidemics considered here) differ from those actually used in the simulations (displayed in Table 2.6) for two reasons. First, the 5 year age-class values calculated in Table 2.5 are merged to produce values for the MEXIPOP age classes. Second, an adjustment to these values is needed because the calculation interval in the model, 0.25, is not vanishingly small. The adjusted values noted in Table 2.6 are equal to

$$4*\{1 - \sqrt[4]{(1 - \text{case fatality values in Table 2.5})}\},$$

and return the correct values for mortality in a simulation where the dt = 0.25.

The morbidity due to smallpox in the initial, 1520, encounter must have been enormous since smallpox is so easily communicated and infectious. Dixon argues for a nearly 100 percent morbidity in virgin-soil populations.[62] In the MEXIPOP simulations, the initial encounter with each disease, such as with smallpox in 1520, is modeled as affecting 90 percent of the population in all age-groups (Table 2.6). The high mortalities noted by Dixon for virgin-soil-like populations may be simulated by assuming high morbidities and historically noted case fatalities.[63]

Gibson identifies "The simplest of all infectious diseases... measles" [64] as *sarampión* in Spanish and *zahuatl tepiton* in Nahuatl (Table 2.4). Using this identification, the first measles outbreak in the Basin occurred in 1531-1532, but there is some uncertainty about this identification since Motolinía, Chimpalphin, and Mendieta also identify *viruelas* in 1531, and Chimpalphin notes *viruelas* for 1532.[65] These identifications notwithstanding, Zinsser and McNeill concur that this epidemic was measles, and it will be so

61   A. S. Benenson, "Smallpox," in A. S. Evans (ed.) *Viral Infections of Humans*, New York and London: Plenum Medical Book Company, p. 492; Crosby, "Virgin Soil Epidemics," p. 292; Dixon, *Smallpox*, p. 171; C. S. Judd, Jr. "Depopulation in Polynesia," *Bulletin of the History of Medicine* 51 (1977), p. 550; A. J. Mercer, "Smallpox and Epidemiological-Demographic Change in Europe: The Role of Vaccination," *Population Studies* 39 (1985), pp. 293, 302; and E. Stearn, and A.E. Stearn. *The Effect of Smallpox on the Destiny of the Amerindian*, Boston: Bruce Humphries Inc., 1945 p. 15.

62   Dixon, *Smallpox*, p. 310.

63   Dixon, *Smallpox*, pp. 207-208.

64   Maxcy quoted in F. L. Black, "Measles," in A. S. Evans (ed.), *Viral Infections* p. 297; and Gibson, *The Aztecs*, p. 448.

65   All cited in Gibson, *The Aztecs*, p. 448.

TABLE 2.6 EPIDEMIC CASE FATALITY AND MORBIDITY VALUES

YEAR	0-1 CF (A)	0-1 MORB (A)	1-5 CF	1-5 MORB	5-15 CF	5-15 MORB	15-45 CF	15-45 MORB	45-60 CF	45-60 MORB	60+ CF	60+ MORB
1520-21	0.636	0.9	0.636	0.9	0.381	0.9	0.408	0.9	0.524	0.9	0.555	0.9
1531-32	0.156	0.9	0.026	0.9	0.026	0.9	0.026	0.9	0.074	0.9	0.126	0.9
1538	0.636	0.9	0.636	0.9	0.381	0.9	0.408	0.1	0.524	0.1	0.555	0.1
1545-48	0.9	1	0.9	0.5	0.9	0.36	0.9	0.24	0.9	0.15	0.9	0.13
(b)	*0.1*	*0.9*	*0.025*	*0.9*	*0.278*	*0.9*	*0.278*	*0.9*	*0.603*	*0.9*	*0.636*	*0.9*
1550	0.005	0.8	0.006	0.8	0.001	0.8	0.001	0.8	0.002	0.8	0.007	0.8
1558	0.005	0.8	0.006	0.8	0.001	0.8	0.001	0.8	0.002	0.8	0.007	0.8
1559	0.9	0.25	0.9	0.1	0.9	0.09	0.9	0.07	0.9	0.04	0.9	0.03
(b)	*0.1*	*0.9*	*0.025*	*0.9*	*0.278*	*0.9*	*0.217*	*0.1*	*0.603*	*0.1*	*0.636*	*0.1*
1563-64	0.156	0.9	0.026	0.9	0.026	0.9	0.052	0.1	0.074	0.1	0.126	0.1
1566	0.005	0.9	0.006	0.9	0.001	0.9	0.001	0.9	0.002	0.9	0.007	0.9
1576-81	0.9	1	0.9	0.5	0.9	0.36	0.9	0.24	0.9	0.15	0.9	0.13
(b)	*0.1*	*0.9*	*0.025*	*0.9*	*0.278*	*0.9*	*0.217*	*0.1*	*0.603*	*0.1*	*0.636*	*0.1*
1587-88	0.005	0.8	0.006	0.8	0.001	0.8	0.001	0.8	0.002	0.8	0.007	0.8
1590	0.078	0.9	0.015	0.9	0.011	0.9	0.024	0.9	0.025	0.9	0.015	0.9
1592-93	0.156	0.9	0.026	0.9	0.026	0.9	0.052	0.5	0.074	0.1	0.126	0.1
1595-97	0.156	0.9	0.026	0.5	0.026	0.1	0.052	0.1	0.074	0.1	0.126	0.1
1601-02	0.005	0.8	0.026	0.8	0.001	0.8	0.001	0.8	0.002	0.8	0.007	0.8
1604-07	0.156	0.9	0.026	0.9	0.026	0.5	0.052	0.1	0.074	0.1	0.126	0.1
1613	0.005	0.8	0.006	0.8	0.001	0.8	0.001	0.8	0.002	0.8	0.007	0.8
1615-16	0.156	0.9	0.026	0.9	0.026	0.7	0.052	0.1	0.074	0.1	0.12	0.1

(a) C F = case fatality; morb = morbidity
(b) upper (roman type) values for pneumonic plague, lower (italic type) values for typhus

assumed here.[66] The next occurrence of measles in the Basin probably dates to 1563-1564, when *zahuatl, sarampión,* and *mataltotonqui* are reported.[67] *Mataltotonqui* is tentatively translated by Gibson as pleurisy.[68] That such a respiratory complaint is noted along with measles is not surprising and does not necessarily indicate that there were multiple epidemics at this date. This is because measles is more like a respiratory disease with a rash than a rash with respiratory complications.[69] Indeed, virtually all observers of virgin-soil measles epidemics stress the importance of the respiratory element, particularly pneumonia, in the epidemics.[70] Measles likely next appeared in the Basin in 1592-1593, when *tlatlacistli,*[71] *sarampión,* and *cocoliztili* were reported with "mortality among children."[72] High mortality concentrated among the young would be expected of a self-immunizing disease such as measles that was presumably absent for nearly 30 years since the older population would have been exposed before. It is reasonable to conclude that the 1592-1593 outbreak was measles since *cocoliztili* is translated by Gibson as a general term referring to any epidemic sickness.[73] "Widespread sickness, ... but with relatively few deaths" *sarampión, paperas,* and *tabardillo* are reported for 1595-1596.[74] It is possible that in addition to measles at this date, mumps (*paperas*) and typhus (*tabardillo*) plagued the Basin.[75] In 1604-1607 *sarampión, cocoliztili,* and diarrhea are noted in the Basin.[76] This outbreak may represent diseases in addition to measles, but diarrheal symptoms are common in the severe measles of West Africa[77] and dehydration (a

---

66 Zinnser, *Rats, Lice and History,* p. 256; and McNeill, *Plagues and Peoples,* pp. 184-185.

67 Gibson, *The Aztecs,* p. 449.

68 Gibson, *The Aztecs,* p. 448.

69 Judd, "Depopulation in Polynesia," p. 591.

70 W. R. Centerwall, "A Recent Experience with Measles in a 'Virgin Soil' Population," In *Pan American Health Organization Scientific Publication #165, Biomedical Challenges Presented by the American Indian,* Washington, DC: Pan American Health Organization, 1968, pp. 78, 79; P. E. Christensen, H. Schmidt, H. O. Bang, V. Andersen, B. Jordal, and O. Jensen. "An epidemic of Measles in Southern Greenland, 1951," *Acta Medica Scandinavica,* p. 144; and A. F. W. Peart, and F. P. Nagler. "Measles in the Canadian Arctic, 1952," *Canadian Journal of Public Health* 45: (1954), p. 151.

71 Translated by Gibson, *The Aztecs,* 448, as influenza.

72 Gibson, *The Aztecs,* p. 449.

73 Gibson, *The Aztecs,* p. 448.

74 Gibson, *The Aztecs,* p. 449.

75 Ibid.

76 Ibid.

77 D. Morley, "The Severe Measles of West Africa," *Proceedings of the Royal Society of Medicine,* 57 (1964), p. 847.

common result of diarrhea) greatly contributed to the mortality in virgin-soil measles epidemics in Amazonia.[78] Hence, diarrhea may well have been present in measles outbreaks in the sixteenth-century. The last measles outbreak (recorded as *sarampión* and *viruelas*) in the first century of Spanish dominion in the Basin is recorded in Mexico City in 1615-1616.[79]

Unlike the situation for smallpox noted above, there is a relatively large literature of epidemic measles in virgin-soil-like populations, indeed measles is among the most studied epidemic diseases. Nevertheless, this richness does not simplify the calculation of simulation mortalities since there is a great range of recorded mortality, even in situations of high morbidity (indicating a relatively virgin population). Nineteenth-century epidemics in Iceland and the Faroes indicate a relatively small community-wide mortality, less than 10 percent, even in situations of high morbidity (Table 2.7). This is in contrast to the 26-50 percent mortalities recorded for presumably virgin-soil nineteenth-century epidemics in Oceania (Table 2.4). There is contemporary, eye-witness evidence, however, supporting the lower mortalities, even in virgin-soil populations (Table 2.4).[80] The best data detailing the age pattern of epidemic measles case fatality is from studies that report lower mortality (Table 2.4).[81] It is from this conservative data that the age-class case fatalities for MEXIPOP are drawn (using the same modification of case fatalities as for smallpox) (Table 2.6). Like smallpox, measles is a very contagious disease because it is spread easily as an aerosol and survives drying.[82] For this reason, it is not unreasonable to posit a 90 percent initial morbidity for the 1531-1532 epidemic. Since measles epidemics returned frequently to the Basin, it is necessary to adjust the age-class morbidity for the subsequent epidemics to account for the fact that the later epidemics would affect primarily the young, who had no previous experience with the disease. For example, Table 2.6 shows that in 1563 only 10 percent of the over 30 age-classes would be infected, while 90 percent of the younger are affected.

---

78   Centerwall, "A Recent Experience with Measles," p. 79.

79   Gibson, *The Aztecs*, p. 449.

80   Centerwall, "A Recent Experience with Measles," p. 79; Christensen *et al.*, "An Epidemic of Measles," p. 442; N. Nuttels, "Medical Problems in Newly Contacted Groups," in *Pan American Health Organization Scientific Publication #165, Biomedical Challenges Presented by the American Indian*, Washington, DC: Pan American Health Organization, 1968, p. 70; and Peart and Nagler, "Measles in the Canadian Arctic," p. 146.

81   T. A. Cockburn, *The Evolution and Eradication of Infectious Diseases*, Baltimore: The Johns Hopkins University Press, 1963, p. 82; and Peart and Nagler, "Measles in the Canadian Arctic," p. 146.

82   Black, "Measles," p. 300.

TABLE 2.7 MEASLES CASE FATALITY AND MORBIDITY RATES

(all rates expressed as percentages)

Case Fatality

AGE-CLASS	CANADIAN ARTIC (A)	GREENLAND (B)	FAROES (C)	AVERAGE
0-1	13.00	2.50	28.60	14.70
1-5	6.00	1.50	0.30	2.60
5-10	6.00	0.00	0.30	2.10
10-15	9.00	0.00	0.20	3.07
15-20	9.00	0.95	0.20	3.38
20-25	11.90	0.95	0.30	4.38
25-30	11.90	0.95	0.30	4.38
30-35	13.40	0.95	1.50	5.28
35-40	13.40	2.40	1.50	5.77
40-45	16.40	2.40	3.10	7.30
45-50	16.40	2.40	3.10	7.30
50-55	9.00	2.40	4.80	5.40
55-60	9.00	12.50	4.80	8.77
60-65	13.40	12.50	7.30	11.07
65-70	13.40	12.50	7.30	11.07
70-75	13.40	12.50	9.00	11.63
75-80	13.40	12.50	9.00	11.63
80+	13.40	12.50	16.30	14.07

Community

REFERENCE	LOCATION & DATE	CASE FATALITY	MORBIDITY	MORTALITY
(A) Peart *et al*. 1954	Canadian Artic 1952	7.00	99.00	6.93
Centerwall 1968	Amazonia 1960	17.10	99.00	16.93
Nutels 1968	Amazonia 1950	26.80	—	—
Crosby 1976	US Civil war white	6.00	—	—
Crosby 1976	US Civil war black	11.00	—	—
(B) Christensen et al. 1953	Greenland 1951	1.80	99.00	1.78
Judd 1977	Fiji 1875	26.60	99.00	26.33
Panum 1940	Faroes 1846	—	—	1.60
Hirsch 1883	Iceland 1882	—	—	4.50
Peart et al. 1954	Faroes 1846	2.80	75.00	2.10
(C) Cockburn 1963	Faroes 1846	—	95.60	—
Gluck 1855	Hawaii 1848	—	—	27.00
Corney 1884	Fiji 1873	—	—	26.00
Tooth et al. 1963	Australia 1961	—	—	3.00
Bridges 1949	Argentina 1884	—	—	50.00

While their severity is unquestioned, the "great pestilence[s]" of 1545-1548 and 1575-1581 are difficult to identify conclusively.[83] Humboldt identified the causal disease of 1545-1548 as *matlazahuatl*.[84] Gerhard, Zinsser, Guerra, and Gibson all identify *matlazahuatl* as typhus (*Rickettsia prowazeki*).[85] Zinsser also argues that the 1576-1581 epidemic was typhus.[86] Kubler argues contra, that the two outbreaks differed, since there is evidence that the mortality of the 1576-1581 epidemic was 2.5 times that in 1545-1548.[87] In contrast, MacLeod identifies both these epidemics as pneumonic plague (*Yersina pestis*).[88] Unfortunately, the recorded symptoms do not serve to unambiguously settle the matter. The most common symptoms, bleeding in the nose and eyes is noted for both dates by Gibson,[89] Zinsser also notes congestion, bloody stools, and fever for the 1545-1548 outbreak, while Kubler lists stomach pains, fever, and violent coughing among the symptoms for the 1576-1581 episode.[90]

Zinsser makes the case for typhus by arguing that these symptoms could be those of typhoid fever or dysentery, but that the mortality of these would not be high enough, and that only plague or typhus would have the requisite mortality and fit the symptoms, but bubonic plague could hardly have been missed.[91] Further, *matlazahuatl* is translated by Zinsser and Guerra as describing a disease in which there are skin eruptions in the form of a net.[92] This description fits well with the most obvious symptom of typhus, its rash.[93] There are no similar skin eruptions for pneumonic plague so it would not be reasonable fit to the description. The other obvious symptom of the sixteenth-century epidemics, bleeding from the nose and eyes, is less commonly noted for typhus, except for bloody

---

83 Gibson, *The Aztecs*, p. 448.

84 As quoted in Gibson, *The Aztecs*, p. 449.

85 Gerhard, *Historical Geography of New Spain*, p. 24; Zinsser, *Rats, Lice and History*, p. 256; Francisco Guerra, "Aztec Medicine," *Medical History*, 10 (1966), pp. 330-331; and Gibson, *The Aztecs*, p. 448.

86 Zinsser, *Rats, Lice and History*, pp. 256-257.

87 Kubler "Population Movements," p. 631.

88 MacLeod, *Spanish Central America*, p. 19.

89 Gibson, *The Aztecs*, pp. 448-449.

90 Zinsser, *Lice and History*, p. 256; and Kubler, "Population Movements," p. 632.

91 Zinsser, *Rats, Lice and History*, p. 256.

92 Zinsser, *Rats, Lice and History*, pp. 257-258; and Guerra, "Aztec Medicine," p. 330.

93 Charles L. Wisseman, Jr. "Rickettsial Diseases," in F. H. S. Top and Paul F. Wehrle (eds.), *Communicable and Infectious Diseases*, Eighth edition. Saint Louis: The C. V. Mosby Company, p. 570: P. F. Zdrodovskii, and H. M. Golinevich, *The Rickettsial Diseases*, Trans. B. Haigt. New York: Pergamon Press, 1960, pp. 221-222; and Zinsser, *Rats, Lice and History*, p. 216.

sputum,[94] probably due to secondary pneumonia, which is involved in many cases.[95]

There is a question as to whether typhus could have been easily transported to the New World, however. Unlike the directly transmitted viruses, smallpox and measles, typhus is transmitted between humans by the body louse (*Pediculus humanus*).[96] The typhus infected louse only survives 12-14 days after feeding on infected blood, thus for *Rickettsia prowazeki* to survive the voyage the infection would have to have been transferred from sailor to sailor, a serious event that Zinsser argues would have been noted.[97] He does argue for the possibility that the infection may be kept alive in ship-board rodents and re-ignited in a human population by the rat flea.[98] This possibility is contradicted by Zdrodovskii and Golinevich who argue that, in contrast to other rickettsial diseases, there is no known non-human reservoir of the typhus fever rickettsiae.[99] Perhaps the difficulty of transport explains the relatively late introduction of typhus, if typhus it was, to a time when more rapid and frequent Atlantic crossings occurred, a point made by Ramenofsky for measles and influenza.[100] However transported, when conditions are favorable among a louse infested population, typhus epidemics are easily ignited.[101] Zinsser agrees that typhus could have readily spread since there is evidence that Amerindians suffered lice, a point amplified by Posey.[102] While lice there may have been, Bernal Díaz commented on the cleanliness of the people and especially remarked on the Amerindian custom of bathing, especially sweat baths.[103] Schendel remarked that the extreme cleanliness of the Aztecs may have protected them from the ravages of many diseases.[104]

Another intriguing possibility is that these epidemics were not due to European typhus at all; a further possibility is that there was an pre-Colombian typhus or typhus-like disease. Zinsser cites Mooser, who

---

[94] Christopher Morris, "The Plague in Britain," *The Historical Journal* 14 (1971), p. 207.

[95] Zdrodovskii and Golinevich, *The Rickettsial Diseases*, p. 223.

[96] Wisseman, "Rickettsial Diseases," p. 570.

[97] Zinsser, *Rats, Lice and History*, pp. 261-262.

[98] Zinsser, *Rats, Lice and History*, p. 262.

[99] Zdrodovskii and Golinevich, *The Rickettsial Diseases*, p. 211.

[100] Ramenofsky, *Vectors of Death*, p. 167.

[101] Zdrodovskii and Golinevich, *The Rickettsial Diseases*, p. 211.

[102] Zinsser, *Rats, Lice and History*, p. 259; and Darrell A Posey, "Entomological Considerations in Southeastern Aboriginal Demography," *Ethnohistory*, 23 (1976), pp. 147-160.

[103] Gordon Schendel, *Medicine in Mexico*, Austin, TX: University of Texas Press, 1968, p. 41.

[104] Schendel, *Medicine in Mexico*, p. 43.

believes that typhus was pre-existent in Mexico because Indians of Michoacán called a typhus-like disease *cocolixtle meco*, or painful spotted fever.[105] Guerra is more confident that *matlazahuatl* was a pre-Colombian diseases since he has "...no doubt [that] they [*matlazahuatl* and *cocoliztili*] were the great killers of the Aztec in pre-Colombian times."[106] He implies that an indigenous fever that the Spanish identified soon after 1519 as typhus, was *matlazahuatl*.[107] Modern epidemiology does not identify an American typhus, however, but there are New World rickettsial diseases that may be confused with typhus (*Rickettsia prowazeki*), particularly, Rocky Mountain Spotted fever (*Dermacentroxenus rickettsi*). Newman also notes the possible existence of pre-Colombian rickettsial diseases.[108] Rocky Mountain Spotted fever is an even better candidate to fit the symptoms Guerra, Gibson, and Zinsser list for *matlazahuatl*,[109] headache, bleeding in the nose and eyes, congestion, bloody stools, fever, severe prostration, rash, mental disturbances, and necrosis, since it is characteristically marked by headache, muscular pain, vomiting, rash, delirium, coma and nose bleeding.[110] Further, Mooser notes that a pre-contact Aztec codex shows a man with a net-like rash who is suffering a bloody nose.[111] It seems quite possible, therefore, that the disease pictured on the Aztec codex and described as *matlazahuatl* or *cocolixtle meco* was not European typhus or an American variant but its American cousin, Rocky Mountain Spotted fever.

This identification is, perhaps, less likely, if only because of the more complex epidemiology of this disease. Unlike typhus, Rocky Mountain spotted fever requires animal hosts for its tick vectors. Since an epidemic of Rocky Mountain spotted fever depends on the density of these vectors and, therefore, their hosts, it is only through changes in the density of these that an epidemic could be credibly conceived. Such circumstances may have been present by mid-sixteenth century, however, when the density of European domestic animals was rapidly increasing relative to the Amerindian population.[112] Domestic animals such as cattle, dogs, and horses can serve as hosts for the wild ticks (who usually inhabit deer, rabbits, wild pigs, and wild rodents).[113] Hence, the "population explosion" of Spanish domesticates may have served to spark a similar explosion of

---

105   Zinsser, *Rats, Lice and History*, p. 257.

106   Guerra, "Aztec Medicine," p. 330.

107   Guerra, "Aztec Medicine," p. 331.

108   Newman, "Aboriginal New World Epidemiology," p. 668.

109   Guerra, "Aztec Medicine," 331; Gibson, *The Aztecs*, pp. 448, 449; and Zinsser, *Rats, Lice and History*, p. 256.

110   Zdrodovskii and Golinevich, *The Rickettsial Diseases*, pp. 282-283.

111   Cited in Zinsser, *Rats, Lice and History*, p. 258.

112   Crosby, *The Colombian Exchange*, p. 75; and Simpson, *Exploitation*.

113   Zdrodovskii and Golinevich, *The Rickettsial Diseases*, pp. 285-286.

Rocky Mountain Spotted fever carrying ticks, and thus an epidemic of the fever. While this possibility is a logical one, there are no data on significantly sized Rocky Mountain Spotted fever epidemics in the literature. Since data with which to calibrate MEXIPOP are therefore missing, this possibility will not be modeled here.

A third possibility is advanced by MacLeod who bases his argument that the great epidemics of 1545-1548 and 1576-1581 were pneumonic plague on the similarity of the recorded symptoms to those describing plague (*Yersina pestis*) in Spain.[114] Specifically, he identifies the nosebleeds, the death after three days sickness, and the *dolores de costado* (literally pains in the side) as being described in the same terms in both the European documents and the colonial texts.[115] These symptoms generally resemble those of pneumonic plague as it is typically described: as a disease with symptoms similar to bronchopneumonia, that is, marked by fever, chest pains, headache, coughing, bloody sputum, and death in 1-3 days.[116]

It is important to note that this argument is for pneumonic plague, not the more widely noted bubonic plague. While the infectious bacilli, *Yersina pestis*, are the same for both varieties, bubonic plague epidemics are more complex since they require both a rodent host (typically domestic rats) and insect vector (usually the rat flea, *Xnopsylla cheopis*) to spread the microorganisms to humans. In contrast, pneumonic plague is spread directly from human to human by aerosols such as those produced in sneezing or coughing. In addition, the most characteristic symptom of bubonic plague, literally its namesake, buboes (infected swellings of the lymph glands nearest the flea bite), are usually not present in pneumonic plague possibly because death from pneumonic plague is so rapid that the victim dies before they can form. This later point is important because the presence of buboes certainly would have enabled the Spanish chroniclers to identify the disease as bubonic plague since it was well known in sixteenth-century Europe.

As with typhus, the complexity of the epidemiology of plague raises questions about its early transmission to the New World. Direct transmission of pneumonic plague from Spain via person to person contact on shipboard, would be virtually impossible since the case fatality of pneumonic plague approaches 100 percent, its infectiousness is very high, and its development time is so rapid—an infected crew would perish in a matter of a few days. The same argument may be made with less vigor for

---

114 MacLeod, *Spanish Central America*, p. 19.

115 MacLeod, *Spanish Central America*, p. 19.

116 Michael W. Dols, *The Black Death in the Middle East*, Princeton: Princeton University Press, 1977, p. 73; L. Fabian Hirst, *The Conquest of Plague*, Oxford: Clarendon Press, 1953, pp. 30, 225; Morris, "The Plague in Britain," p. 207; R. Pollitzer, *Plague*, World Health Organization Monograph Series No. 22. Geneva: World Health Organization, 1954, p. 441; and J. F. D. Shrewsbury, *A History of Bubonic Plague in the British Isles*, Cambridge: Cambridge University Press, 1970, p. 6.

the bubonic form, since it requires an epizootic in rodents, is less virulent, slower to kill, and less infective. These points notwithstanding, direct transmission seems unlikely. More likely, plague bacilli were transported to the New World in infected rat fleas. This is certainly possible since infected fleas may survive for 50-or-more days without rat hosts in fodder, cloth, grain, or hides.[117] Upon their arrival in Mexico, these now very hungry fleas may have spread plague to domestic or wild rodents or directly to humans. Other vectors are possible since wild rodent fleas and the Old World human flea, *Pulex irritans* (capable of inhabiting domesticated animals such as dogs as well as wild rabbits or rodents as well as humans), both can serve as vectors of plague, albeit with less efficiency than the rat flea, *Xnopsylla cheopis*.[118] Indeed, Hirst and Morris argue that passage of plague through wild rodents or their fleas imbues the plague bacillus with a pneumonic tendency.[119] Further, Morris notes that there may be some tendency for plague to manifest itself in the pneumonic form in virgin-soil outbreaks such as would have been the case in sixteenth century Mexico.[120]

Since the identity of the pathogen for these important periods of epidemic is uncertain, two differing models of epidemic history for the Basin have been prepared, one assumes typhus, the other pneumonic plague for the 1545-1548, 1559, and 1576-1581 epidemics (see Table 2.6). Dealing first with typhus, specific data for typhus mortalities are scarce and what there are variable. Scrimshaw and colleagues note that this variability may be a function of nutrition since typhus is more common and severe in poorly nourished populations, but Rotberg and Rabb argue that the data for typhus' nutritional dependence is equivocal.[121] Ramenofsky and Wisseman set the general range for typhus mortality at 10-40 percent.[122] Fiset is more specific and notes case fatalities for severe typhus of about 10 percent for those aged less than 20 years and greater than 50 percent for those older than 50 (Table 2.8).[123] These estimates generally agree with Wisseman's argument that even severe typhus is relatively mild for those less than 15

[117] Hirst, *The Conquest of Plague*, pp. 314, 324; and R. Pollitzer, *Plague*, p. 385.

[118] Pollitzer, *Plague*, pp. 333, 357, 378, 380.

[119] Hirst, *The Conquest of Plague*, p. 222; Morris, "The Plague in Britain," p. 207.

[120] Morris, "The Plague in Britain," p. 207.

[121] N. S. Scrimshaw, C. E. Taylor, and J. E. Gordon. *Interactions of Nutrition and Infection*, Geneva: World Health Organization, 1968, 67; and R. I. Rotberg and T. K. Rabb, "The Relationship of Nutrition, Disease, and Social Conditions: A Graphical Presentation," in R. I. Rotberg and T. K. Rabb (eds.), Hunger and History. Cambridge: Cambridge University Press, 1983, p. 308.

[122] Ramenofsky, *Vectors of Death*, p. 156; and Wisseman, "Rickettsial Diseases," p. 570.

[123] Paul Fiset, "Clinical and Laboratory Diagnosis of Rickettsial Diseases of Man," in Gueh-Djen Hsiung and Robert H. Green (eds.), *Virology and Rickettsiology*, Volume 1 Part 2. CRC Handbook Series in Clinical Laboratory Science. West Palm Beach, Fla: CRC Press, Inc., 1978, p. 361.

years of age but sharply increases in virulence with age.[124] More specific typhus case fatality rates, derived form nineteenth-century Russian data, are summarized in Table 2.8. Examining the case fatality values for the typhus epidemics (1545-1548, 1559, 1576-1581) tabulated in Table 2.6 shows that the 0-1 age-class is given a higher case fatality rate, 10 percent, than would be implied by the data in Table 2.8. The simulation value is set at one-half of the 15-45 age-class rate using the argument that if more than 25 percent of mothers (aged 15-45) perished in the epidemic, at least half of their infants would perish as well.

TABLE 2.8 TYPHUS CASE FATALITY RATES

(all rates expressed as percentages)

Age-class	Case fatality (a)	Case fatality §	Case fatality (b)	Case fatality §	Average
0-10	10.00	2.50	2.00	3.00	4.38
10-20	10.00	2.50	2.00	3.00	4.38
20-30	—	5.50	9.00	4.00	6.17
30-40	—	20.00	19.00	12.40	17.13
40-50	—	48.50	31.00	23.20	34.23
50-60	50.00	63.60	37.00	43.00	48.40
60-70	50.00	62.50	37.00	52.30	50.45
70-80	50.00	100.00	—	47.10	65.70

(a) Fiset 1978
(b) Zdrodovskiii & Golinevich 1960

Morbidity rates for insect-vectored typhus is more difficult to estimate than those for the aerosol-spread diseases, smallpox and measles, because the rate of human infection is dependent on the population density of lice as well. Posey and Zinsser note that lice were certainly present in Amerindian populations and that they were probably quite prevalent.[125] Assuming that this was the case, it is not unreasonable to posit that the initial typhus epidemic also had a 90 percent morbidity rate. As for the diseases noted above, infection by the typhus rickettsiae conveys a long-lived immunity to further infection so morbidity rates for the subsequent epidemics are adjusted by age class to reflect this fact (Table 2.6).[126]

Despite its historical importance as a serious epidemic killer, historical statistics on plague case fatalities are scarce. If the plague outbreaks in the Basin were primarily of the pneumonic form, however, this lacuna is not

---

124 Wisseman, "Rickettsial Diseases," p. 570.

125 Posey, "Entomological Considerations"; and Zinsser, *Rats, Lice and History*, p. 259.

126 Wisseman, "Rickettsial Diseases," p. 571; and Zdrodovskii and Golinevich, *The Rickettsial Diseases*, p. 486.

significant since pneumonic plague case fatalities are most always reported as approximately 95-100 percent.[127] Thus, figuring conservatively, the case fatality rate for the 1545-1548 and 1576-1581 pneumonic plague outbreaks in the Basin is set at 90 percent (Table 2.6).

Serious as these epidemics were, the population of the Basin did not virtually disappear in these epidemics (as would have been the case with a disease with a 90 percent morbidity rate and a 90 percent case fatality rate). Hence, the morbidity rate could not have been as high for the pneumonic plague epidemics as for the others considered here. Estimating the morbidity rate for pneumonic plague is more involved than for the other diseases since direct data are lacking. There is, however, a study that computes the age-class mortality due to a plague epidemic in London in 1603 from which it is possible to calculate morbidity rates.[128] Since mortality is the product of morbidity and case fatality, it is possible to calculate age-class morbidity from these published mortalities and assumed case fatalities (Table 2.9). In Table 2.9, age-class morbidities in column C result from dividing the age-class mortalities in column A by the assumed case fatalities in column B. While it is reasonably certain that those who contract plague and survive are resistant to further infection,[129] the very small proportion who do survive infection render it unnecessary to adjust the morbidity figures for subsequent epidemic outbreaks (Table 2.6). The epidemic in 1559, however, is not reported as a severe one, and since it is identified as having the same symptoms as the 1545-48 and 1576-1581 pestilences, it is modeled using roughly 25 percent of the morbidity given to the more severe events Table 2.6).[130]

While the epidemics of smallpox, measles, pneumonic plague, and typhus represent most of the epidemics with significant demographic effects in the first 100 years of Spanish occupance of the Basin, there remain a number of years in which there were other epidemics significant enough to be reported. *Paperas* (mumps) was reported for 1550 and death and famine were noted for 1558.[131] Similarly, general illness, *cocoliztili*, was recorded for 1566, 1587-1588, 1601-1602, and 1613.[132] Further the disease Gibson

---

[127] Dols, *The Black Death in the Middle East*, p. 73; Hirst, *The Conquest of Plague*, p. 229; T.H. Hollingsworth, *Historical Demography*, Ithaca, NY: Cornell University Press, 1969, p. 365; and Shrewsbury, *A History*, p. 6.

[128] Mary F. Hollingsworth and T. H. Hollingsworth, "Plague Mortality Rates by Age and Sex in the Parish of St. Botolph's without Bishopsgate, London, 1603," *Population Studies*, 25 (1971), pp. 131-146.

[129] Pollitzer, *Plague*, pp. 137-138.

[130] Gibson, *The Aztecs*, p. 449.

[131] Ibid.

[132] Ibid.

TABLE 2.9 PNEUMONIC PLAGUE MORBIDITY RATES

(all rates expressed as percentages)

Age-class	Mortality (a)	Case fatality (assumed)	Morbidity
0-1	68.00	90.00	75.56
1-4	37.40	90.00	41.56
5-9	32.50	90.00	36.11
10-14	23.90	90.00	26.56
15-19	25.30	90.00	28.11
20-24	25.70	90.00	28.56
25-29	16.70	90.00	18.56
30-34	16.90	90.00	18.78
35-39	20.40	90.00	22.67
40-44	14.40	90.00	16.00
45-49	15.50	90.00	17.22
50-54	16.00	90.00	17.78
55-59	5.80	90.00	6.44
60-64	8.10	90.00	9.00
65-69	3.20	90.00	3.56
70-74	20.50	90.00	22.78
75-79	21.00	90.00	23.33
80+	1.60	90.00	1.78

(a) Hollingsworth and Hollingsworth 1971

identifies as influenza, *tlatlacistli*, was reported for 1590.[133] Aside from the mumps, these, presumably more minor and less well-defined epidemics pose a problem in identification and simulation. For the purposes of this study, all these episodes will be modeled as influenza-pneumonia outbreaks. These identifications are by no means certain, however, if for no other reason than many diseases' symptoms resemble those of influenza and pneumonia is a very common secondary condition.

It is conceivable that epidemic influenzas (type A orthomyxoviruses) could have accompanied the original Amerindians over the Bering land bridge, but this is unlikely since influenza needs congregated human populations to be viable.[134] Feral ducks or other migratory waterfowl may also have transmitted influenza to the Americas at a later date, although there is no evidence for type A influenza in the New World before Columbus.[135] It seems reasonably certain that epidemic influenzas were transported to the New World in the sixteenth century. McBryde and Beveridge note that there were influenza pandemics in the Old World in 1510 and world-wide in

---

133   Ibid.

134   K. David Patterson, *Pandemic Influenza 1700-1900*. Totowa, NJ: Rowman & Littlefield, 1986, p. 6.

135   Patterson, *Pandemic Influenza*, p. 6.

1557-1558.[136] The latter episode was quite severe and Spanish cities were reported to be nearly depopulated by the disease.[137] Like smallpox and measles, influenza is an aerosol spread viral disease of high communicability.[138] Unlike those diseases, however, influenza's many antigenic forms insure that even those with previous experience with one-or-more varieties of "flu" can be infected anew by a new strain.[139] This latter fact along with the fact that many influenza victims do not show clinical symptoms ensures that during outbreaks of a new variety influenza morbidity is high, even if its case fatality is usually low. Hence, the presence of influenza in Spain, its high communicability, and its myriad of types (insuring a large susceptible population) argue for its introduction to the Americas. The relatively late date of influenza's introduction to the Americas may be due to the facts that since the incubation period for flu is short (1-3 days), early crew sizes were small, and voyage durations were long, a ship-board "flu" outbreak would be completed before land-fall in the Caribbean.[140]

Morbidity and case fatality data are difficult to obtain for influenza since minor influenza infections often may be passed off as "colds" (Rhinoviruses) and deaths ultimately due to influenza are usually attributed to complications such as pneumonia and bronchitis.[141] It is for this reason that much of the data on influenza epidemics before this century consists only of general estimates of morbidity (Table 2.10). Indeed, the most common measure of the impact of an influenza epidemic is the "excess mortality" due to respiratory problems that are observed above the usual expected for the place and season.[142] Such figures have been converted to mortality rates for a few well-studied nineteenth-century influenza epidemics (columns D, E, and F in Table 2.11). Studies of the great pandemic of influenza of 1918-1919 provide somewhat more firm data as well (Table 2.10 and columns B and C in Table 2.11).

There is great variance in the recorded values for influenza-induced case fatality and doubtless this reflects the variety of differing strains of

---

136   William Ian Beveridge, *Influenza: The Last Great Plague*, New York: Prodist, 1978, p. 26: and F.W. McBryde, "Influenza in America During the Sixteenth Century, (Guatemala: 1523, 1559-62, 1576)," *Bulletin of the History of Medicine*, 8 (1940), p. 297.

137   Beveridge, *Influenza*, p. 26.

138   F. M. Davenport, "Influenza Viruses," in A. S. Evans (ed.), *Viral Infections of Humans*, New York and London: Plenum Medical Book Company, 1976, p. 287.

139   Patterson, *Pandemic Influenza*, p. 5.

140   Ramenofsky, *Vectors of Death*, p. 167.

141   Andrew D. Cliff Peter Haggett, and J. Keith Ord, *Spatial Aspects of Influenza Epidemics*, London: Pion Limited, 1986, p. 20; and Davenport, "Influenza Viruses," p. 275.

142   Ibid.

TABLE 2.10 INFLUENZA EPIDEMICS

(all rates expressed as percentages)

LOCATION	DATE	CASE FATALITY	Community MORBIDITY	MORTALITY
Tonga (a)	1918-19	—	—	10.00
Samoa (a)	1918-19	—	—	25.00
Tahiti (a)	1918-19	—	—	30.00
USA (b)	1918-19	—	—	0.50
Iceland (c)	1918-45	0.96	0.77	0.01
Iceland (c)	1918-19	0.69	7.96	0.05
Iceland (c)	1920-45	0.47	—	—
Iceland (c)	1918-19	0.98	—	—
Reykjavik (c)	1918-19	1.70	—	—
World (e)	1918-19	2.50	20.00	0.50
W. Samoa (e)	1918-19	—	—	19.70
Rome (d)	1781	—	67.00	—
Britain (d)	1781	—	75.00	—
Java (d)	1831	1.30	23.50	0.31
Memel (d)	1833	—	80.00	—
Konigsberg (d)	1833	—	58.00	—
Stockholm (d)	1833	—	25.00	—
Edinburgh (d)	1833	—	50.00	—
London (d)	1833	—	80.00	—
Paris (d)	1833	—	80.00	—
Europe (d)	1836	—	50.00	—
Britain (d)	1836	2.00	—	—
Europe (d)	1889	1.42	42.00	0.60
Ireland (d)	1892	—	—	7.80
Ireland (d)	1900	—	—	11.00
Guatemala (f)	1918-19	—	—	13.00
Oceana	1950	3.30	100.00	3.30
Averages	—	1.34	47.09	3.09

(a) Judd 1977 (b) Beveridge 1978 (c) Cliff *et al.* 1986
(d) Patterson 1986 (e) Crosby 1977 (f) Shattuck 1933

different virulence. Some patterns emerge, however. Compared to the other diseases noted thus far, influenza generally is less virulent; even if the most serious recent epidemic, that of 1918-1919, is considered. Further, the 1918-1919 epidemic data suggests that this influenza strain was more virulent in isolated, virgin-soil-like regions than elsewhere (Table 2.10). This generality may not apply to other strains, however, since the 1918-1919 variety was notably more virulent than its immediate, nineteenth-century, predecessors (see columns G and H in Table 2.11). These differences suggest that case fatalities derived from the so-called "Spanish influenza" of 1918-1919 be used to simulate the more severe flu-like

TABLE 2.11 INFLUENZA AGE-CLASS MORTALITY RATES

(all rates expressed as percentages)

AGE-CLASS	USA (a) 1918-19 MORBIDITY	Iceland (b) 1918-19 CASE FATALITY	Paris (c) 1889-90 MORTALITY	England (c) 1891 (D) MORTALITY	London (c) 1891 (E) MORTALITY	19th C AGE-CLASS MORTALITY	1918-19 AGE-CLASS MORTALITY
0-1	35.00	21.70	—	0.03	0.75	0.39	7.60
1-5	35.00	4.30	—	—	0.75	0.75	1.51
5-10	35.00	4.30	—	—	0.10	0.10	1.51
10-15	35.00	2.15	0.10	—	0.10	0.10	0.75
15-20	35.00	2.15	0.20	—	0.10	0.10	0.75
20-25	35.00	7.40	0.20	—	0.10	0.15	2.59
25-30	35.00	7.40	0.20	—	0.10	0.15	2.59
30-35	35.00	7.40	0.20	—	0.10	0.15	2.59
35-40	27.00	7.40	0.20	0.06	0.10	0.12	2.00
40-45	27.00	12.75	0.25	0.06	0.30	0.20	3.44
45-50	27.00	12.75	0.30	0.08	0.30	0.23	3.44
50-55	20.00	12.75	0.30	0.08	0.30	0.23	2.55
55-60	20.00	12.75	0.40	0.16	0.30	0.29	2.55
60-65	20.00	9.76	0.50	0.16	0.80	0.49	1.95
65-70	15.00	9.76	0.70	0.32	0.80	0.61	1.46
70-75	10.00	9.76	1.25	0.32	0.80	0.79	0.98
75-80	—	—	1.50	0.55	0.80	0.95	—
80-85	—	—	—	0.75	1.50	1.13	—
85+	—	—	—	—	1.50	1.50	—

(a) Beveridge 1978 (b) Cliff et al. 1986 (c) Patterson 1986
(d) Influenza only (e) Influenza and pneumonia

disease of 1590 and data from the lesser nineteenth-century epidemics be used to simulate the outbreaks of 1550, 1558, 1566, 1587-1588, 1601-1602, and 1613 (Tables 2.4 and 2.6).

While the "flu" generally is a less frightening disease because of its relatively low case fatality, its high morbidity is characteristic. Davenport argues that the morbidity from a new variety of influenza ranges from 20-40 percent.[143] The higher values noted by Patterson for nineteenth-century epidemics (see column D Table 2.10) are probably due to the congregated nature of the population for most of his cases and to the rather rudimentary nature of sanitation. Since there is evidence that repeated infection of individuals by various strains of influenza viruses produces a broadened antibody response to strains not previously encountered, high values for European morbidities argue for even higher morbidity values in virgin-soil populations.[144] Indeed, Brown and colleagues found a virtually 100 percent morbidity rate for a virgin-soil Pacific island population.[145] Since all three; relatively congregated populations, virgin-soil population, and low-level sanitation, were present in sixteenth-century Mexico, it is not unreasonable to posit a 90 percent morbidity rate for each of the influenza epidemics noted above (Table 2.6). The high morbidity for each event is warranted because to be serious enough to generate comment each event must have involved a new strain of influenza virus since "repeat" attacks would have been relatively easily dealt with by the population and little mortality would have occurred. Further, Beveridge argues that a general characteristic of influenza is that it attacks all types of people, "the weak and spoiled...the youngest as well as the oldest."[146] Thus, influenza susceptibility is most likely uniform across age classes, and the differences noted in the literature probably reflect socio-culturally determined exposure rates rather than differing biological susceptibility (see column B Table 2.11). With this in mind, the simulation morbidity has been set uniformly across the age-classes (Table 2.6).

MORTALITY INTERACTIONS

Background Mortality Interactions

The calculation of community background mortality is more complicated than that for epidemic mortality. For epidemic mortality there can be both an absence of epidemic crises, leading to an absolute minimum, 0.0, mortality, or an absolute maximum mortality, 1.0, in the presence of an epidemic that completely wipes out the population. For background

---

143   Davenport, "Influenza Viruses," p. 280.

144   P. Brown, D. C. Gajdusek, and J. A. Morris, "Epidemic A2 Influenza in Isolated Pacific Island Populations Without Pre-Epidemic Antibody to Influenza Types A and B, and the Discovery of Other Still Unexposed Populations," *American Journal of Epidemiology* 83 (1966), p. 184.

145   Brown *et al.*, "Epidemic A2 Influenza," p. 179.

146   Beveridge, *Influenza*, p. 26.

mortalities, however, there is always present a level of mortality that corresponds to the nutritional and epidemiological situation at the time.

Nowhere are these complications more evident than in the interaction between malnutrition and disease. Especially important are those for the endemic mortalities and malnutrition. In any population the effects of the interactions of these infirmities are complex and often not well understood. In general, however, the interactions between malnutrition and infection may be synergistic or antagonistic. But in human populations, synergy is the rule.[147] Synergy occurs when "infections of almost any degree of severity worsen nutritional status by interfering with food intake and by causing an increased loss of essential nutrients from the body. Conversely, the commonest types of malnutrition, even when subclinical, affect one or more of the mechanisms of resistance to infections or to the resulting infectious disease."[148] The effects of various forms and levels of malnutrition on infections have been widely studied, yet specific information is scarce and often equivocal. Yet, in a general sense, it seems clear that synergy is most important for children below 5 years of age since their immune system is less developed and their nutritional needs are greatest.[149] Synergistic effects also seem to be less important for mild to moderate cases of protein-calorie-malnutrition than for severe famine.[150] In the case of severe and widespread malnutrition, famine, there are additions to these bio-medical synergies, and these additions may powerfully affect the community experience with food shortfalls. Social factors such as the breakdown of traditional sanitation practices, and the tendency of populations to mix and migrate may serve to provoke severe outbreaks of otherwise relatively latent endemic diseases.[151]

There is evidence that malnutrition may interfere with normal resistance in four ways: (1) by reducing the immunoglobulin production in the mucosa, tears, and saliva, thus increasing the possibility of infection;[152] (2)

---

[147] C. E. Taylor and C. DeSweemer, "Nutrition and Infection," in M. Rechcigl (ed.), *Food, Nutrition and Health, World Review of Nutrition and Dietetics*, Basel: Karger, 1973. Vol. 16, p. 206.

[148] N. S. Scrimshaw, "Interactions of Malnutrition and Infection: Advances in Understanding," in R. E. Olson (ed.), *Protein Calorie Malnutrition*, New York: Academic Press, 1975, p. 353.

[149] A. R. Frisancho, "Nutritional Influences on Human Growth and Maturation," in K. A. Bennett (ed.), *Yearbook of Physical Anthropology*, Vol. 21. Washington, DC: American Association of Physical Anthropologists, 1978, pp. 180-181; and Taylor and DeSweemer, "Nutrition and Infection," p. 206.

[150] L. J. Mata, "Malnutrition-Infection Interactions in the Tropics," *The American Journal of Tropical Medicine and Hygiene*, 24 (1975), p. 568.

[151] F. B. Bang, "Famine Symposium—The Role of Disease in the Ecology of Famine," *Ecology of Food and Nutrition* 7 (1978), pp. 1, 7.

[152] Frisancho, "Nutritional Influences," pp. 180-181; and Rotberg and Rabb, "The Relationship of Nutrition, Disease, and Social Conditions," p. 307.

by inhibiting or decreasing antibody production[153] (3) by reducing cell-mediated immune responses;[154] and (4) by reducing humoral immune responses.[155] All of this is made much more complex by considering specific nutritional problems such as protein deficiency, since different classes of infection respond differently to different nutritional states.

Infections trigger malnutrition primarily by altering the bodily mechanisms that regulate the nitrogen (from proteins) balance.[156] These include: (1) the increased loss of protein that accompanies the increased adrenocortical activity; (2) the increased caloric expenditure that accompanies illness (e.g., fever); (3) the reduced food intake that results from general malaise, diminished appetite, and the tendency for care givers to withdraw solid foods (especially those high in protein) from the sick; and (4) the changes in the gastro-intestinal tract that reduce absorption.[157]

The relationship between nutrition and disease is antagonistic when the combined effect of malnutrition and a specific disease is less than would be expected from the sum of the individual effects. It has been identified only in cases where a very specific nutritional deficiency in the host limits the viability of the infectious agent to cause clinical symptoms in the host.[158] This phenomena has been observed for malaria, however, with both severe general malnutrition[159] and with ascariasis (infestations of intestinal worms) that deprives the host and plasmodium of essential nutrients.[160]

Proceeding beyond the general arguments over synergy and considering the situation for indigenous Amerindian diseases, it is evident that many of the diseases that are synergistic with malnutrition are among those found in the pre-Columbian New World. Among these are intestinal

153   Frisancho, "Nutritional Influences," p. 217; Rotberg and Rabb, "The Relationship of Nutrition, Disease, and Social Conditions," p. 307; and Scrimshaw, et al., Interactions, p. 13.

154   Frisancho, "Nutritional Influences," pp. 180-181; Rotberg and Rabb, "The Relationship of Nutrition, Disease, and Social Conditions," p. 307; and Scrimshaw, "Advances in Understanding," p. 354.

155   Rotberg and Rabb, "The Relationship of Nutrition, Disease, and Social Conditions," p. 307; and Scrimshaw, "Advances in Understanding," p. 354; but see Frisancho, "Nutritional Influences," pp. 180-181, who argues contra.

156   Taylor and DeSweemer, "Nutrition and Infection," p. 207.

157   W. R. Beisel, "Synergism and Antagonism of Parasitic Diseases and Malnutrition," Reviews of Infectious Diseases 4 (1982), p. 749; Rotberg & Rabb, "The Relationship of Nutrition, Disease, and Social Conditions," p. 307; Scrimshaw, "Advances in Understanding," p. 354; Scrimshaw, et al., Interactions, pp. 26, 27-28, 29, 34; and Taylor and DeSweemer, "Nutrition and Infection," p. 207.

158   Taylor and DeSweemer, "Nutrition and Infection," p. 205.

159   Beisel, "Synergism and Antagonism," p. 749.

160   J. Murray, A. Murray, M. Murray, and C. Murray, "The Biological Supression of Malaria: an Ecological and Nutritional Interrelationship of a Host and Two Parasites," The American Journal of Clinical Nutrition, 31 (1978), pp. 1363-1366.

parasitic diseases, especially infestations of worms. These strongly compromise the host's nutrition while they render the poorly nourished host more susceptible to additional infections.[161] Similarly, other intestinal disorders such as protozoan, amoebic, and bacillary dysentery and bacillary diarrhea both interfere with the nutritional status of the host and are made more serious by malnutrition.[162] Respiratory infections such as tuberculosis, streptococcus and staphylococcus infections, and others causing pneumonia and bronchopneumonia are more prevalent and virulent in malnourished hosts and are implicated in reducing the host's nutritional integrity, though, perhaps to a lesser degree.[163] There is also evidence of some synergy in the rickettsial diseases and some trypanosome infections.[164]

The argument for synergy between malnutrition and endemic disease is reinforced by examining the age-class specific mortalities due to endemic diseases and famines. Examination of Figure 2.10, which shows age-class famine mortalities in a contemporary Bangladesh famine, and Preston's "typical" endemic disease mortality pattern highlights the similarities of pattern between the two (i.e., the similarities in the proportions of mortalities for the same age-group).

Since these age specific mortality patterns are similar and there are important synergies between nutritional status and endemic disease, it is sensible to model the mortality due to either cause as a complex of endemic disease and nutritional status. Endemic disease *per se* does not appear as a separate variable in Figure 2.4, however. In situations where the nutritional stress is at its "usual" levels, (i.e., when *nutr_disc* is equal to its usual, 0.0, level) the levels of endemic disease are determined by the "usual" values of the background age-class case fatality (e.g., $B\_CF\_0\_1$) and background age-class morbidity (e.g., $B\_morb\_0\_1$) variables (Figure 2.6). Reduced levels of nutrition (i.e., situations in which weight ratios are less than 1.0) increase the age-group background morbidities (e.g., $B\_morb\_0\_1$), that is, poor per-capita nutrition will result in a greater proportion of the population suffering from the various background infirmities, while improved nutrition will decrease the age-group background morbidities. At

---

161 Beisel, "Synergism and Antagonism," p. 749; Rotberg and Rabb, "The Relationship of Nutrition, Disease, and Social Conditions," p. 308; Scrimshaw, *et al.*, *Interactions*, p. 34; and Taylor and DeSweemer, "Nutrition and Infection," p. 208.

162 Mata,"Malnutrition-Infection Interactions," p. 566; Rotberg and Rabb, "The Relationship of Nutrition," p. 308; Scrimshaw *et al.* 1968, pp. 26, 29; and Taylor and DeSweemer, "Nutrition and Infection," pp. 207, 209.

163 Mata, "Malnutrition-Infection Interactions," 566; Rotberg and Rabb, "The Relationship of Nutrition, Disease, and Social Conditions," p. 308; Scrimshaw, *et al.*, *Interactions*, pp. 26, 29; and Taylor and DeSweemer, "Nutrition and Infection," pp. 207, 209.

164 Scrimshaw, *et al.*, *Interactions*, p. 30, 33.

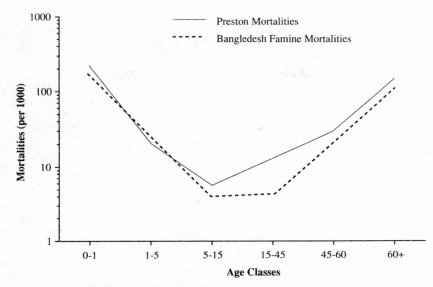

Sources: Preston 1976: 91; Watkins & Menken 1985: 655

Figure 2.10 Preston and Bangladesh Mortalities Compared

the same time, malnutrition also increases the likelihood of death due to these illnesses, hence a decrease in the values of the weight ratios will increase the age-class background case fatalities, (e.g., $B\_CF\_0\_1$) and, conversely, improved nutrition will decrease the age-class background case fatalities. The modeling is the same in the case of severe malnutrition, since in that case mortality may not be due to simple starvation, but rather, victims typically succumb to endemic respiratory or gastro-intestinal complications.[165] Similarly, many endemic infections, especially those of the gastro-intestinal tract, trigger severe malnutrition, even in the presence of adequate food.[166]

These associations are operationalized in the simulation of the background mortality through the systemic connections of the variables that track the nutrition state of the population (i.e., *nutr-disc*). It is necessary to set limits to define these relationships. In situations where the level of per-capita nutrition improves, the resulting level of improved background mortality (i.e., morbidity and case fatality) is uncertain, but it is unlikely to exceed a 25 percent improvement. To set the limit in the opposite situations, of famine, a *nutr_disc* equal to 0.0 would signify that there was no food for a year, and would result in mortality rates of virtually 1.0. This has not been a common situation in any historical circumstance; to gain a more

---

[165] Peny Kane, "The Demography of Famine," *Genus* 18 (1987), p. 52.

[166] Beisel, "Synergism and Antagonism," p. 749; Scrimshaw, *et al.*, *Interactions*, pp. 26, 27-28; and Taylor and DeSweemer, "Nutrition and Infection," p. 207.

reasonable idea of the true ranges of famine induced mortality, it is helpful to examine the additional mortality noted in a number of historical famines (Table 2.12). The figures in the right-hand column reflect the famine peak multiplication of the pre-famine crude mortality rates. A simple mean of these figures is 4.4x, but this figure may be too large to characterize severe famines since Watkins and Menken argue that famines that doubled the crude death rates were rare.[167] But, the calculation of this multiplier is very dependent on the spatial scale of the reported famine. A very severe local famine will not alter the regional statistics significantly, and it seems reasonable to argue that the most severe famines may have been less wide-spread.

TABLE 2.12 FAMINE MORTALITY EXTREMES

Location	Date	Mortality Multiplier
China	1877-78	2.1-3.0
Italy	1376	13.3
Finland	1676	5.0-6.6
Bengal	1700	6.6
England	1597	1.52
Bangledesh	1971-72	1.39
Bangledesh	1974-75	1.52-1.6
China	1958-61	1.72-2.0
Ireland	1845	2.06

Sources: Hugo 1984: 13; Watkins & Menken 1985: 650; Kane 1987:51; Boyle & O'Gráda 1986: 562.

This issue is more complex than the discussion in the previous paragraph implies, however. While Watkins and Menken may be right in arguing for a 2x upper limit on the community-level, crude death rates in the most severe famines, such a limit does not help much in calculating each age-group's mortality rate at different levels of *nutr_disc*. Since each age-class has different mortality rates at *nutr_disc* = 1.0, but the same mortality, 1.0, at *nutr_disc* = 0.0, simply multiplying each age-class's usual (*nutr_disc* = 1.0) mortality by a constant (at any value of the *nutr-disc*) to set a new value, may exaggerate the mortality experienced by some age-groups (at this level of *nutr-disc*) and understate it for others. A slightly different situation applies for setting lower, "good times" limits on mortalities. Here, it is assumed that for *nutr_disc* = 1.5, the minimum mortality (equal to 75% of the "usual," *nutr_disc* = 1.0, level) for each age-class is obtained. For each age-class, the resulting mortality is modeled as a curvilinear function of *nutr_disc*, over the range of *nutr_disc* from 0.0 - 1.5 (see Figure 2.6 for an example of these age-specific mortality curves).

---

[167] Watkins and Menken, "Famines in Historical Perspective," p. 653.

Spanish *congregaciones* (forced resettlements) may have further altered background mortality. This is because actions that alter the local disease environment, the contact frequency of human hosts and disease causing organisms, or the food production system will alter the morbidity of a population.[168] *Congregaciones,* likely had the effect of disrupting usual sanitary arrangements, consequently increasing the exposure of local populations to parasitic diseases of the gastro-intestinal tract. The movement itself is likely to have increased the possibility of spread of air-borne infectious diseases such as those of the respiratory tract. Further, such disruption may have upset the usual food production routine. Because of their timing, near the end of the period examined here, and the small population thereby put at risk, these effects are not modeled in MEXIPOP.

Similarly, background case fatality is increased in times of crisis. Since episodes of wide-spread epidemic or famine morbidity would interfere with the ability of care-givers to adequately care for their dependents, even if the care is simple and non-medical (e.g., fetching food and water for the victim or keeping the patient warm), such episodes would also increase the likelihood of mortality from these background infirmities. Joralemon and Crosby argue that the epidemic crises that affected large numbers of post-conquest Amerindians reduced their ability to care adequately for those taken ill and so contributed to increased mortality.[169] These arguments are based on documented, twentieth-century "virgin soil" epidemics in isolated Pacific islands, Polynesia, and in the Canadian Arctic.[170] While this effect is well documented for increased case fatality for the epidemic diseases themselves, it is important to note that especially vulnerable in such times are the young or aged dependent age-groups, who are the most susceptible to background mortality in the first place. This is tricky, however, since the background case fatality consists of a number of different kinds of deaths: accidental, infant diarrhea, death in childbirth, death in old age due to accumulated infirmities, deaths due to other indigenous diseases, and so on. Nevertheless, examination of Figure 2.8 shows that the most demographically important of these causes of death are those due to indigenous diseases that affect the elderly and youth disproportionally (i.e., infant diarrheas, dysenteries, and respiratory problems).

These effects (increased mortality for populations in which everyone is simultaneously ill) are captured in the models through the multiplication of the *care_factor* variable (which ranges from 1.0 to 1.25) with the age-class background mortality variables, to produce higher mortalities in situations of high morbidity (Figure 2.4). The magnitude of the *care_factor* multiplier

---

168 Sinnecker, *General Epidemiology*, p. 24.

169 D. Joralemon, "New World Depopulation and the Case of Disease," *Journal of Anthropological Research,* 38 (1982), p. 113; and Crosby, "Virgin Soil Epidemics," p. 295.

170 Brown *et al.*, "Epidemic A2 Influenza," p. 181; Judd, "Depopulation in Polynesia," p. 591; and Peart and Nagler, "Measles in the Canadian Arctic," p. 153.

is determined from the level of community-wide morbidity by using a graphical function of *morb_sum*, itself the sum of the total background morbidity *(Bkgd_morb)* and the total epidemic morbidity *(E_morb)*. The community-level background morbidity, *Bkgd_morb*, is calculated from the age-class morbidities by multiplying each age-class' population by its corresponding morbidity (e.g., *B_morb_0_1 * pop_0_1*), summing the resultant numbers of ill in each age-group, and dividing this sum by the total population (Figure 2.4).

Since it is important to know the community-wide epidemic morbidity, *E_morb*, it is necessary to calculate the community-level morbidity from the age-class morbidities. This is accomplished in the simulation by noting that the community level of morbidity is equal to the sum of the numbers of affected in all the age-classes divided by the total population. Since the number affected in each age-group is equal to the age-class morbidity multiplied by the age-class population, the community morbidity = Σ (age-class morbidities * age-class populations)/total population. This simple calculation is noted in the right hand portion of Figure 2.7.

Epidemic Mortality Interactions

Epidemic mortality is the "extra" mortality imposed on the community by the crises of introduced infectious disease (neglecting potential epidemics of indigenous diseases). In some ways modeling this mortality is less complicated than that for background mortality. This is because, with some important exceptions, the mortality of introduced epidemic disease is relatively less intimately connected with the state of nutrition than is indigenous, endemic disease. For example, among the infectious diseases introduced in the sixteenth century, only chicken pox, cholera, and measles are believed to be strongly synergistic.[171] Minimal synergy with malnutrition is noted for smallpox, malaria, plague, typhoid, tetanus, yellow fever, and poliomyelitis.[172] Variable or equivocal interactions are reported for typhus, diphtheria, and influenza.[173]

There is another phenomena acting to produce a synergy between infections. Cockburn notes that a population exposed to a heavy infection may respond poorly to an exposure of some other pathogen since there is a "crowding out" phenomena where heavy production of one antibody can inhibit the production of another.[174] This may not be important here since the interactions we are concerned with involve alien pathogens, and the

---

[171] Beisel, "Synergism and Antagonism," p. 746; A. Keys, J. Brozek, A. Henschul, O. Mickelsen, and H. L. Taylor, *The Biology of Human Starvation*, Vol. 1. Minneapolis: University of Minnesota Press, 1950, p. 235; and Rotberg and Rabb, "The Relationship of Nutrition" p. 308.

[172] Scrimshaw, *et al.*, *Interactions*, pp. 30, 33, 61; and Taylor and DeSweemer, "Nutrition and Infection," p. 208.

[173] Rotberg and Rabb, "The Relationship of Nutrition, Disease, and Social Conditions," p. 308.

[174] Cockburn, *The Evolution and Eradication of Infectious Diseases*, p. 76.

Amerindian populations are less likely to have been very efficient in producing antibodies for the introduced diseases in any case.

Nevertheless, there are connections within the health ecology of the affected groups. As noted above, there is ample evidence that high levels of morbidity (due to either indigenous disease, severe malnutrition, epidemic disease, or a combination of all three) increases the case fatality of all, even the highly fatal introduced diseases. This effect is captured in the models using the *care factor* variable to modify the epidemic mortalities analogously to the way it was used to increase the background mortalities above (Figure 2.4).

Just as forced *congregaciones* may have served to increase the likelihood of mortality due to malnutrition or indigenous disease, they may have multiplied the mortality due to introduced infections since the contact frequency of possibly infectious individuals was increased and the proportion of possibly susceptible individuals was artificially increased in the new settlements.[175] Nevertheless, this interaction is not modeled in MEXIPOP because the major *congregaciones* did not take place until late in the century, well after most of the population loss had occurred.[176]

An important difference between the introduced epidemic diseases and the indigenous diseases is that indigenous diseases were endemic in the populations and, for that reason, their prevalence was primarily a function of local epidemiological conditions and was, therefore, relatively independent of particular dates. This is in contrast to the incidence of European, epidemic, infections, since their effect was highly localized in time. This dependence on date is modeled in Figure 2.7, where both the age-class epidemic morbidities (e.g., $E\_morb\_60\_99$) and age-class epidemic case fatalities (e.g., $E\_CF\_60\_99$) are shown as functions of date.

General Interactions

The general components of mortalities, epidemic and background, must be merged into age-group-specific total mortalities. Since the mortality of a population age-group is comprised of both background and epidemic mortalities, each age-class mortality in the model diagram is logically connected with both a background and a epidemic mortality variable (Figure 2.4). Age-class background mortalities (e.g., BM_0_1 in Figures 2.3 and 2.4) connect to and partially determine the age-class mortalities (e.g., $mort\_0\_1$ in Figure 2.3). Similarly, age-group epidemic mortalities (e.g., $ttl\_EM\_0\_1$ in Figure 2.4) also connect to and partially determine the age-group mortalities (e.g., $mort\_0\_1$ in Figure 2.3).

The age-class mortalities are not simple sums of the two component mortalities, however. Such simple sums would overstate the total mortality since, in general, an epidemic mortality episode would be more likely to "kill off" the infirm before the healthy. But, this infirm group includes those

---

175 Sinnecker, *General Epidemiology*, pp. 145, 152.

176 H.F. Cline, "Civil Congregations of the Indians in New Spain, 1598-1606," *Hispanic American Historical Review*, 29 (1949), pp. 349-369.

who would be expected to die from the background mortality in the course of a year. Using only the largest component mortality (usually epidemic mortality) assumes that every one of those who would be expected to die in a normal situation would succumb to the crisis and this procedure understates the total since there will be some "normal" background mortality in addition to the epidemic mortality. For these reasons, I have calculated the total age-class mortalities as the sum of the largest component of mortality (usually, but not always a epidemic mortality) plus 1/2 of the other mortality component. However, the simplicity of this, admittedly rough, calculation obscures the complexity of the interactions between different causes of death.

Turning to the interconnections of the health of a population and its food production system, Bang has aptly noted that to understand the genesis of famine, it is necessary to examine where breakdowns interfere with the flow of energy within the productive system.[177] Fundamental to the flow of food energy to a population is the provision of agricultural labor, and it is here that the health of the population influences agricultural production. This effect is captured in MEXIPOP by the relationship that determines the available labor (Figure 2.7). Since potential agricultural laborers are adults (i.e., those in the 15-45 and 45-60 age-groups), and those who are sick cannot contribute productive labor, the number of laborers available is diminished by the number of sick laborers. The simplifying assumption, that all ill adult laborers do not contribute productive work, overstates the effect of illness. In periods of epidemics especially, the number of potentially ill workers in these age-groups may be large (indeed the numbers affected will be large for all age-classes in some situations) and in these cases their ailments are more likely to be serious, thus preventing them from contributing. The number of available laborers is ascertained in the *well_labor* variable by first multiplying the respective epidemic morbidities by a constant whose value may be set in a range of 0.0-0.5. This diminishment of epidemic morbidities is necessary since epidemics are complex spatial and temporal events and cannot affect everyone in an area the size of the Basin at the same time. More importantly, we do not know the exact timing of epidemics in sixteenth-century Mexico. Some must have been concurrent with key planting or harvest times and these must have diminished production severely. Others may have fallen at relatively less important dates in the agricultural season and affected the total harvest very little. This degree of synergy between epidemic illness and agricultural output is controlled in alternate simulation runs by altering this constant. Adding the epidemic and background morbidities for each age-class (i.e., for the 15-45 and 45-60 age-classes) and subtracting the resulting sum from 1.0 yields the proportion of each age-group not affected by epidemic illness. This is then multiplied by the respective age-group population to yield the total number of available

---

[177] Bang, *The Role of Disease*, p. 11.

laborers at the key periods in each age-group. The sum of these two "healthy" labor age-classes represents the *well_labor*.

Since the Hispanic conquerors demanded labor tribute that resulted in a withdrawal of labor available to contribute to the flow of food to the Amerindian community, not all of the "healthy" laborers were available for work in the Indian economy at all times. This phenomena is captured by the *trib_labor_fract* variable, which diminishes the *total_labor* variable (equal to *well_labor*) producing the *labor_available_fract* variable (Figure 2.7). Since labor tribute varied over time, it is modeled as a function of *date*. The *labor_avail_fract* variable is the ratio of the *labor_available* to the total available labor, the sum of the *pop_45_60* and *pop_15_45* age-classes.

The Production Sub-system

GENERAL DEMAND MODEL

To clarify the MEXIPOP production sub-system, it is helpful to discuss the general structure that underlies the simulation of agricultural production in general. Agricultural production strategy is determined by demand. That is to say, the demands felt by individual agricultural households are reflected in their production goals. In these cases, the total demand is restricted to four sources, for household consumption, for tribute payment to support the conquers, for trade to support the urban population, and for surplus to store against calamity. Hence, as allowed by access to land, labor, and other productive capital and technology, increased total demand forces the agricultural household to increase production. This assumption reflects the prevalent view of primarily consumption, neolithic technology, agriculture.[178]

Embedded in this assumption of Amerindian agricultural production is another: production levels are a product of the labor and technology applied to a specified area such that "standard" yields can be expected. Thus, in principle, increases in demand result in increases in output that are produced by a complex interaction of increased labor, different technology and cultigens, and enhanced procedures applied to a fixed area, leading to increases in land productivity and/or expansion of the area cultivated. While perhaps all of these options were practiced by Amerindian agriculturalists during Spanish colonization, the evidence of major technological changes in

---

[178] Ester Boserup, *The Conditions of Agricultural Growth*, Chicago: Aldine, 1966; Harold C. Brookfield, "Intensification and Disintensification in Pacific Agriculture: A Theoretical Approach," *Pacific Viewpoint,* 13 (1972), pp. 30-48.; A. V. Chayanov, "Peasant Farm Organization," in D. Thorner, B. Kerblay and R. E. F. Smith (ed.), *A.V. Chayanov in the Theory of Peasant Economy*, Homewood, IL: R. D. Irwin, 1966; and B. L. Turner, II, and S. B. Brush, "Purpose, Classification, and Organization," in B. L. Turner II and S. B. Brush, (eds.) *Comparative Farming Systems*, New York: The Guilford Press, 1987, p. 7.

cropping in Amerindian systems in the sixteenth century, either by way of "landesque" capital or by changes in cultigens is slim.[179] For these reasons and for the sake of efficiency in the models, I have simplified these relationships by setting the area cultivated by each agriculturalist as a component that is responsive to the level of demand. All else equal, a given level of demand draws forth a production area necessary to meet the demand up to specified limits and according to the land productivity. This simplification neglects the possibility of long-term environmental degradation.

The issues of intensification and de-intensification for early colonial period agriculture in the Basin are complex. Population declined, even as productive lands passed out of Amerindian control. Further, environmental thresholds and opportunities constrained the options for agricultural change. These complications are particularly evident in the Basin since several distinctive types of agriculture (each with a different land-use intensity and labor input demand) were practiced in suitable regions. Details of treatment of these issues are found below.

The model uses the logic of household-level production noted above to set the production response, although, the simulation tracks the total production. This is done by assuming that similar households react similarly to demand, hence by multiplying the number of similar households by the household demand yields a total projected production.

For the Basin, the "household" that is assumed to be the basic unit of production and residence, was likely not a nuclear family. In calculating the size and number of such aggregations, production units (PUs) here, it is clear that they must not be a constant, since changes in population size must have changed the size of families, and of PUs. To accommodate this and to use the population data generated by MEXIPOP (i.e., the population of specific age-groups), I have defined the number (and size) of the PUs in terms of the numbers of adults in the 15-45 and 45-60 age-groups. The logic is as follows. Half of the sum of the 15-45 and 45-60 age-class populations is deemed to represent the possible number of married couples and this is also the number of extended families, since each extended family consists of a married couple and children and related kin. This assumes that the members of the 60-99 age-class are no longer the heads of extended families in this sense and comprise part of the related kin. But not all of these people (i.e., not all of half of the sum of the 15-45 and 45-60 age-classes) are couples; there must be allowances for those not married, or for

---

[179] Landesque capital refers "...to any investment in land with an anticipated life well beyond the present crop, or crop cycle." See P. Blakie, and H. Brookfield. "Defining and Debating the Problem," in P. Blakie and H. Brookfield (eds.), *Land Degradation and Society*, London: Methuen, 1987, p. 9. The creation of landesque capital involves savings of labor and other inputs for future production.

85

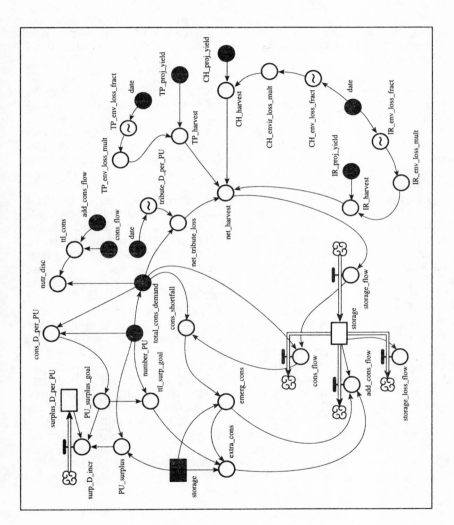

Figure 2.11 Post-harvest Production Sub-system

widows and widowers. I assume that 80 percent of the maximum number of extended families is a realistic figure for the number of extended families. Hence, the sum of the population of the 15-45 and 45-60 age-classes by 0.4 (0.8/2) is equal to the number of families. Dividing the total population by the number of families yields the average family size. The size of an average PU differs between the regions (see below for specific calculations) and is a multiple of the size of the average family. Similarly, the number of production units is equal to the total population divided by the number of production units.

Consumption Demand

To assess the first of the "demands" noted above, consumption demand generated by a production unit (PU), it is necessary to determine the demand of individuals within age-classes. Having determined these age-group values (below), it is a simple task to calculate the total annual consumption demand by multiplying the population numbers in each age-class by the age-class' average annual demand. The average PU consumption demand, *cons_D_per_PU*, is the total annual demand divided by the number of production units (Figure 2.11).

The age-group consumption demands for the two most important dietary components are calculated using values for recommended intakes for daily energy (kcal) and protein (gm) intakes. Column A of Table 2.13 uses values for daily needs prepared for the contemporary Mexican population and averaged across age classes to determine average needs for the age-groups in MEXIPOP. Since Mexican maize varieties average 3,610 kcal/kg and 96 gm protein/kg, it is straightforward to calculate the amounts of maize, if eaten alone, necessary to meet daily energy or protein needs (Table 2.13).[180] The upper section (columns E-F) of Table 2.13 displays these calculations extended throughout a year. The amount of maize required to satisfy energy demands is not the same as that required to satisfy protein needs since the amount of maize necessary to meet daily energy needs fails to provide the necessary protein for all but the 1-5 age-class. This deficit, calculated on an annual basis, is displayed in column H in Table 2.13. And even for the 1-5 year-olds, it is unlikely that these young children could ingest the full 1/3 kg of maize daily necessary to meet their energy or protein needs. Further, for the older age-classes to meet protein needs by maize alone would require eating an large amount, even assuming that the maize was treated with lime in the traditional manner and thus had an enhanced protein quality.[181] We need not be overly concerned by this deficit, however, because, as is noted below, much of the dietary variety available in the Basin served to enhance protein consumption.

180   M. Hernández, A. Chávez, and H. Bourges, *Valor Nutritivo de los Alimentos Mexicanos: Tablas de uso Práctico*, Mexico: Publicaciones de la División de Nutrición L 12, 6a Instituto Nacional de la Nutrición, 1974, pp. 5-6.

181   S. H. Katz, M. L. Hediger, and L.A. Valleroy, "Traditional Maize Processing Techniques of the New World," *Science,* 184 (1974), pp. 765-773.

TABLE 2.13 NUTRITIONAL NEEDS CALCULATIONS

	A	B	C	D	E	F	G	H
AGE CLASS	ENERGY (A) NEEDS (KCAL/DAY)	PROTEIN (A) NEEDS (GM/DAY)	DAILY MAIZE ENERGY (KG/DAY)	DAILY MAIZE PROTEIN (KG/DAY)	YEARLY MAIZE ENERGY (KG/YR)	YEARLY MAIZE PROTEIN (KG/YR)	YEARLY MAIZE (B) /YR (KG)	PROTEIN DEFICIT (-)(C) OR SURPLUS/YR (KG)
0-1	n/a	n/a	n/a	n/a	n/a	n/a	n/a	n/a
1-5	1250	33	0.35	0.34	126.39	125.47	82.15	0.92
5-15	2350	67	0.65	0.70	237.60	254.74	154.44	-17.14
15-45	2275	77	0.63	0.80	230.02	292.76	149.514	-62.74
45-60	1975	77	0.55	0.80	199.69	292.76	129.80	-93.07
60-99	1975	77	0.55	0.80	199.69	292.76	129.80	-93.07

Assumes 1 kg maize = 3610 kcal & 96 gm protein
(a) after Hernández, Chávez, & Bourges. 1974: 5, 6
(b) if maize = 65% of kcal needs
(c) assumes maize eaten to satisfy energy needs

ALTERNATIVE CALCULATIONS

	I	J	K	L	M	N	O	P
AGE CLASS	ENERGY NEEDS (D) (KCAL/DAY)	TOTAL MAIZE PER YEAR (KG)(G)	ENERGY NEEDS (KCAL/DAY) (E)	TOTAL MAIZE PER YEAR (KG) (G)	PROTEIN NEEDS (F) (GM/DAY)	ENERGY NEEDS (F) (KCAL/DAY)	DAILY MAIZE NEEDS (KG)	TOTAL MAIZE PER YR (G) (KG)
0-1	n/a	n/a	n/a	n/a	n/a	n/a	n/a	n/a
1-5	1270	83.46	1075	70.65	45	1400	0.39	92.01
5-15	1270	83.46	2021	132.82	66.25	2467	0.68	162.13
15-45	2370	155.76	1956.50	128.58	76.25	2925	0.81	192.231
45-60	2370	155.76	1698.50	111.63	65	2925	0.81	192.23
60-99	2370	155.76	1698.50	111.63	65	2750	0.76	180.73

(d) after Cook & Borah 1973: 157-8;
(e) Column A above x 0.86
(f) after National Research Council 1945;
(g) if maize = 65% of kcal needs

Even though these arguments show that it is improbable that the Amerindian populations obtained all their needs through the consumption of maize alone, it is frequently asserted that maize contributed from 50-80 percent of the total dietary energy supply.[182] Taking a middle figure, column G in Table 2.13 shows the annual consumption of maize if it was consumed (and available) to satisfy 65 percent of the dietary *energy* needs. While these figures seem reasonable, it is useful to explore some of the other estimates that have been offered as to Amerindian maize consumption.

Cook and Borah also estimate the average dietary energy supply needed by sixteenth-century Amerindians (Table 2.13, column I).[183] The annual maize consumption implied by these daily consumption figures (again assuming maize used to satisfy 65 percent of total energy needs) is displayed in Table 2.13, column J. These figures are a good deal larger than those derived form Hernández and colleagues (compare columns G and J in Table 2.13). Further, it is intriguing to note that these estimates assume a lighter population than those derived from Hernández and colleagues. They assume an adult woman of 55 kg, and an adult man of 65 kg in computing their recommendations, while Cook and Borah use an average man of 53.6 kg and an average woman of 49.6 kg.[184]

A modified figure for annual maize consumption may be calculated by noting that the ratio of Cook and Borah's adult average (i.e., men averaged with women) weight to Hernández and colleagues' is 0.86. While the basis of Hernandez and colleagues weight estimates is unclear, Cook and Borah's date from studies published in the 1930s-1950s.[185] Assuming that these, presumably earlier, measurements may be better representative of sixteenth-century conditions, multiplying the columns G and A estimates by 0.86 yield a set of even smaller annual needs estimates (Table. 2.13, columns K-L). In accepting these figures, it is assumed that the best estimate will be derived from using the Mexican consumption data and Cook and Borah's size data.

Gibson notes three estimates of sixteenth and seventeenth-century maize consumption. In the first, for 1555-1556, the daily ration of maize for workers (presumably male adults) was 1/48 *fanega*.[186] Since a *fanega* totals about 35.45-38.18 kg, this is equal to about 0.74-0.80 kg/day.[187] He also records a 1618 document that sets the weekly ration of maize for

---

182   Cook and Borah, *Essays in Population History*, Vol. 2, p. 163, 165; Hassig, *Trade, Tribute, and Transportation*, pp. 18, 20; Sanders, *et al.*, *The Basin of Mexico*, 233; and R. S. Santley, and E. K. Rose. "Diet, Nutrition, and Population Dynamics in the Basin of Mexico," *World Archaeology*, 11 (1979), p. 194.

183   Cook and Borah, *Essays in Population History*, Vol. 3, pp. 157-158.

184   Hernández *et al. Valor Nutritivo*, 5; and Cook and Borah, *Essays in Population History*, Vol. 3, p. 151.

185   Cook and Borah, *Essays in Population History*, Vol. 3, pp. 144-154, 149.

186   Gibson, *The Aztecs*, p. 311.

187   Ibid.

workers at 1/12 *fanega* (about 0.42-0.45 kg/day).[188] In the third estimate, Gibson cites colonial estimates that show that 1.0 *fanega* would support a laborer for 50-75 days (this approximates 0.47-0.71 kg/day).[189] These assessments are all greater than the estimate for 15-45 year-olds derived in Table 2.13, column G, 149.514 kg/year (equal to 0.4096 kg/day). It is difficult to compare this estimate with Gibson's since his are presumably for males alone and may represent more than 65 percent of the total dietary energy. If Gibson's estimates are for all of the daily requirements, they approximate those necessary to meet the total energy or protein needs as estimated in Table 2.13, columns C-D.

A set of protein and energy need estimates used by Anderson and colleagues to evaluate the nutritional status of contemporary Otomi Indians in Mexico, give rise to even higher estimates of daily and annual energy needs and roughly similar protein needs than does the Mexican data (compare columns G, and P, Table 2.13).[190]

But there are problems here as well. Without detailing the controversy surrounding the "small but healthy hypothesis," several nutritional experts maintain that it is incorrect to apply nutritional standards developed for modern Western societies to populations that have adapted to different physical and socioeconomic conditions. In general, these critics insist that proposed energy and protein requirements are set higher than necessary for the relatively smaller stature populations in the developing world.[191] Since Cook and Borah, Newman, and others provide ample evidence of the small stature of early twentieth-century Amerindian groups, this argument has some validity, especially in evaluating the estimates used by Anderson and colleagues.[192] For this reason, and because the Hernández and colleagues'

---

[188] Ibid.

[189] Ibid.

[190] R.K. Anderson, J. Calvo, G. Serrano, and G. C. Payne, "A Study of the Nutritional Status and Food Habits of Otomi Indians in the Mezquital Valley of Mexico," *American Journal of Public Health*, 36 (1946), pp. 889-900.

[191] D. Seckler, "The 'Small But Healthy?' Hypothesis: A Reply to Critics," *Economic and Political Weekly*, (1984), pp. 1886-1888.

[192] Cook and Borah, *Essays in Population History*, Vol. 3, pp. 141-149; and M. T. Newman "Adaptations in the Physique of American Aborigines to Nutritional Factors," *Human Biology*, 32 (1960), pp. 288-313.

standards were developed for the Mexican situation, I reject the Anderson and colleagues standards.[193]

Santley and Rose provide a lower estimate for average daily protein needs, 35 gm/day, and the daily and annual maize consumption implied by these assumptions (based on maize offering 65 percent of the total dietary protein), 0.365 kg maize/day and 86.50 kg maize per year, is much smaller than that implied by the Mexican data.[194] Unlike the figures posited by Cook and Borah or Hernández and colleagues, the values used by Santley and Rose are averages across the entire population, and this presents a problem in evaluating their data since they presume a particular, unstated, population composition, since the relative numbers of people at different ages determines the total quantities of food consumed. Without knowing this population assumption it is difficult to compare Santley and Rose's figures with the others. Thus, while their figures may be comparable, they are not sufficiently aggregate for use in the models.

Santley and Rose stress the importance of other protein sources in a mostly grain diet.[195] Examination of the wide variety of vegetable and animal protein sources available in the Basin points to the richness of these sources. Important indigenous vegetable protein sources include beans, grain amaranths, and seeds from mesquite. The most well known of these are *Phaseolus spp.*: both the common bean (*P. vulgaris*) and the lima bean (*P. lunatis*). Sanders and colleagues note that beans were commonly intercropped in the Basin to restore soil fertility (a practice universally recognized), but also served as a dietary supplement.[196] Santley and Rose posit a conquest-era diet that includes 10 percent beans by weight, and note that such an addition improves the raw protein of the diet from 2-5 times.[197] Beans alone may have been sufficient to complement the maize

---

[193] See E. Messer, "The Small but Healthy Hypothesis: Historical, Political, and Ecological Influences on Nutritional Standards," *Human Ecology*, 14 (1986), pp. 57-75, for a discussion of this debate and of the politics involved in all this. It should be noted here that the small stature (by comparison with the large stature of modern North American and Western European populations) of some "developing nations" populations, and of sixteenth century Amerindians, may be the result of *chronic* malnutrition, especially during the critical growing years. It is not clear, however, that this chronic shortage, if it exists and produces this effect, results in a population that is likely to experience significantly different infectious disease mortality (Seckler, "Small But Healthy"). It is more likely that it is relatively *acute* nutritional shortfalls that are implicated in the synergistic effects noted above. Of course, a marginally nourished population is more likely to fall into a state of acute malnourishment in times of crisis. In any case, by using the Mexican standards to define adequacy, it is likely that this chronic effect will be minimized (Hernández, *et al. Valor Nutritivo*).

[194] Santley and Rose, "Diet, Nutrition, and Population Dynamics," p. 198.

[195] Santley and Rose, "Diet, Nutrition, and Population Dynamics."

[196] Sanders, *et al.*, p. 239-240.

[197] Santley and Rose, "Diet, Nutrition, and Population Dynamics," p. 194.

based diet, but the grain amaranths (*Amaranthus spp.*) were also important since their productivity rivals maize, but they have both a higher protein yield and a higher protein score.[198] Another likely source of gathered or cultivated vegetable protein in Amerindian diets are the seeds from mesquite (*Prosopis spp.*). *Mizquitl* in the Aztec language, mesquite seeds are also high in protein.[199]

In addition to these relatively common proteinaceous foods, the Basin provided another near-unique aquatic protein food, *tecuitlatl*, or blue-green algae (*Spirulina geitleri*). When processed, this cheese-like foodstuff is over 60 percent protein by weight, and its addition to the diet, even in small quantities, virtually removes any protein shortage limit that may have existed without it.[200]

Plant foods were not the sole sources of protein supplementation. Larger fauna protein sources include: white tailed deer (*Odocoileus spp.*), cotton tailed rabbits (*Sylvilagus spp.*), domesticated dogs (*Canaris familiarius*), domesticated turkeys (*Meleagris gallopavo*), aramadillos (*Dasypus sexcintus*), various rodents, fish, frogs, snakes, and waterfowl.[201] In addition, smaller fauna protein sources were commonly eaten (and relished) in the Basin, these include: agave worms (*Hypopta agavis* and *Aegiale hesperiarus*); various aquatic insects (*Azayacatl*), their larvae, and their eggs (*Ahuauhtl*); various fresh water shrimp; and larval water salamanders (*Axolotl*).[202]

After the conquest, Spanish cultigens increased the variety of food stuffs available. The variety of these additions is impressive. They include: wheat, barley, lettuce, radishes, carrots, cabbage, apples, quinces, oranges,

---

198 K. Hindley, "Reviving the Food of the Aztecs," *Science News* 116 (1979), p. 169; B. Ortíz de Montellano, "Aztec Cannibalism: An Ecological Necessity?" *Science*, 200 (1978), p. 612; Ortíz de Montellano, personal communication; and Santley and Rose, "Diet, Nutrition, and Population Dynamics," p. 194.

199 Ortíz de Montellano, personal communication.

200 W. V. Farrar, "Tecuitlatl; A Glimpse of Aztec Food Technology," *Nature*, 211 (1966), pp. 341-342; Hassig, *Trade, Tribute, and Transportation*, p. 129; Ortíz de Montellano, personal communication; Sanders, *et al., The Basin of Mexico*, pp. 290-291; and Santley and Rose, "Diet, Nutrition, and Population Dynamics," p. 291.

201 M. D. Coe, "The Chinampas of Mexico," *Scientific American*, 211 (1964), p. 95; Gibson, *The Aztecs*, p. 339, 341; Francisco Guerra, "Aztec Science and Technology," *History of Science*, 8 (1969), p. 38; Ortíz de Montellano, "Aztec Cannibalism," p. 612; Ortíz de Montellano, personal communication; Sanders, *et al., The Basin of Mexico*, pp. 282-285; Santley and Rose, "Diet, Nutrition, and population dynamics," p. 193; and Soustelle, *The Daily Life of the Aztecs*, p. 15.

202 Gibson, *The Aztecs*, p. 341; Guerra, "Aztec Science and Technology," p. 38; Ortíz de Montellano, "Aztec Cannibalism," p. 612; Ortíz de Montellano, personal communication; Soustelle, *The Daily Life of the Aztecs*, 15; and G.C. Wilken, "The ecology of gathering in a Mexican farming region," *Economic Botany* 24 (1970), p. 291.

lemons, peaches, apricots, walnuts, bananas, and peanuts.[203] As food sources for Amerindians, however, they were not as important as their number indicates. The Spanish grains, wheat and barley, were not readily accepted by the indigenous population since they required different production techniques from maize and demonstrated less productivity than did maize, at least in the best areas.[204]

Introduced animal foods met with greater acceptance. Cattle, sheep, swine, goats, European bees, and chickens were all early additions.[205] Chicken and swine were quickly and widely accepted by Amerindian families.[206] Indeed, Gibson argues that after maize, chickens were the most important item of tribute, testifying to their wide-spread acceptance.[207] Cattle and sheep were apparently less important initially as Amerindian food sources. Simpson argues that cattle and sheep were important, however, in the cultural ecology of New Spain since their numbers were large and overgrazing led to accelerated erosion that had negative effects, such as increased siltation within the lacustrine system in the Basin.[208]

Perhaps this negative impact, along with Spanish disapproval, helps explain the reduction in Amerindian consumption of insects, chia, amaranth, and algae over time.[209] Thus, the dietary benefits conveyed by these dietary additions may have been counter-balanced by a progressive reduction in the variety of indigenous foods.[210]

Surplus Demand

In MEXIPOP, the second demand, the production of surplus in excess of immediate needs for use in an emergency, is simulated by setting a goal for surplus, *PU_surplus_goal*, that is a proportion of the consumption demand, cons_D_per_PU (Figure 2.11). Comparison of this goal with the amount remaining in surplus (the value of the *surplus* variable) yields an annual surplus demand for each PU, *surplus_D_per_PU* (Figure 2.11). While it is clear that different segments of the population had differing needs for and capabilities of storing surplus, I argue here that it is reasonable to average the amount of surplus demanded by different segments of the population so that an average, per PU, surplus demand may be used.

203 Cook and Borah, *Essays in Population History*, Vol. 3, pp. 167-168.

204 Cook and Borah, *Essays in Population History*, Vol. 3, p. 170; and Hassig, *Trade, Tribute, and Transportation*, p. 224.

205 Cook and Borah, *Essays in Population History*, Vol. 3, pp. 167-168.

206 Cook and Borah, *Essays in Population History*, Vol. 3, p. 171; Gibson, *The Aztecs*, p. 344; and Hassig, *Trade, Tribute, and Transportation*, pp. 221-222.

207 Gibson, *The Aztecs*, p. 344.

208 Simpson, *Exploitation*.

209 Cook and Borah, *Essays in Population History*, Vol. 3, p. 173; and Hassig, *Trade, Tribute, and Transportation*, p. 229.

210 Soustelle, *The Daily Life of the Aztecs*, pp. 148-149.

It is important to note that production for surplus was not a Spanish innovation—it was of considerable importance in the Aztec world as well. Indeed, the large urban populations of Tenochtitlan and other centers in the Basin were dependent on surplus produced in their surrounding hinterlands.[211] The Aztec empire extracted tribute, some in the form of agricultural surpluses, from subjugated groups throughout central Mexico.[212]

Tribute Demand

Similarly, production units planned additional production to accommodate a third demand, for annual grain tribute. Unlike its use in much of the literature, "tribute" is not used here to refer to that portion of the harvest diverted to the large cities in the Basin for the support of the urban population. Here, tribute is assumed to pass out of the Amerindian economy, since it is assumed to be used to support the Spanish, and their numbers are not tracked here. Since tribute demands, *tribute_D_per_PU*, varied from year to year, *tribute_D_per_PU* is modeled as a function of date (Figure 2.11).

The food production and consumption subsection of MEXIPOP is calibrated in units of kilograms of maize. Thus, the consumption, tribute, and surplus demands, the production levels, and the resulting food provision are all in the same maize units. This simplification is justified by considering that while Amerindian cultigens were many and diverse, maize constituted from 50 to over 80 percent of the total diet in terms of weight and of calories of food energy, and in terms of land area devoted to its cultivation in the two regions in question.[213] Further, Sanders and colleagues argue that since there was such great dietary diversity available in the Basin, there was no nutritional limiting factor, such as protein or micronutrients may be in some diets and, therefore, it is reasonable to use the staple grain as surrogate for agricultural production in general.[214]

---

211   Coe, "The Chinampas of Mexico," p. 90; Hassig, *Trade, Tribute, and Transportation*, pp. 21-28; and J. R. Parsons, "The Role of Chinampa Agriculture in the Food Supply of Aztec Tenochtitlan," in C. E. Cleland (ed.), *Cultural Change and Continuity: Essays in Honor of James Bennett Griffin*, New York: Academic Press, pp. 247-248.

212   R. H. Barlow, *The Extent of the Empire of the Culhua Mexica*, Ibero-Americana 28. Berkeley: University of California Press, 1949; F. F. Berdan, "A Comparative Analysis of Aztec Tribute Documents," *Actas XLI Congreso Internacional de Americanistas, 1974, vol. 2* (1976), pp. 251-252; Hassig, *Trade, Tribute, and Transportation*, pp. 105-110; and Parsons, "The Role of Chinampa Agriculture," pp. 251-252.

213   Cook and Borah, *Essays in Population History*, Vol. 3, pp. 163, 165; Hassig, *Trade, Tribute, and Transportation*, pp. 18, 20; Sanders, *et al.*, *The Basin of Mexico*, p. 233; and Santley and Rose, "Diet, Nutrition, and population dynamics," p. 194.

214   Sanders, *et al.*, *The Basin of Mexico*, p. 373.

MEXIPOP PRODUCTION SUB-SYSTEM

Basin Agriculture

The Basin offers a variety of climatic and agro-ecozones, and several distinct types of agriculture were practiced at the time of the conquest. Since the effects of disease on agricultural labor may have had differing effects on the production in these different agricultural systems, a simple average will not suffice to characterize the agricultural productivity in the Basin.[215] A brief description of this diversity will help provide background for the model description that is to follow. Sanders and colleagues identify nine different agro-ecozones in the Basin; the lake system, the saline lakeshore, the deep soil alluvium, the thin soil alluvium, the upland alluvium, the lower piedmont, the middle piedmont, the upper piedmont, and the sierra. While these regions differ in soil erodibility, soil depth, soil fertility, and soil texture as well as in aspect and slope, the fundamental distinction they share is altitude.[216] This is important in the Basin because growing-season rainfall and the probability of early frost is positively correlated with elevation.

It is possible to distinguish three basic agricultural strategies to overcome the primary environmental problems of frost, erosion, and moisture management. In the freshwater lakes and on their margins the primary environmental limitation is drainage, hence raised-field and drainage techniques were used.[217] A particularly important type of raised-field agriculture is the *chinampa* technique, literally the use of artificially constructed islands within freshwater lakes as intensively cultivated agricultural fields. To cope with the problem of erosion, virtually the entire better-watered southeast quadrant (exclusive of the drainage technique areas) and the low, middle, and upper piedmont of the central and northern areas of the Basin were terraced in some fashion.[218] Terracing also aids in the conservation of soil moisture in less well-watered areas.[219] In the areas without need for or access to irrigation water, the areas of *temporal* agriculture, the moisture necessary for plant growth was derived from seasonal rainfall and soil moisture storage. Problems of frost and the timing and adequacy of moisture are interrelated for most of the agricultural areas of the Basin. Simply stated, the problem is to plant early enough to enable a

---

215   Sanders, *et al.*, *The Basin of Mexico*.

216   Sanders, *et al.*, *The Basin of Mexico*, pp. 84-88.

217   Sanders, *et al.*, *The Basin of Mexico*, pp. 273-281. It should be noted that raised-fields are not a drainage technology *per se*, and are included here only for simplicity of exposition.

218   R. A. Donkin, *Agricultural Terracing in the Aborginal New World*, Tucson, Arizona: The University of New Mexico Press for the Wenner-Gren Foundation for Anthropological Research, Inc., 1979, p. 41; and Sanders, *et al.*, *The Basin of Mexico*, p. 251.

219   Sanders, *et al.*, *The Basin of Mexico*, p. 243.

harvest before the killing frosts in the Fall, yet to have adequate rainfall during the critical growing periods of maize. For much of the Basin, the solution was to plant early and to use pre-planting irrigation water, from seasonal or permanent water sources, to raise the soil moisture levels to enable the maize to survive until the summer rains.[220] In favored areas with permanent water sources, permanent irrigation was also used to supplement the growing season rainfall.[221]

The distinctions among these agricultural practices are important because the productivity of the differing systems varies. To simplify, I distinguish three distinctive types of agricultural systems in the Basin. The most productive by far was *chinampa*. Sanders and Parsons estimate sixteenth-century *chinampa* productivity at 3,000 kg/ha/yr of maize.[222] This high productivity is offset by the small area devoted to *chinampa* cultivation, which is estimated at a maximum of 12,500 ha per annum by Sanders and colleagues, at 9,000 ha per annum by Armillas, and at 9,500 ha per annum by Parsons.[223] [224] The second general variety encompasses flood water and pre-planting irrigated agriculture, and while its productivity varies by type and location, an average of Sanders' and Sanders and colleagues' estimates of maize productivity for all irrigation-based agriculture in all eco-zones is 1,100 kg/ha/yr of maize.[225] Far larger is the area of potential irrigation cultivation (both flood water and canal), possibly 121,000 ha cultivated each year out of a total of over 143,000 ha, summing over all eco-zones.[226] The third major type of agriculture is *temporal,* or rainfed, agriculture. It is estimated to have an average (over all eco-zones and soil types) maize productivity of 350 kg/ha/yr.[227] A system of *temporal*

---

220 Sanders, *et al., The Basin of Mexico*, p. 230.

221 W. E. Doolittle, *Canal Irrigation in Prehistoric Mexico.* Austin: University of Texas Press, 1990, pp. 115-135; and Sanders, *et al., The Basin of Mexico*, pp. 252-253.

222 Sanders, "The Agricultural History of the Basin," p. 144; and Parsons, "The Role of Chinampa Agriculture," p. 224.

223 Sanders, et al., *The Basin of Mexico*, 380; Pedro Armillas, "Gardens on Swamps," *Science,* 174 (1971), p. 660; and Parsons, "The Role of Chinampa Agriculture," p. 243.

224 Calneck argues that the chinampas ringing part of Tenochtitlan were used mostly for the provision of garden vegetables since their small size would have produced only 15 percent of a household's grain needs: Edward E. Calneck, "Settlement Patterns and Chinampan Agriculture at Tenochtitlan," *American Antiquity,* 37 (1972), p. 112. For this reason, these chinampas have been excluded in these calculations.

225 Sanders, "The Agricultural History of the Basin," p. 144; and Sanders, *et al., The Basin of Mexico*, p. 256.

226 Sanders, *et al., The Basin of Mexico*, p. 380.

227 Sanders, "The Agricultural History of the Basin," p. 144.

agriculture may have occupied as much as 94,000 ha, of which nearly 46,000 ha may have been cultivated annually.[228]

Less specific are Cook and Borah, who estimate an overall-Basin maize productivity average of 700-1,200 kg/ha/yr.[229] This is similar to a pan-Basin weighted average, 1,040 kg/ha/yr, calculated from Sanders and colleagues on the basis of estimates of total area cropped and productivity.[230] Both Sanders and colleagues' and Cook and Borah's estimate are based on contemporary (1940s and 1950s) Basin practice.

Sixteenth-century productivity data cited by Gibson generally support Cook and Borah's and Sanders and colleagues' pan-Basin maize productivity averages.[231] Gibson notes that the official *fanega de sembradura*, the area planted with 1.0 *fanega* of seed, was computed to be 3.23 hectare (8.8 acres).[232] Since a *fanega* is interpreted to be about 35-38 kg (78-84 lbs), each hectare would have been planted with about 11-12 kg seed.[233] Since productivity ratios, measured as a ratio of seed to harvest, of from 1:100-1:200 were considered good in the colonial period; good land productivity, then, would have ranged from 1,100-2,400 kg/ha.[234] These figures presumably apply to well-managed irrigated or *chinampa* agriculture. In contrast, Gibson cites a calculation for *chinampa* productivity, of from 567 kg/ha to 611 kg/ha, that is notably low compared to Sanders' and Parsons' estimate.[235] This estimate is at odds with Gibson's general productivity estimates as well, and for that reason, it is likely to be in error, or represent a particularly poorly producing *chinampa*.

Other sixteenth-century data challenge Sanders' widely cited figures. Offner confronts them, citing postconquest (1530s and 1540s) productivity data that suggest much smaller yields, in the range of 67-116 kg/ha/yr for locations in the Teotihuacán Valley, for locations south and east of Texcoco, and in the far north of the Basin.[236] Much depends on how these lands were cultivated, and it is unclear under what agricultural regime these lands were subject, or whether there was adequate labor to sustain better productivity. Nevertheless, these yields are small even for *temporal*

---

228 Sanders, *et al.*, *The Basin of Mexico*, p. 380.

229 Cook and Borah, *Essays in Population History*, Vol. 3, pp. 166-167.

230 Sanders, *et al.*, *The Basin of Mexico*, p. 380.

231 Gibson, *The Aztecs*, pp. 309-310; Cook and Borah, *Essays in Population History*, Vol. 3, pp. 166-167; and Sanders, *et al.*, *The Basin of Mexico*, p. 380.

232 Gibson, *The Aztecs*, p. 309.

233 Ibid.

234 Gibson, *The Aztecs*, p. 310.

235 Sanders, "The Agricultural History of the Basin," p. 144; and Parsons, "The Role of Chinampa Agriculture," p. 224.

236 J.A. Offner, "Archival Reports of Poor Crop Yields in the Early Postconquest Texcocan Heartland and their Implications for Studies of Aztec Period Populations," *American Antiquity* 45 (1980), pp. 848-856.

cultivation (according to Sanders' estimates), unless on particularly poor lands. Better yields, 439-447 kg/ha/yr, were noted for "very good" lands in the original documents that Offner explored.[237] As provocative as these data are, they are insufficiently detailed to use as a basis for agricultural productivity in MEXIPOP.

One aspect of the Basin's productive system that is assumed to be the same for all types of production is the size of production units. While there is general agreement that sixteenth-century social, productive, and residential organization of the Basin was generally collective (i.e., was not based on the nuclear family), there is little agreement as to specifics. Based on colonial maps and other archival sources, Calneck argues that residential units in Tenochtitlan housed joint families of 2-6 closely related nuclear families including extended family members.[238] He estimates that such households were populated by from 2-30 individuals, with an average of 10-15.[239] For a rural area in the sixteenth-century Basin, Carrasco reports that 54 percent of the households were nuclear families but that there was an average of 5.4 persons and 1.4 couples in the sample households.[240] He notes a more complex pattern in the 1540s in another area of the Basin where 61.7 percent of the households were joint families, and 36.7 percent were single families (single in this sense probably means extended as opposed to joint).[241] The household populations in this sample averaged 8.2, comprised of an average of 1.9 couples (i.e., families).[242] Offner cites documents suggesting that in yet another Basin community the early sixteenth-century household pattern was even more complex: while 29.5 percent of his sample households included nuclear families, 10.5 percent were simple joint families, 22.0 percent were nuclear families with extended family relations, 13.0 percent were more complex joint family arrangements, and 21.0 percent were joint families without extended kin relations.[243] In this document, the average household size is 6.0, composed

---

237 Offner, "Archival reports," p. 853.

238 Calneck, "Settlement Patterns," p. 111.

239 Ibid.

240 Pedro Carrasco, "Social Organization of Ancient Mexico," in R. Wauchope (ed.), *Handbook of Middle American Indians*, Austin: University of Texas Press, 1971. Vol. 10, pp. 368-369.

241 Pedro Carrasco, "The Joint Family in Ancient Mexico: The Case of Molotla," in Hugo G. Nutini, Pedro Carrasco and James M. Taggert (eds.), *Essays on Mexican Kinship*, London: The University of Pittsburgh Press, 1976, p. 47.

242 Carrasco, "Tenochtitlan," pp. 45-46.

243 Jerome A. Offner, "Household Organization in the Texcocan Heartland: The Evidence in the Codex Vergara," in H. R. Harvey and H. J. Prem (eds.), *Explorations in Ethnohistory. Indians of Central Mexico in the Sixteenth Century*. Albuquerque: University of New Mexico Press, 1984, pp. 136-137.

of 1.3 couples.[244] Cook and Borah used *Suma de Visitas de Pueblos* documents, dated in the 1540s, to calculate average household sizes.[245] For their Mexico-Hidalgo region (encompassing the Basin and other valleys), they argue that the mean number of *casados* (married men with living spouses) per house was 1.93, while the total number of persons per house averaged 6.05.[246] Viewed as a production unit, Sanders and colleagues use an average "extended family" of 7.0 as the basic unit of production and consumption in their calculations of Basin agriculture.[247]

Since the proportions of people at different ages within these compound households is not known, and the data make clear that there was a good deal of variance in the totals as well, an average figure must be used for the size of the "production units," or *PU*s. To estimate this figure, I averaged Carrasco's two estimates of household size with Offner's and Cook and Borah's to get an average of 6.41 persons per household. A similar average of the number of couples (families) within the households yielded 1.63. I neglected Sanders and colleagues' estimate since it was not explicitly documented and was probably the result of a similar averaging. Calneck's estimate for the Tenochtitlan metropolis is of less interest since it likely represents a particular urban pattern, and my interest in this calculation is for the rural, agricultural pattern. Thus, the size of the production unit is 1.63 times the size of the average family size as calculated above. Similarly, the number of production units is equal to the total population divided by the number of production units.

MEXIPOP Model Logic

Returning to the general structure of MEXIPOP, the total production is modeled as the sum of three independent production flows, that for the *temporal* system, *TP_proj_production*, that for the *chinampa* system, *CH_proj_production*, and that for the irrigation agriculture, *IR_proj_production* (Figure 2.11). While the assumption of independence of the agricultural types facilitates the simulation, it should be noted that probably only the *chinampa* system functioned independently. Many other agriculturalists were probably involved in both *temporal* and irrigation agriculture simultaneously by cultivating multiple plots, some located in areas where they could use irrigation water, and others farmed on a dry-land basis.

Assuming the independence of these three agricultural flows, that the relative decline in population was the same for each agricultural system, and that there was no net rural/urban population migration, leads to the conclusion that the *average* agricultural intensity (for the Amerindian agricultural economy) summed for the Basin as a whole remained stagnant.

---

244 Offner, "Household Organization," p. 138.

245 Cook and Borah, *Essays in Population History*, Vol. 1, pp. 123-124.

246 Ibid.

247 Sanders, *et al.*, *The Basin of Mexico*, p. 372.

This result is counter intuitive and counter to arguments made by Hassig and Cook and Borah that population decline led to the abandonment of the least productive lands (in this case most likely the *temporal* lands) in favor of better watered areas.[248] If such a shift did take place, it would have had the effect of increasing the average output intensity and labor productivity of the Basin as a whole. This abandonment (and/or seizure by the Spanish) of agricultural lands is controlled in MEXIPOP by the available area variables (e.g., *IR_avail_area*) described below. These production flows are derived from three identical (in all but the numerical details) logical chains in Figure 2.12. The resulting total flow of maize is compared with the nutritional needs of the population and the degree of shortfall or excess is calculated in the *nutr_disc* variable (Figure 2.10). It is this variable that affects the mortalities in the logic of Figure 2.4. For simplicity's sake, I will only describe the production logic of irrigated cultivation since the logic for the other two is the same, although the specific values differ.

The first step in calculating production is to determine the total demand experienced by the agricultural households. As noted above, each household (PU) has to plan production to meet consumption, tribute, and surplus demands. This is symbolized in MEXIPOP by the summation of the values of *surplus_D_per_PU*, *tribute_D_per_PU*, and *cons_D_per_PU* in the *per_PU_demand* variable (Figure 2.12). Further, since a large proportion of the Basin's population (e.g., urban artisans and nobility) was probably not engaged directly in staple grain production, the agricultural households also produced additional grain for consumption by the non-agricultural households. Sanders and colleagues estimate that perhaps 20 percent of the Basin's population was clustered in the large urban constellation of Tlatelolco-Tenochtitlán and nearby towns.[249] This population was probably not directly involved in staple production. Thus, the demand felt by each of the agricultural PUs' as well as the resulting production output will be larger than that needed for on-farm consumption alone. To simplify, it is assumed that the demands for consumption, tribute, and individual PU surplus are the same for all PUs (i.e., for those engaged in agriculture and for those that are not) and that any change affected each equally.

This logic neglects the role of imported staples (i.e., maize and other staple grains imported into the Basin from areas outside) in the provisioning of the urban population. This omission may not be important since Gibson and Anderson and Barlow argue that much maize could not have been transported to the Basin from distant points.[250] Hassig agrees and

---

248 Hassig, *Trade, Tribute, and Transportation*, p. 181; and Cook and Borah, *Essays in Population History*, Vol. 3, p. 168.

249 Sanders, *et al.*, *The Basin of Mexico*, p. 403.

250 Gibson, *The Aztecs*, p. 312; and Edgar Anderson and R. H. Barlow, "The Maize Tribute of Moctezuma's Empire," *Annals of the Missouri Botanical Gardens*, 30 (1943), p. 418.

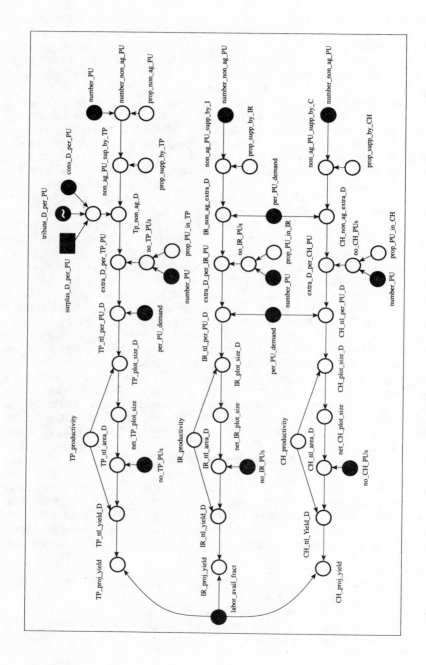

Figure 2.12 Pre-harvest Production Sub-system

calculates that, for the Basin in pre-Colombian times, the lack of transport technology (e.g., animals and carts), the economic costs (provisions for the human carriers), and the rugged nature of the environment constrained the distance for the economic shipment of bulk commodities such as grains to less than 30 km.[251] Indeed, Berdan's examination of Aztec tribute documents shows that bulk staples (maize, beans, and chia) were a small part of the more than 50 different types of extra-Basin tribute items.[252] This figure is for overland transport only, since the water-borne transport in canoes was very much more efficient within the lakes of the Basin. This calculation suggests that the role of imported grain in the total must have been small. Sanders and colleagues corroborate this assertion by providing figures that imply that imported staples may have supported only 4 percent of the total population and less than 10 percent of the urban population (about 40,000-50,000 people in a Basin population estimated at 1,100,000).[253]

During the sixteenth century, as Spanish roads, draft animals, and carts became more prevalent, however, food provision for the Basin was increasingly linked to nearby areas outside the Basin.[254] Nevertheless, the importance of local (i.e., Basin) production in the provisioning of cities in the colonial period is highlighted by the mid-sixteenth-century regulations that abolished markets within 10 leagues (about 42 km) of Mexico City.[255] The intent of these laws was to insure that sufficient grain flowed to the capital. If imported grain was significant, such market regulation probably would not have been necessary. It is also unclear to what extent any importation benefited the Indian population since much of it must have been in Spanish-preferred foods for the growing Spanish population of the capital.

To calculate the total urban (i.e., non-agricultural) demand, it is necessary to estimate the proportion of the population that was not engaged in agricultural production. It is assumed that the proportion of non-agricultural PUs is a constant over time. This is equivalent to assuming that there was no rural to urban (or urban to rural) net migration, and that the rate of natural decrease (or increase) of population was the same for the rural and urban sectors. This assumption is likely to have been violated in specific instances and for short periods, but such imbalances are likely to have been compensated for by imbalances in the opposite direction in other times, so that the net effect is constancy. Hassig notes that during the early colonial period, Mexico City grew in relative size to the other regional

251 Hassig, *Trade, Tribute, and Transportation*, p. 40.

252 Berdan, "Comparative Analysis."

253 Sanders, *et al.*, *The Basin of Mexico*, p. 176.

254 Hassig, *Trade, Tribute, and Transportation*, pp. 202, 248-249.

255 Hassig, *Trade, Tribute, and Transportation*, p. 239.

centers, but he does not speculate as to whether the net urban proportion changed.[256]

Further, it is not reasonable to assume that each agricultural type in the Basin supported the same proportion of non-agricultural population to agricultural population, however, since the productivity of each agricultural system differs. One way to calculate these proportions is to estimate the total number of PUs that could have been supported by each agricultural type and to subtract the number of PUs needed to produce that total. This difference is the number of non-agricultural PUs supported by each agricultural regime. The relative proportions of non-agricultural PUs supported by each agricultural regime is then calculated by ratio with the total number of non-agricultural PUs. This technique assumes that the relative numbers of PUs in each class is constant.

Such a method offers only a rough approximation, since the uncertainty at each stage of the calculation is large. Nevertheless, such an approximation is necessary and may be calculated from assumptions already detailed along with estimates provided by Sanders and colleagues (Table 2.14). Using the previously calculated values for age-group annual consumption (Table 2.13) and a population based on Coale and Demeny's "level 8 West" population, an approximate annual maize consumption may be calculated (Table 2.14).[257] A rough estimate of the per-PU consumption level follows by dividing the total annual consumption by the number of PUs (Table 2.14). Using Sanders and colleagues' estimates of the total amounts of agricultural land under different agricultural regimes and the average estimates of land productivity calculated above, the total annual production for each agricultural regime may be calculated (Table 2.14).[258] Dividing these totals by the per-PU consumption yields the total number of PUs supported in each regime (Table 2.14). Again utilizing Sanders and colleagues' estimates of average plot size per household for the different regimes, the number of agricultural plots (or PUs) in each regime may be calculated (Table 2.14).[259] Subtracting these PUs from the total number supported in each regime yields the total number of non-agricultural PUs supported by each agricultural technique (Table 2.14). The ratio of each regime's non-agricultural PUs to the total determines the proportion of the total each regime supported (Table 2.14).

Further, the non-agricultural proportions of the population may be estimated by dividing the total of non-agricultural PUs by the total number of PUs supported (Table 2.14). This figure, 0.298, is the urban-non-agricultural proportion of the Basin's population and is represented in Figure 2.12 by *prop_non_ag_PU*. Thus, the number of non-agricultural

256   Hassig, *Trade, Tribute, and Transportation*, p. 257.

257   Coale and Demeny, *Model Life Tables*.

258   Sanders, *et al.*, *The Basin of Mexico*, p. 380.

259   Ibid.

TABLE 2.14 BASIN AGRICULTURAL PRODUCTION

Age-class	Population Porportion	Total Population	Demand Per Year	Total Annual Demand (kg maize)
0-1	0.024	26,180	n/a	n/a
1-5	0.080	87,670	80	7,013,600
5-15	0.183	201,300	150	30,195,000
15-45	0.457	502,920	150	75,438,000
45-60	0.156	171,270	130	22,265,100
60-99	0.101	110,660	130	14,385,800
Total				149,297,500
pop 15-60*0.4 = number of families =				269,676
size of family = total pop/number of families =				4.08
size of PU = 1.53 * size of families =				6.24
number of PUs = total pop/PU size =				176,259
per PU demand = total demand/number of PUs =				847.04

Ag type	Total area available (ha)	Cultivated area/year	Per ha product	Total annual product	Total PUs supported
Chinampa	12,500	12,500	3,000	37,500,000	44,272
Irrigated	143,200	121,175	1,100	133,292,500	157,364
Temporal	93,900	45,700	350	15,995,000	18,884
Total	249,600	179,375		186,787,500	220,519

Ag type	Average plot size (ha)	Agricultural PUs	Non-Ag PUs	Proportion of total non-ag PUs (%)
Chinampa	0.485	25,773	18,499	28
Irrigated	1.100	110,159	47,204	72
Temporal	2.420	18,884	0	0
Total	n/a	154,816	65,703	n/a

After: Sanders 1976: 144; and Sanders *et al.* 1976: 380.

PUs, *number_non_ag_PU*, is equal to the number of PUs, *number_PU*, multiplied by the proportion non-agricultural, *prop_non_ag_PU* (Figure 2.12).

This calculation assumes a situation of maximal agricultural intensity and extension, since that is the assumption underlying the figures used.[260] This may not be a problem since it is reasonable to assume that the proportion of non-agricultural PUs supported by each agricultural regime is likely to have been constant, even if the extent of each agricultural technique changed over time.

Having calculated the necessary proportions, it is possible to calculate the total demand for each agriculture-based production unit. Again using the

---

260   Sanders, *et al.*, *The Basin of Mexico*, p. 308.

irrigated agricultural regime as indicative of the general pattern, the logic of these calculations is represented in Figure 2.12 by the string of converters that begins by calculating the number of non-agricultural PUs supported by the irrigated regime, *non_ag_PU_supp_by_I*, from the product of the proportion of non-agricultural PUs supported by irrigation, *prop_supp_by_IR*, and the total number of non-agricultural PUs, *number_non_ag_PU*. Multiplying this product by the total demand for each PU, *per_PU_demand*, yields the total amount of "extra" demand felt by the agricultural PUs working within irrigated agriculture, *IR_non_ag_extra_D*. Similarly, the number of PUs employed in irrigation agriculture, *no_IR_PUs*, is obtained from the product of the total number of PUs, *number_PU*, multiplied by the proportion of PUs in irrigated agriculture, *prop_PU_in_IR*. Thus the extra demand "felt" by each of the irrigation PUs due to the proportion of the urban demand that they supply is simply equal to the total extra demand, *IR_non_ag_extra_D*, divided by the number of irrigation-based PUs, *no_IR_PUs*. The total demand, then, for each irrigation PU is the sum of the extra demand, *extra_D_per_IR_PU*, and the standard per PU demand, *per_PU_demand*.

On the assumption that the plot size cultivated by an average irrigation PU is determined by the demand for output (i.e., it will not be larger than necessary to meet the demand, nor smaller, since demand would not be met in that case), the plot size that is implied by the demand on individual irrigation PUs, *IR_plot_size_D*, is equal to the total demand per irrigation PU, *IR_ttl_per_PU_D*, divided by the productivity that the farmer can expect from the land, *IR_productivity* (Figure 2.12). The land productivity is assumed to be a constant; for irrigation agriculture it is equal to 1,100 kg/ha (see above for a discussion of the issues surrounding this assumption). But there is a limit to the size of plot that can be cultivated by a production unit, even if the demand soars, due to the constraints of land, technology, and labor. For that reason, the *IR_plot_size_D* variable is constrained not to exceed 1.18 ha, about 15 percent above the usual size, regardless of the total demand by the *net_TP_plot size* variable (this limit is equal to 2.71 ha for *temporal*, and 0.554 ha for *chinampa*) (Figure 2.12). Over time, the Spanish appropriated lands for their own purposes, especially for grazing cattle and sheep.[261] Certainly this land use change reduced the area available for Indian cultivation. Nevertheless, the vastly diminished Indian populations certainly needed much less agricultural land, hence this withdrawal in and of itself probably did not affect the sizes of Indian *milpas*—as it would have done if the population had not declined precipitously. The effects of the introduction of cattle and appropriation of lands previously used for agriculture for grazing may have indirectly diminished Indian agricultural production by displacing Indian holdings to less desirable locations, thus diminishing their productivity, and by the predatory effects of the cattle on Indian milpas.

---

261   Simpson, *Exploitation*.

Now the total area given over to irrigation agriculture, *IR_ttl_area_D*, is the product of the average plot size, *net_IR_plot_size*, and the number of irrigation PUs, *no_IR_PUs* (Figure 2.12). Similarly, the total production that is expected to result from this area, *IR_ttl_yield_D*, is also a simple product of the total area, *IR_ttl_area_D*, by the average productivity of the land, *IR_productivity*.

This resulting figure does not take into consideration the health of the labor force, however. It is here that the fraction of labor that is available for work (i.e., those that are not sick), *labor_avail_fract*, that was calculated above is multiplied by the total expected production, *IR_ttl_yield_D*, to produce the actual product, *IR_proj_yield* resulting from the labor. This relatively crude approximation of the effect of morbidity in the labor force is necessitated by the fact that model iterations are constrained to a time resolution of a single year. Thus, the timing of illness, clearly an important consideration in figuring the effect of that illness on production, cannot be accurately simulated here. By using the morbidity rate for agricultural labor to diminish directly the agricultural production, it is assumed that for some producers the effects of illness will not matter much and for others the effects will be profound, but the average, tracked here, will render a suitable approximation of the total effects.

Perhaps more subtle is the assumption that equal labor morbidity will depress production by equal proportions in each of the agricultural regimes (Figure 2.12). By assuming that land productivity is a constant for each agricultural regime, a labor withdrawal, such as that initiated by illness, is equivalent to a reduction in the area cultivated. Thus, a similar proportional labor reduction in all cultivation regimes is equivalent to a similar proportional reduction in cultivated area for each regime, and will result in a similar proportional reduction in total output for each regime.

Turning to Figure 2.11, the irrigation regime projected output flow is symbolized by the variable *IR_proj_yield*. But this projected output was not the actual harvest in many years, since environmental hazards such as frosts and droughts reduced the actual total in specific years (Table 2.15). These effects are modeled in MEXIPOP by the *IR_env_loss_fract* and *IR_env_loss_mult* variables Figure. 2.11). Accordingly, the net harvest, *IR_harvest*, is the difference between the production that would have occurred in the absence of environmental problems, *IR_proj_yield* and the amount of loss due to those problems. This amount is modeled as a proportion of the projected production, *IR_env_loss_fract*, and is a function of *date*. Table 2.15 records these estimated yield losses for each agricultural regime for the dates where mention is made of agro-climatic problems.

From this harvested total, tribute contributions are removed by subtracting the total tribute from the *net_harvest* (the sum of the harvests from all 3 sectors) using the *net_tribute_loss* variable. The total amount of tribute, *net_tribute_loss*, is modeled as a product of the number of tribute payers, *number_PU*, by the amount of tribute owed by each PU,

TABLE 2.15 AGRO-ENVIRONMENTAL CONDITIONS

| DATE | DESCRIPTION | Yield Loss (percentage) | | |
		CHINAMPA	IRRIGATED	TEMPORAL
1528	heavy rains ruin maize	10	10	10
1541	severe early frost => loss of maize and wheat	20	20	20
1543	drought, frost => shortage of maize, wheat	10	20	20
1544-51	shortages and rise in prices	—	—	—
1557	locust plagues	10	10	10
1558	locusts; frosts; shortages	10	20	20
1559	locusts in April	10	10	10
1573	shortages of maize and wheat	—	—	—
1576	drought and prolonged heat; limited yields	0	10	10
1577	rains April-November; wet fields; small harvests	10	10	10
1579	maize shortage; great famine	—	—	—
1587	late rains in July; famine in Mexico City in September	0	10	20
1590	continuous heavy rains injure wheat	10	10	10
1591	early rains followed by drought	5	10	20
1592	locusts in May	5	10	10
1594	drought and frost	10	10	20
1597	drought and frost; poorer than expected harvests	10	10	20
1598	shortages of wheat and maize in Mexico City	—	—	—
1599	rains delayed in spring; early autum frosts	10	10	20
1600	heavy rains, but scant harvest	5	10	10
1601	abundundance, good harvests everywhere	—	—	—
1604	maize desiccated	0	5	5
1606	rains in July; early harvests	—	—	—
1609	limited harvests; short supplies	5	10	10
1615	shortage of maize and wheat	—	—	—
1616	late rains; drought; and extreme shortage	10	20	30
1617	abundant harvests of maize and wheat	—	—	—
1618	drought in July	0	10	20
1620	drought; great shortages	10	20	30

after Gibson (1964: 452-454)

tribute_D_per_PU. This variable, in turn, is modeled as function of *date* since the amount of tribute varied over time. The *storage_flow* variable transfers the remaining harvest to the *storage* stock (Figure 2.11) .

There are three pathways by which maize is consumed in the model. The first represents the usual situation in which the remaining harvest (after environmental and tribute losses are subtracted), *storage_flow*, is adequate to meet the consumption needs of the population, *total_cons_demand* (Figure 2.11). In this first path, the *cons_flow* variable represents the flow of maize used for consumption, leaving (in some cases) a residual in the *storage* stock. In some cases, however, the flow of maize from the harvest will not be sufficient to meet the total consumption demand. This is the second case, in which the stored maize (from previous harvests) is also eaten until the basic consumption demand is satisfied or until the stored maize is exhausted. In the model, the amount of this extra consumption is determined by the set of convertors that determine: (1) the shortfall (i.e., the *cons_flow* subtracted from the *total_cons_demand*), *cons_shortfall*; (2) the ratio of the shortfall and the amount in storage, *emerg_cons*; and (3) the fraction of the stored maize that will be consumed to meet the basic needs. This extra consumption is symbolized by the *add_cons_flow* variable (Figure 2.11). The third case, the opposite of the second, is a situation in which there is more than enough harvest flow and reserves in storage to satisfy the basic consumption demands and leave a desired amount in storage. In this case, the additional stored stocks are also consumed, providing extra food, until the amount remaining is storage is equal to the desired amount. This logic is symbolized in MEXIPOP by another similar set of convertors that determine: (1) the extent of the additional maize (i.e., it subtracts the desired surplus from the total in storage); (2) the ratio of this available maize to the amount in storage; and (3) the fraction of the stored maize that will be consumed in addition, *extra_cons*. This additional consumption is also symbolized by the *add_cons_flow* variable (Figure 2.11).

In addition to the additional consumption outflows, the amount in *storage* is diminished annually by *storage_loss_flow*. Annual *storage_loss_flow* is set equal to a constant proportion (15 percent) of the remaining *storage*.[262]

The tripartite paths of maize consumption are re-united in determining the total maize consumption. Accordingly, the total consumption, *ttl_cons*, is equal to the sum of the *cons_flow* variable and the *add_cons_flow* variables (Figure 2.11). Comparison of this total with the total needed for consumption, *total_cons_demand*, yields a ratio, *nutr_disc*, that represents the average state of nutrition of the whole population in each simulation

---

[262] Board on Science and Technology for International Development, Commission on International Relations, and The National Research Council. *Post Harvest Food Losses in Developing Countries*, Washington, DC: National Academy of Sciences, 1978, p. 76.

year. In making this simple calculation it is presupposed that at any given level of shortfall (or excess) the nutritional change for each age-class is the same. One should note that this situation is not realistic, since societies do not tend to apportion food, especially in times of scarcity, in equal proportions to all ages; the productive members usually have superior access. It is uncertain, however, how this appropriation operated in New Spain, and for that reason (and to avoid complexity), it is assumed that each age-group received the same proportion of food rations (e.g., if the nutritional discrepancy was equal to 80 percent of the normal, each age-group would receive 80 percent of its normal ration).

Summary

Because of its importance and complexity, a brief summary of the dynamic simulation model developed in this chapter is useful. This simulation technique posits a complex of mutually affecting variables so that change in one variable affects the level of others. Since the value of each variable is recalculated after a specified time step, the dynamic pattern of these variable's values are simulated in an iterative fashion. The simulation model detailed here, MEXIPOP, examines population size as part of such an interactive system. This complex system is usefully divided into three sections or sub-systems; the demographic, the health, and the production.

Starting with the demographic sub-system, the dynamics of a population of given age structure are determined by the contributions of the basic demographic variables; fertility, mortality, and migration. The non-crisis values of these basic demographic variables are a part of the assumed demographic structure of the population. These values are modified in times of crisis through interactions in the health sub-section.

In this sub-section, the health condition of the population is modeled using two segments, a "background," indigenous part and an introduced, "epidemic" part. The state of each of these health components affect the mortality and fertility variables. The state of epidemic health also affects the migration component. The level of background health in non-crisis situations is assumed to be compatible with the levels of mortality and fertility in the demographic sub-section. Epidemic health is modeled as a function of the date and assumed morbidity and case fatality rates. Since the epidemic morbidity rate affects the labor inputs to agriculture, epidemics affect agricultural production. Agricultural production, by determining nutritional sufficiency, affects the quality of indigenous health, and indirectly the mortality and fertility rates.

The production sub-system is linked to the rest of the model in another way as well. Since production levels are determined in MEXIPOP using a general demand model, and the major component of that demand is the consumption demand, production levels are a function of population numbers. In addition, production levels reflect demands for surplus and tribute. The production possibilities are modeled to take into account the differing productivity of the three major agricultural types within the Basin.

Chapter 3

HISTORICAL AND SIMULATION COMPARISONS

The detailed structural description and justification of MEXIPOP provided in the previous chapter was undertaken in order to provide details of a relatively independent methodology with which it is possible to "test" certain of the historically compiled statistics of the sixteenth-century Amerindian population in the Basin of Mexico. The task in this chapter is first, to execute the simulations, and second, to compare the simulated populations with historical estimates of the Basin's sixteenth-century Amerindian population. To accomplish this goal, it is necessary to match the historical reconstructions with particular simulation runs.

The general method utilized in these comparisons involves a four step process. The first step identifies and quantifies historical Basin population estimates. The second step arranges individual estimates by date into groups that reflect a similar set of assumptions about the sixteenth-century depopulation. This step is not necessary for some cases that consist of many estimates spanning a considerable part of the century. The third step necessitates creating a simulation run that closely "mimics" the population dynamics of a group of historical reconstructions. The last step examines the assumptions underlying such simulation results. After these preliminary steps, interpretations as to the validity or probability of these historical estimates are offered.

Historical Population Estimates

While there have been numerous estimates of the sixteenth-century central Mexican population,[1] the most detailed and thorough post-conquest central Mexican estimates were produced by the so-called "Berkeley School" starting in the late 1940s.[2] These estimates and some modifications of them by critics form the bulk of historic estimates examined here.

---

[1] See Dobyns, "Estimating," for a thorough review.

[2] Whitmore and Turner, *Population Reconstruction of the Basin of Mexico*, p. 14.

There are ten separate works from which Basin populations are extracted in this study; several consist of a time-series (or group) of estimates, while others are point-in-time estimates only. Of those treated here, only two works develop Basin-specific populations, the rest calculate "Central Mexico" or "New Spain" estimates that must be modified to yield Basin estimates.[3] Regardless of the spatial scale, these estimates are based on the use of surrogate documentary data. Such surrogates are colonial documents that do not explicitly record whole population numbers; rather they include tax and tribute records, journalistic impressions, ecclesiastical documents, and military records.[4] It is primarily in their choice of documents and in their interpretations that these studies differ.

Original Estimates

The first "Berkeley School" estimate that encompassed the Basin of Mexico was *The Population of Central Mexico in the Sixteenth Century*.[5] This monograph uses 15 Spanish secular and ecclesiastical records to establish central Mexican populations for four sixteenth-century dates. These documents reflect conditions for as early as 1531, but the bulk of data was compiled for the 1540s and the 1570s.[6] They use the relatively rich documentation for the decade of 1560-1570 to construct a well-supported 1565 figure that is used, in turn, to produce or support estimates for the less well documented dates of 1519, 1540, and 1597.[7]

Cook and Simpson basically calculate the 1565 population for each community listed in the surviving documents by multiplying by four one of the following (depending on the nature of the source document): the number of household tributes paid (i.e., the community tribute amount divided by the per-household tribute amount); the number of married men; or the number of tribute payers.[8] Raw figures for tributary numbers from communities with only sparse data from less authoritative texts are augmented by a complex use of ratios obtained from communities with better data. The total population of their central Mexican region in 1565 is the sum of these adjusted local estimates. The estimate for 1540 was derived by computing a ratio of the relative 1540 and 1565 community

3 New Spain in this instance refers generally to Central Mexico.

4 Whitmore and Turner, *Population Reconstruction of the Basin of Mexico*, p. 15.

5 Cook and Simpson, *The Population of Central Mexico in the Sixteenth Century*.

6 Cook and Simpson, *The Population of Central Mexico in the Sixteenth Century*, pp. 1, 3.

7 Cook and Simpson, *The Population of Central Mexico in the Sixteenth Century*, pp. 1-2.

8 Cook and Simpson, *The Population of Central Mexico in the Sixteenth Century*, p. 13.

TABLE 3.1 SIXTEENTH-CENTURY SITES WITHIN THE BASIN OF MEXICO *

Acolhuacan	Huixquilucan	Teotlalpa
Acolman	Ixtapalapa D. F.	Tepetlaoxtoc
Apaxco	Jilotzingo	Tepexpan
Atlapulco	Mexicalcingo D. F.	Tepotzotlan
Atzcapotzaloco D. F.	Milpa Alta D. F.	Tequisistlan
Axapusco [1]	Mixquic	Tequixquiac
Chalco [2]	Nextlalpa	Texcoco
Chicoloapa	Otumba	Tlahuac
Chiconauhtla	Tacuba	Tlanalapa
Chimalhuacán	Tacubaya	Tlalnepantla
Churubusco D. F.	Talasco	Tlapanaloya
Coatepec	Teacalco	Tultitlan
Coatitlan [3]	Tecama	Xaltocan
Coyoacán	Tecamac	Xochimilco D. F.
Coyotepec	Tecoloapan & Calcoyuca	Zacualpa
Cuautitlán	Temascalapa	Zitlaltepec
Culhuacan	Tenayuca	Zumpango
Huehuetoca	Tenochtitlan & Tlateloco	
Huexotla	Teoloyucan	
Hueypoxtla	Teotihuacan	

[1] including Zacualpan
[2] including Amecameca, Tlamanalco, Tenango
[3] including Acaluacan and Ecatepec
* All lie within the modern state of México except those labeled D.F. that lie within the Federal District

Sources: Cook and Simpson 1948, Gibson 1964, Sanders 1970, and Gerhard 1972

populations for locales where data for both dates were available and using this ratio to calculate 1540 figures for communities without sufficient 1540 data.[9] For 1519, the central Mexican population is estimated three ways: by using clerical estimates of baptisms; by use of military estimates of the population size and of military strength; and by means of a ratio derived by comparing the few town size estimates for 1519 with those derived for

---

9   Cook and Simpson, *The Population of Central Mexico in the Sixteenth Century*, pp. 39-43.

112

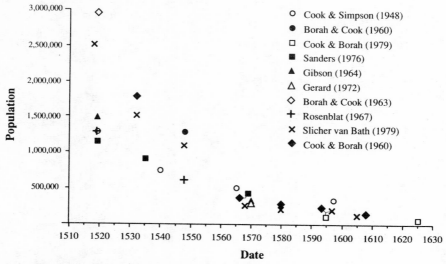

Figure 3.1 Basin Population Estimates

1565.[10] The last sixteenth-century estimate, for 1597, was also based on three methods of estimate: one based on the stated population loss; a second on a 1597-1565 ratio; and a third utilizing the relationship between encomienda and royal towns.

Since Cook and Simpson tabulated their 1565 population estimates by community, it is possible to create a Basin-only estimate by identifying the Basin communities. These are identified and treated separately by using Cook and Simpson's list of towns with 1565 populations and their map of town locations; Gerhard's maps and descriptions; Sanders' list of Basin communities; and Gibson's maps (Table 3.1).[11] By summing Cook and Simpson's estimates for the Basin sites, a 1565 population of the Basin is obtained. Basin-only estimates for 1519, 1540, and 1597 are obtained by multiplying the 1565 Basin-only total by the appropriate ratio of the central Mexico population for these dates divided by the 1565 central Mexico

10 Cook and Simpson, *The Population of Central Mexico in the Sixteenth Century*, pp. 10-16.

11 Cook and Simpson, *The Population of Central Mexico in the Sixteenth Century*, appendices I and III; Gerhard, *Historical Geography of New Spain*; William T. Sanders, "The Population of the Teotihuacan Valley, the Basin of Mexico, and the Central Mexican Symbiotic Region in the 16th Century," in *The Natural Environment, Contemporary Occupation and 16th Century Population of the Valley*. The Teotihuacan Valley Project Final Report. Vol. 1. University Park, PA: Department of Anthropology, 1970, pp. 414-415; and Gibson, *The Aztecs*, pp. 14, 48, 88-89.

population (Figure 3.1).[12] Table 3.2 summarizes the results of these calculations and of those detailed in the following sections.

TABLE 3.2 POPULATION ESTIMATES FOR THE BASIN OF MEXICO

Date	Source/Calculation	Population
1518	(Slicher van Bath 1978) = [a] x 0.85	2,514,708
1519	(Cook & Simpson 1948) = [d] x 2.50	1,293,652
1519	[a] (Borah & Cook 1963) Aztec tribute lists	2,958,480
1519	(Rosenblat 1967) modified Aztec figure	1,280,519
1519	(Gibson 1964) mid-point estimate	1,477,602
1519	(Sanders 1970 & 1976) mid-point estimate	1,155,050
1530-35	(Sanders 1970 & 1976) mid-point estimate	912,068
1532	[b] (Cook & Borah 1960) = [e] x 4.68	1,772,494
1532	(Slicher van Bath 1978) = [b] x 0.85	1,506,620
1540	(Cook & Simpson 1948) = [d] x 1.46	755,493
1548	[c] (Borah & Cook 1960) direct calculation	1,288,253
1548	(Rosenblat 1967) = [c] x 0.475	611,788
1548	(Slicher van Bath 1978) = [c] x 0.85	1,095,015
1565	[d] (Cook & Simpson 1948) datum population	517,461
1568	[e] (Cook & Borah 1960) datum population	378,738
1568	(Slicher van Bath 1978) = [e] x 0.85	264,444
1568	(Sanders 1970 & 1976) mid-point estimate	405,108
1570	(Gibson 1964) direct calculation	328,356
1570	(Gerard 1972) direct calculation	295,590
1580	[f] (Cook & Borah 1960) = [e] x 0.72	273,449
1580	(Slicher van Bath 1978) = [f] x 0.85	232,474
1595	[g] (Cook & Borah 1960) = [e] x 0.45	170,810
1595	(Cook & Borah 1979) direct calculation	169,413
1595	(Slicher van Bath 1978) = [g] x 0.85	145,189
1597	(Cook & Simpson 1948) = [d] x 0.65	346,698
1605	(Slicher van Bath 1978) = [h] x 0.85	129,735
1608	[h] (Cook & Borah 1960) = [e] x 0.40	152,629
1620-25	(Cook & Borah 1979) direct calculation	73,314

Utilizing essentially the same methods, but with additional data, Cook and Borah re-calculated the population of central Mexico for dates from 1532 to 1608.[13] In this monograph they utilize 19 documents, but among the most important are the *Suma de visitas de pueblos por orden alfabético* (1547-1551) documents, that record tribute amounts paid for about half of the principal towns in central Mexico for the 1530s and 1540s.[14] Because this early source records significantly smaller numbers of tribute payers

12 Cook and Simpson, *The Population of Central Mexico in the Sixteenth Century*, pp. 38, 43, 46.

13 Cook and Borah, *The Indian Population of Central Mexico*.

14 Whitmore and Turner, *Population Reconstruction of the Basin of Mexico*, p. 18.

than later compilations do and because Cook and Borah incorporate a smaller multiplier (3.3 instead of the 4.0 used in the previously cited study) to determine the total population from the tributary population, the estimates in this study reflect a far more rapid decrease in population than does the 1948 Cook and Borah study (Table 3.2 and Figure 3.1).[15]

Since Cook and Borah also calculate their regional totals from community values, the list of Basin communities in Table 3.1 was used to extract a Basin-only 1568 estimate from this work (Table 3.2 and Figure 3.1).[16] Since they recognize regional differences in Indian mortality, there are 10 differing ratios used to calculate the degree of depopulation for dates other than 1568.[17] The ratios for region I, the Central Plateau, are used here to calculate the population at 1532, 1580, 1595, and 1608 from the 1568 estimate (Table 3.2 and Figure 3.1).[18]

TABLE 3.3 POPULATION ESTIMATE FOR THE BASIN OF MEXICO: 1548

517,461	the 1565 Basin population (see Table 3.2)
- 29,629	the 1565 population of the 5 communities
487,832	the 1565 Basin population without the 5 communities
x 1.4	Borah & Cook's (1960) derived ratio
682,964	the 1548 tribute population without the 5 communities
+ 13,389	the 1548 tribute population of the 5 communities
696,353	the total tribute population of the Basin
+ 348,482	add 50 percent for tribute exempt commoners
+ 243,723	add 35 percent for tribute exempt aristocracy
1,288,253	the total 1548 Basin population.

(Calculated from various Cook, Simpson, and Borah documents)

The third work examined here, *The Population of Central Mexico in 1548*,[19] derives a 1548 central Mexico population solely from the *Suma de visitas de pueblos por orden alfabético* documents noted above. Because Borah and Cook believe that these documents reflect a population with a lower proportion of tribute payers to total population, they engage in a complex adjustment to the number of tributaries so that the implied total population is consistent with their other studies (Table 3.2 and Figure

---

[15] Cook and Borah, *The Indian Population of Central Mexico*, p. 38.

[16] Cook and Borah, *The Indian Population of Central Mexico*, Appendix.

[17] Cook and Borah, *The Indian Population of Central Mexico*, p. 48.

[18] Cook and Borah, *The Indian Population of Central Mexico*, pp. 33, 48.

[19] Borah and Cook, *The Population of Central Mexico in 1548*.

3.1).[20] Since only 5 communities in the Basin appear in the *Suma* documents the calculation of the Basin population is a complex application of Borah and Cook's method; Table 3.3 details the derivation of this figure.

An alternative eve-of-the-conquest (1519) estimate was produced from analysis of Aztec tribute rolls.[21] This monograph produces an even greater initial population than the Cook and Simpson study and reflects a pattern of gradual inflation of depopulation rates in later monographs as Borah and Cook extended their analysis. Since this study was not sufficiently disaggregate to calculate a Basin-only total in the same manner as the previous studies, a more indirect method was used whereby the 1519 central Mexico total population, 25.2 million, was multiplied by the proportion of this total presumed to reside in the Basin, 11.74 percent,[22] to yield a Basin-only total of 2.97 million (Table 3.2 and Figure 3.1).

The last of the Cook and Borah studies considered here uses reports made for the Royal Inspector General's visits (reflecting the situation in the first twenty years of the seventeenth century) to estimate the populations at the end of the first one hundred years of Spanish occupancy, in 1595 and 1620-1625.[23] They calculate the population using the same basic procedures as in their earlier works, but with reduced tributary multipliers of 2.8 and 3.3.[24] The results of these calculations for the Basin communities are also displayed in Table 3.2.

Using Rosenblat's modified values for Borah and Cook's[25] 1519 and 1548 estimates for central Mexico, it is possible to calculate two Basin estimates for these dates, albeit rather speculatively for the early date. For 1519, he re-examines Borah and Cook's Aztec documents and obtains a central Mexico total of 10,907,317 (in contrast to the 25.2 million obtained by Borah and Cook).[26] Applying the same 11.74 percent proportion multiplier we used to convert Borah and Cook's total (above), another, much smaller, 1519 Basin estimate is obtained (Table 3.2 and Figure 3.1). Rosenblat is equally severe in re-calculating the 1548 central Mexican

---

20 Borah and Cook, *The Population of Central Mexico in 1548*; see Whitmore and Turner, *Population Reconstruction of the Basin of Mexico*, pp. 19-20 for details on this calculation for the Basin of Mexico.

21 Borah and Cook, *Aboriginal Population of Central Mexico*.

22 Derived from Cook and Simpson, *The Population of Central Mexico in the Sixteenth Century*, appendix; and representing the Basin proportion in 1565.

23 Cook and Borah, *Essays in Population History*. Vol. 3.

24 Whitmore and Turner, *Population Reconstruction of the Basin of Mexico*, p. 21.

25 Rosenblat, "The Population of Hispañola"; Borah and Cook, *The Population of Central Mexico in 1548*; and Borah and Cook, *Aboriginal Population of Central Mexico*.

26 Rosenblat, *La Población*, p. 71; and Borah and Cook, *Aboriginal Population of Central Mexico*.

population from Borah and Cook.[27] He accepts Borah and Cook's basic *Suma* figure, but reduces their various modifications of it to produce a central Mexico sum of 3.2 million that is slightly less than half (0.475 x) that of Borah and Cook.[28] Applying this ratio to the 1548 Basin population calculated above yields a new 1548 figure of 611,788 (Table 3.2 and Figure 3.1).

Another critic of the reconstructions derived by Cook, Borah, and Simpson, Slicher van Bath, argues that, as a first approximation, the total population figures need to be adjusted downward about 15 percent since they double count married men and married couples.[29] Basin-only estimates can be constructed by applying Slicher van Bath's 15 percent reduction to the figures calculated from Cook and Borah and Borah and Cook above (Table 3.2 and Figure 3.1).[30]

In his valuable account of the sixteenth- and seventeenth-century Basin, Gibson independently derives Basin populations for 1519 and 1570 (as well as for seventeenth-century dates beyond the scope of this study).[31] He calculates the 1570 population as roughly 2.8 times the number of tributaries in López de Velasco's 1570 survey (Table 3.2 and Figure 3.1).[32] His 1519 total is calculated as a multiple (4.0-5.0 times that) of the 1570 figure (Table 3.2 and Figure 3.1). A second 1570 Basin estimate may be derived using Gibson's 2.8 x multiplier and Gerhard's estimate of Basin tributaries (Table 3.2 and Figure 3.1).[33]

A second group of Basin-specific estimates for 1519, 1530-1535, and 1568 has been assembled by Sanders.[34] While he criticizes the methodology and conclusions derived in Borah and Cook, Sanders accepts Cook and Borah's 1568 population figures as the earliest substantially

---

[27] Rosenblat, *La Población*, p. 70; and Borah and Cook, *The Population of Central Mexico in 1548*.

[28] Rosenblat, *La Población*, p. 70; and Borah and Cook, *The Population of Central Mexico in 1548*.

[29] Slicher van Bath, "The Calculation of the Population of New Spain"; and Whitmore and Turner, *Population Reconstruction of the Basin of Mexico*, p. 24.

[30] Slicher van Bath, "The Calculation of the Population of New Spain," p. 92; Cook and Borah, *The Indian Population of Central Mexico*; Borah and Cook, *The Population of Central Mexico in 1548*; and Borah and Cook, *Aboriginal Population of Central Mexico*.

[31] Gibson, *The Aztecs*.

[32] Gibson, *The Aztecs*, pp. 137, 140-141.

[33] Gerhard, *Historical Geography of New Spain*, pp. 76-78, 100-102, 178-180, 180-183, 226-228, 247-250, 273-275, 311-314.

[34] Sanders, "The Population of the Teotihuacan Valley"; and Sanders, "The Population of the Central Mexican Symbiotic Region."

correct estimates.[35] Sanders uses Borah and Cook's figures to derive a slightly higher range of estimates for 1568 than the figure independently calculated here (see Table 3.2).[36] Using this estimate and tax documents from the Basin, he multiplies the 1568 figures by a 2.0-2.5 x factor to produce a range of figures for the period 1530-1535 (Table 3.2 and Figure 3.1).[37] Similarly, a range of estimates for 1519 results from applying a 2.7-3.0 x multiplier to the 1568 range (Table 3.2 and Figure 3.1).[38] For all three of these estimates the mid-point of the range of estimates is displayed in Table 3.2.

Grouped Estimates

Since several of the estimates derived above are for only a single date[39] and the others ("families") are simple multiples of a single date estimate,[40] it is not reasonable to compare them separately with MEXIPOP simulations. Further, several estimates and "families" of estimates cluster relatively closely at key dates.[41] Such comparison is facilitated if the historical estimates are divided into groups on the basis of the relative severity of their implied depopulation and each resulting "group" is mated with a MEXIPOP simulation run.

Examination of Figure 3.1 suggests three groupings of estimates, here labeled "severe," "moderate," and "mild." These groupings are described immediately below, and in greater detail later in the chapter (see Figure 3.2 and Table 3.4 throughout).

---

35   Sanders, "The Population of the Central Mexican Symbiotic Region"; Borah and Cook, *The Population of Central Mexico in 1548*; Borah and Cook, *Aboriginal Population of Central Mexico;* and Cook and Borah, *The Indian Population of Central Mexico.*

36   Sanders, "The Population of the Central Mexican Symbiotic Region," p. 130.

37   Ibid.

38   Ibid.

39   See Borah and Cook, *Aboriginal Population of Central Mexico.*

40   See Cook and Simpson, *The Population of Central Mexico in the Sixteenth Century*; or Cook and Borah, *The Indian Population of Central Mexico.*

41   See Gibson, *The Aztecs;* and Sanders, "The Population of the Central Mexican Symbiotic Region," for 1519 and 1570.

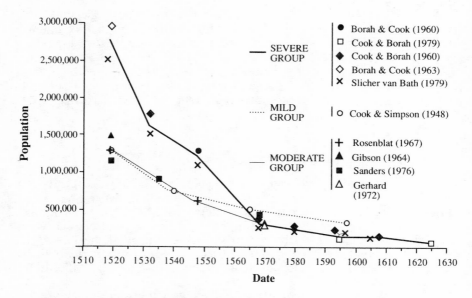

Figure 3.2 Basin Population Estimate Groups

Severe Group
    The estimates derived from Cook and Borah, Borah and Cook, and Slicher van Bath comprise this clustering (Figure 3.2).[42] These 16 estimates span the entire post-contact sixteenth century and include the only post-1600 estimates considered here. These form an internally consistent set since, with the exception of those by Slicher van Bath (who only modifies the Berkeley scholars' figures by 15 percent), they are all made by the same team and may be presumed to reflect a relatively consistent methodology and outlook. This group embodies the most severe depopulation estimates (Table 3.4). From a pre-conquest total of 2,736,594 in 1519, a virtually complete, 97.23 percent, depopulation is implied by their 1625 figure of 73,314 (Table 3.4). Even as early as mid-century (1568) the population numbers derived for this group indicate a 94.09 percent loss.

---

[42] Cook and Borah, *The Indian Population of Central Mexico*; Cook and Borah, *Essays in Population History*, Vol. 3; Borah and Cook, *The Population of Central Mexico in 1548*; Borah and Cook, *Aboriginal Population of Central Mexico;* and Slicher van Bath, "The Calculation of the Population of New Spain."

TABLE 3.4 GROUPED HISTORICAL RECONSTRUCTIONS GROUP WITH BEST-FIT LINE VALUES

DATE	Mild Group		Moderate Group		Severe Group	
	FITTED LINE	IMPLIED DEPOPULATION*	FITTED LINE	IMPLIED DEPOPULATION*	FITTED LINE	IMPLIED DEPOPULATION*
1519	1,293,652	100.00	1,304,390	100.00	2,736,594	100.00
1532	—	—	—	—	1,639,557	59.91
1535	—	—	912,068	69.92	—	—
1540	755,493	58.40	—	—	—	—
1547	—	—	611,788	46.90	—	—
1548	—	—	—	—	1,191,634	43.54
1565	517,461	40.00	—	—	—	—
1568	—	—	—	—	321,591	11.75
1569	—	—	343,018	26.30	—	—
1580	—	—	—	—	252,962	9.24
1595	—	—	—	—	161,804	5.91
1597	346,698	26.80	—	—	—	—
1607	—	—	—	—	141,182	5.16
1625	—	—	—	—	73,314	2.68

* Percentage of initial (1519) population remaining at date.

Moderate Group

This diverse group of estimates comprises those derived from Gerhard, Rosenblat, Sanders, and Gibson (Figure 3.2).[43] Unfortunately, this group does not include any post-1570 estimates. The ultimate provenance of both Rosenblat's and Sanders' estimates is the body of Cook and Borah's work, especially Borah and Cook, and Cook and Borah, but these reconstructions differ significantly from those of Borah and Cook.[44] Rosenblat directly modifies Borah and Cook to reflect his interpretation of the basic tributary data,[45] while Sanders utilizes Cook and Borah[46] as the starting point for his 1568 datum population. The other estimates in this group are more directly related since the population figure derived from Gerhard's count of tributaries is determined using Gibson's estimate of the whole population to tributary population fraction. Compared with the severe group, the moderate group implies a lower immediate pre-conquest population, 1,304,390, and reflects a level of depopulation at mid-century (1569), 73.7 percent, that is far lower (Table 3.4).

Mild Group

This group comprises those derived from Cook and Simpson's "family" of estimates and encompass the entire sixteenth century (Figure 3.2).[47] While these estimates do not differ greatly from the "moderate" group for the first two decades of Spanish occupance, they diverge increasingly so that by mid-century the absolute difference and trend of change, are both significantly different. While this mild group has a pre-conquest population of 1,293,652 that is similar to that of the moderate group, it generates a somewhat smaller depopulation percentage, 60 percent, for mid-century (1565) (Table 3.4). This is far smaller that the corresponding severe group depopulation for the similar period, 88.25 percent (Table 3.4). Similarly, the severe group's end of century (1595) depopulation figure, 94.09 percent, far overshadows that for the mild group, a 73.2 percent loss by 1597 (Table 3.4).

---

43 Gerhard, *Historical Geography of New Spain*; Rosenblat, *La Población*; Sanders, "The Population of the Central Mexican Symbiotic Region", and Gibson, *The Aztecs.*

44 Borah and Cook, *The Population of Central Mexico in 1548*; Borah and Cook, *Aboriginal Population of Central Mexico;* and Cook and Borah, *The Indian Population of Central Mexico.*

45 Rosenblat, *La Población*; Borah and Cook, *The Population of Central Mexico in 1548*; and Borah and Cook, *Aboriginal Population of Central Mexico.*

46 Cook and Borah, *The Indian Population of Central Mexico.*

47 Cook and Simpson, *The Population of Central Mexico in the Sixteenth Century.*

Simulation Calibration Runs

In a simulation as complex as MEXIPOP it is fruitless to attempt to perform simulations with different values for each key variable because the possible number of combinations would be unmanageably large. For that reason, I have simplified the calibration of MEXIPOP in two ways. First, in the previous chapter, I established two "families" of demographic sub-models, two epidemic history sub-models, and an environmental history sub-model. In addition, the basic parameters of agricultural productivity and nutritional demand were set. This simplification greatly reduces the universe of possible variables. Second, in the sections to follow, I shall perform a series of sensitivity tests to determine the relative importance of other variables in MEXIPOP. With the the simulation process thus streamlined, the pairing of simulations to historical reconstruction groups will proceed in the last section of this chapter.

In order to determine the responsiveness of the population output of MEXIPOP to differing specific inputs (i.e., to determine the sensitivity of MEXIPOP to changes in these variables), it is necessary to establish a basis from which to measure. This is accomplished by first setting key variables to "baseline" values, performing a simulation, and noting the resultant population dynamics. The result of these procedures are eight baseline simulations, corresponding to the eight possible combinations of demographic and epidemic sub-models, each with the same set of baseline assumptions for the other key variables. In the section that immediately follows, the "baseline" assumptions for each of the key MEXIPOP variables are noted. Using the baseline values as a foundation, a further section examines systematic alteration of these key variables one-at-a-time to determine the sensitivity of the MEXIPOP baseline simulations' output to alterations in these key variables

BASELINE SIMULATION ASSUMPTIONS

The first of the baseline simulation variables consists of the two "families" of demographic sub-models, corresponding to levels "8 west" (hereafter labeled "8W") and "3 west" (hereafter labeled "3W") in Coale and Demeny's model life tables (see previous chapter for a fuller description).[48] Further, each demographic "family" consists of two "branches," one assuming a virtually zero population growth rate (in the absence of crises) (hereafter labeled "zpg") and one assuming an approximately 0.5 percent intrinsic growth rate (hereafter labeled "+"). Thus, these four demographic sub-models are designated as 3W +, 3W zpg, 8W +, and 8W zpg (see Tables 2.12, 2.13, and 2.14).

While the standard demographic sub-models address the fertility and mortality of the population, they do not address the third potentially important demographic characteristic of a population, its mobility. Out-migration (or in-migration) from (or to) the Basin may have dramatically

---

48 Coale and Demeny, *Model Life Tables*.

altered the population size and composition. Also since the demographic sub-models do not specifically address widespread homicide, it is modeled here as an out-migration.[49] As a baseline assumption, migration into or out of (and therefore, homicide) the Basin is presumed to be zero. Since migration that includes all age classes in equal proportion has a direct affect on the population size, it is not necessary to probe its sensitivity *per se*, only its timing. The effects of age-specific migration such as that may have been occasioned by warfare homicide or relocation (i.e., loss of reproducing age adults) does have a complex effect that will be examined, however.

The second of the baseline simulation variables are the two models of epidemic disease developed above (see Tables 2.4 and 2.6). These models are identical except in their treatment of the important crisis periods of 1545-1548, 1559, and 1576-1581. One model, "Typhus," assumes the episodes in question reflect typhus epidemics, while the other, "Plague," assumes that pneumonic plague was responsible for these crises.

The third baseline simulation variable is the model of environmental affects on agriculture (Table 2.15). In subsequent tests, the level of agricultural losses due to these crises will be altered to determine the sensitivity of the model's population output to differing levels, but for the present the level of these effects is taken as a given.

Of course, MEXIPOP could not be run without specifying values for a number of other key variables. Two of these, the intrinsic desire of the populace to plan for, produce, and store surplus above their immediate needs (against a calamity) and the interaction of epidemics with agricultural production are integral to the behavior of the system and interact with values generated using the basic assumptions.

The planning for and setting aside of a surplus in excess of anticipated demand(s) is a near-universal in advanced agrarian societies such as existed in the Basin of Mexico. Since the very rationale for this "set-aside" is to temper the effects of a poor harvest or other calamity, the amount of surplus is important in determining the effect of a crisis that leads to reduced harvest yields. For example, if a farming family has a stored surplus equal to 10 percent of the family's yearly needs, a poor harvest that results in a 10 percent shortfall has virtually no effect—in contrast to the situation obtaining for a family in the same crisis with no surplus. The effects of differing amounts of surplus, expressed in MEXIPOP as a percentage of a PU's annual consumption needs, will be explored below; but set initially at zero (Table 3.5).

---

49 Of course, the life tables from which these demographic sub-models were prepared reflect all the causes of death in the sample populations from which they were drawn, and thus, include homicide. It is the excess homicide that may have been occasioned by the initial war of conquest and subsequent Spanish occupance that is modeled here as out-migration.

TABLE 3.5 BASELINE SIMULATION ASSUMPTIONS

Standard simulation	T 3W zpg	P 3W zpg	T 3w +	P 3W +	T 8W zpg	P 8W zpg	T 8W +	P 8W +
Demographic model	3W zpg	3W zpg	3W +	3W +	8W zpg	8W zpg	8W +	8W +
Epidemic model	Typhus	Plague	Typhus	Plague	Typhus	Plague	Typhus	Plague
Environmental loss	Standard	Standard	Standard	Standard	Standard	Standard	Standard	Standard
Migration	0 %	0 %	0 %	0 %	0 %	0 %	0 %	0 %
Surplus	0 %	0 %	0 %	0 %	0 %	0 %	0 %	0 %
Ag-epidemic synergy	20 %	20 %	20 %	20 %	20 %	20 %	20 %	20 %
Labor loss	0 %	0 %	0 %	0 %	0 %	0 %	0 %	0 %
Maize loss	0 %	0 %	0 %	0 %	0 %	0 %	0 %	0 %

Agricultural-epidemic interaction is a key interactive variable because the mortality of an epidemic is multiplied if it greatly disrupts the agricultural round, and produces additional deaths by famine in subsequent months. Since we know little about the seasonal timing of the Basin's epidemics and of their simultaneity for different communities within the Basin, the best that can be achieved in modeling the differential impacts of diseases assumes that all disease events of the same morbidity had the same proportional affect on agriculture (see Chapter 2 for a fuller discussion of how these effects are modeled). It is unlikely that severe epidemics had no impact on agricultural production since famines accompanied epidemics. Initially, it is assumed that 20 percent of the laborers stricken ill will not be able to complete a harvest (Table 3.5). Thus, for a disease with a 50 percent morbidity rate for those in the adult labor age classes (i.e., ages 15-60), and assuming that 20 percent of these households will not garner a harvest, the total production loss is $0.2 \times 0.5 = 0.1$, or 10 percent.

A further diminishment of Amerindian agricultural production was occasioned by the commandeering of Indian labor by the Spanish. Again, we know little about the potential scale of this effect, although it is not likely to have been very great since initially the Spanish were dependent on Amerindian agricultural production, and they probably arranged their labor drafts with the agricultural production season in mind. For purposes of setting a baseline, therefore, this effect is set at zero (Table 3.5).

Similarly, the Spanish withdrew maize from the Amerindian economy, but the scale of this withdrawal is not clear. As the Spanish population grew, the scale of withdrawal must have increased, especially as a proportion for each household, since the number of Amerindian households diminished even as the number of Spanish to be supported increased. Clearly, this variable strongly interacts with Amerindian productive capacity, since as long as Amerindian production was sufficient to meet both subsistence needs and the Spanish demand, there was no immediate shortfall. Nevertheless, such withdrawal—even if it were small—placed the Amerindian households at greater risk to other perturbations of grain production such as environmentally produced losses or losses due to epidemics. Again, to establish a baseline, the scale of Spanish withdrawal is initially set at zero (Table 3.5).

There are, therefore, eight possible baseline cases (each with identical assumptions as to environmental loss, migration, surplus, synergy, labor loss, and maize loss [Table 3.5]): a "3 west" zero growth population acted on by either a typhus or plague epidemic model (hereafter these basic configurations are labeled "Typhus 3W zpg" and "Plague 3W zpg"); a "3 west" 0.5 percent growth population acted on by the same two epidemic models (hereafter "Plague 3W +" and "Typhus 3W +"); an "8 west" zero growth population acted on by either epidemic model (hereafter "Plague 8W zpg" and "Typhus 8W zpg"); and finally, an "8 west" 0.5 percent growth population subject to the same pair of epidemic models (hereafter "Plague 8W +" and "Typhus 8W +") (Table 3.5).

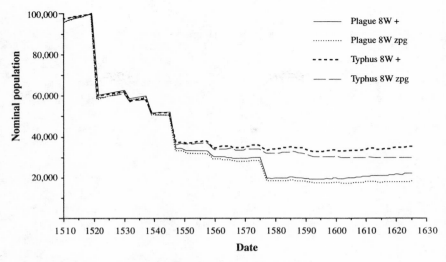

NOTE: All Runs are Based on an Initial Nominal Population of 100,000 in 1519.

Figure 3.3 8W Demographic Sub-Model Baseline Runs

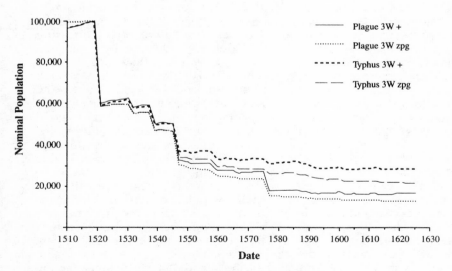

NOTE: All Runs are Based on an Initial Nominal Population of 100,000 in 1519.

Figure 3.4 3W Demographic Sub-Model Baseline Runs

TABLE 3.6 BASELINE SIMULATIONS: SURVIVING POPULATION PROPORTIONS

(displayed as percentage of initial population)

Date	Plague 3W +	Plague 3W zpg	Plague 8W +	Plague 8W zpg	Typhus 3W +	Typhus 3W zpg	Typhus 8W +	Typhus 8W zpg
1519	100.0	100.0	100.0	100.0	100.0	100.0	100.0	100.0
1529	62.1	59.5	62.3	61.8	61.5	59.5	61.5	61.0
1539	49.9	47.0	51.5	50.5	49.0	47.0	51.1	50.2
1549	32.3	29.8	34.1	33.0	37.3	34.1	37.3	36.8
1559	28.6	25.8	31.2	30.1	34.3	30.7	36.0	35.0
1569	26.9	23.5	29.5	28.1	32.8	28.6	35.2	33.7
1579	17.6	15.0	19.7	18.4	31.2	26.3	34.0	32.0
1589	17.5	14.5	20.0	18.4	31.1	25.4	34.6	32.1
1599	16.7	13.6	19.7	17.6	29.3	23.5	33.5	30.4
1609	16.3	13.3	20.5	17.8	28.8	22.5	33.9	30.0
1619	16.4	13.0	21.5	18.1	28.5	21.7	34.7	29.9

Figures 3.3 and 3.4 display plots of population dynamics for the simulations that incorporate these initial premises. The assumptions underlying these runs are detailed in Table 3.5, and a numeric tabulation of the results of these baseline runs are summarized in Table 3.6. Since the purpose in this section is to examine the relative effect differing assumptions make as compared to the baseline simulations, the population numbers used in the plots are demonstrative only, that is to say, the simulations are calibrated so that the initial, 1519, population is 100,000 in each case. Examination of these baseline simulations indicates that: (1) the simulations using populations with a propensity to grow (labeled as "+") decline less proportionally overall than those with no propensity to grow (labeled as "zpg"); (2) the simulations using the 3W demographic regime decline more proportionally overall than those using the 8W assumption; and (3) the simulations using the plague epidemic sub-model decline proportionally more overall than those using the typhus epidemic sub-model. The last observation is a result of the dramatically different shape of the population curves after the 1545-1548 epidemics (the first to use the alternative assumptions). Hence, the most severe baseline assumption is one using the 3W zpg demographic sub-model acted on by the plague epidemic sub-model, "Plague 3W zpg," while the least severe baseline case is the 8W + demographic sub-model acted on by the typhus epidemic sub-model, "Typhus 8W +" (Figures 3.3 and 3.4 and Table 3.6). Since the full range of variation can be encompassed by using only 2 of these baseline simulations, the "Typhus 8W +" case and the "Plague 3W zpg" case, only these two need be considered in the subsequent sensitivity tests.

TABLE 3.7 COMPARISON OF LABOR TRIBUTE EFFECTS

| | T 8W + | | | | | | P 3W zpg | | | | | |
| | BASELINE | | LABOR TRIBUTE = 0.1 | | LABOR TRIBUTE = 0.2 | | BASELINE | | LABOR TRIBUTE = 0.1 | | LABOR TRIBUTE = 0.2 | |
Date	nominal pop.	% initial	nominal pop.	% initial	nominal pop.	% initial	nominal pop.	% initial	nominal pop.	% initial	nominal pop.	% initial
1519	112,498	100.00	112,435	100.00	112,264	100.00	102,304	100.00	102,196	100.00	102,020	100.00
1529	69,198	61.51	67,861	60.36	64,888	57.80	60,865	59.49	59,567	58.29	56,852	55.73
1539	57,525	51.13	55,320	49.20	50,432	44.92	48,090	47.01	46,057	45.07	41,930	41.10
1549	41,971	37.31	39,247	34.91	33,677	30.00	30,471	29.78	28,246	27.64	24,297	23.82
1559	40,455	35.96	36,361	32.34	28,745	25.60	26,343	25.75	23,553	23.05	18,898	18.52
1569	39,633	35.23	34,702	30.86	25,725	22.91	24,060	23.52	20,929	20.48	15,896	15.58
1579	38,214	33.97	32,907	29.27	23,546	20.97	15,305	14.96	13,061	12.78	9,523	9.33
1590	38,297	34.04	32,213	28.65	21,935	19.54	14,808	14.47	12,331	12.07	8,570	8.40
1599	37,689	33.50	30,788	27.38	19,558	17.42	13,888	13.58	11,148	10.91	7,146	7.00
1609	38,113	33.88	30,323	26.97	18,158	16.17	13,604	13.30	10,595	10.37	6,362	6.24
1619	38,986	34.65	30,170	26.83	17,013	15.15	13,329	13.03	10,063	9.85	5,672	5.56

SENSITIVITY TESTS

Four simulations, designed to determine the sensitivity of MEXIPOP's population output to changes in the level of tribute labor withdrawal, were performed. The results indicate that decreasing the level of available labor to 90 percent of normal (i.e., setting labor tribute equal to 10 percent) significantly reduced the simulated population as compared to the baseline case (Table 3.7 and Figure 3.5). The result was more pronounced for a 20 percent withdrawal (Table 3.7 and Figure 3.5). And while the population total remaining at each date was far smaller in the "Plague 3W zpg" cases over the "Typhus 8W +" cases, the relative impact of the changes in labor tribute is roughly equal for these two extreme baseline cases. This useful result suggests that the affect of variables such as labor tribute are relatively independent of the choice of extreme baseline cases.

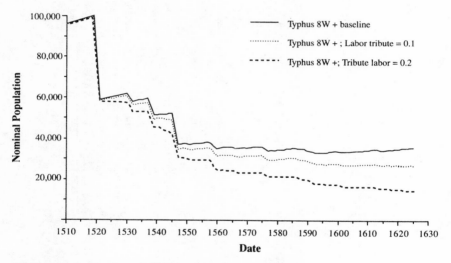

NOTE: *All Runs are Based on an Initial Nominal Population of 100,000 in 1519.*

Figure 3.5 Labor Tribute Comparison

Since labor tribute is set here as a constant for each year, it reduces food production by a constant proportion each year—good year or bad. This result is born out by Figure 3.5, where the population decline in the crisis years is relatively equal between the cases, but the rate of growth (indeed, of decline for the 20 percent case) between the crisis years varies inversely with the amount of labor tribute extracted. As we would expect, the second 10 percent of labor withdrawn affects the population's mortality more than the first 10 percent (Table 3.7). This is because mortality is not a linear function of nutritional sufficiency; a small shortfall (as would be occasioned by the first 10 percent withdrawal) will not drive up mortalities very significantly, but when the shortfall is increased (as it is when the labor withdrawal is increased to 20 percent) mortalities are increased by a larger proportion. As will be shown below, this property of affecting the non-crisis years is shared by the other "withdrawal" variable, maize tribute. The simulations in Figure 3.5 were performed with the surplus variable set to zero. Had the surplus variable been set to a level sufficient to cover the losses imposed by the labor withdrawal there would have been no extra mortality and no additional decline in population such as is shown in Figure 3.5.

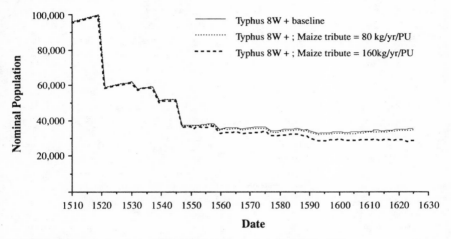

NOTE: All Runs are Based on an Initial Nominal Population of 100,000 in 1519.

Figure 3.6 Maize Tribute Comparison

Like the labor tribute variable discussed above, maize tribute is simulated by "removing" a set amount of maize from each production unit's household economy each year, starting in 1519. Maize tribute is unlike labor, however, since each production unit's decision logic (used to determine each subsequent year's planting area) is based on its experience with the past year's harvest amount, surplus level and desired level, and the amount of maize lost to tribute. Thus, for small amounts, each PU can compensate for the seized grain and produce more the following year. This clearly is the case when the tribute level is set at about 10 percent of a PU's annual consumption needs (80 kg/year). Since such a withdrawal leads to virtually no change in the mortality of the nominal population, it declines at virtually the same pace as the baseline (Figure 3.6). When the withdrawal reaches about 20 percent of the annual consumption needs (160 kg/year), the situation is different since there is not sufficient areal expansion possible to accommodate the demand (Figure 3.6). At such a high level, maize tribute has an impact roughly equal to that when labor tribute is set at 10 percent (compare Figures 3.6 and 3.5). Further, the maize tribute "removal" does not result in a great alteration of the impact of epidemics in the major crisis years (noted by the abrupt falls in population at certain dates in Figure 3.6). This result seem reasonable since the extra mortality imposed by the maize tribute variable is small in any year, especially as compared with the large mortalities incurred in the major epidemic years. Hence, its impact in the epidemic years is negligible except that it forces families up against limits of productivity (i.e., the availability of extra land) or in combination with other factors such as labor lost to epidemics or to tribute. Although, the constant erosion of population due to such small changes, even in the non-crisis years, adds up to significant numbers if continued for 100 years. Because these withdrawal variables (both maize and labor) virtually constitute a multiplication of the background mortality, they will not be utilized in compiling initial attempted "fits" to the historical reconstructions, rather they will be used, where necessary, to "fine tune" the fit of a simulation to a historical reconstruction group.

The effect of the agricultural production-epidemic synergy variable is fundamentally different than that of the tribute-withdrawal variables discussed above because the "synergy" variable is only called into play in epidemic years—it exerts no direct affect at any other time. The end result of increasing synergy is proportionally more rapid depopulation (i.e., the relationship in non-linear) (Figures 3.7 and 3.4). This result is similar to that obtained using the tribute variables and stems from the same reason. Because it only increases mortalities during epidemics, small values of synergy (e.g., synergy = 0.1, 0.2, and 0.3) have little effect on the overall depopulation (Table 3.8 and Figs 3.7 and 3.4), but larger values have profound effects—so large that at synergy = 0.6 the nominal population becomes virtually extinct (Figures 3.7 and 3.4). This pattern suggests that a reasonable range of possible synergy effects is from 0.2 to 0.5. This range encompasses the situation in which epidemic disease had little additional mortality effect through famine (the 0.2 case) to the situation in which crisis mortality was significantly multiplied by famine (the 0.5 case). While there are small differences, there is no fundamental difference in the scale of famine effects engendered by the synergy variable between the two extreme baseline scenarios, Typhus 8W + and Plague 3W zpg.

TABLE 3.8 AGRICULTURAL PRODUCTION–EPIDEMIC SYNERGY COMPARISONS

(a) Plague 3W zpg Baseline

DATE	BASELINE		SYNERGY = 0.1		SYNERGY = 0.3		SYNERGY = 0.4		SYNERGY = 0.5		SYNERGY = 0.6	
	Nominal pop.	% initial	Nominal pop.	% initial	Nominal pop.	% Initial	Nominal pop.	% initial	Nominal pop.	% initial	Nominal pop.	% Initial
1519	102,304	100.00	102,304	100.00	102,304	100.00	102,304	100.00	102,304	100.00	102,304	100.00
1529	60,865	59.49	60,980	59.61	60,729	59.36	60,185	58.83	58,229	56.92	35,803	35.00
1539	48,090	47.01	48,287	47.20	47,676	46.60	46,417	45.37	39,907	39.01	13,233	12.93
1549	30,471	29.78	30,639	29.95	30,179	29.50	29,392	28.73	25,346	24.78	8,488	8.30
1559	26,343	25.75	26,772	26.17	25,602	25.03	23,945	23.41	17,856	17.45	2,720	2.66
1569	24,060	23.52	24,526	23.97	23,164	22.64	21,190	20.71	13,925	13.61	1,065	1.04
1579	15,305	14.96	15,613	15.26	14,728	14.40	13,490	13.19	8,891	8.69	649	0.63
1589	14,808	14.47	15,155	14.81	14,142	13.82	12,789	12.50	8,124	7.94	305	0.30
1599	13,888	13.58	14,282	13.96	13,103	12.81	11,492	11.23	6,223	6.08	79	0.08
1609	13,604	13.30	14,078	13.76	12,691	12.41	10,890	10.64	5,362	5.24	28	0.03
1619	13,329	13.03	13,831	13.52	12,343	12.07	10,464	10.23	4,960	4.85	9	0.01

(b) Typhus 8W + Baseline

DATE	BASELINE		SYNERGY = 0.1		SYNERGY = 0.3		SYNERGY = 0.4		SYNERGY = 0.5		SYNERGY = 0.6	
	Nominal pop.	% initial	Nominal pop.	% initial	Nominal pop.	% Initial	Nominal pop.	% initial	Nominal pop.	% initial	Nominal pop.	% Initial
1519	112,498	100.00	112,498	100.00	112,498	100.00	112,498	100.00	112,498	100.00	112,498	100.00
1529	69,198	61.51	69,262	61.57	69,074	61.40	68,751	61.11	67,586	60.08	58,113	51.66
1539	57,525	51.13	57,678	51.27	57,196	50.84	56,313	50.06	52,168	46.37	27,166	24.15
1549	41,971	37.31	42,126	37.45	41,655	37.03	40,830	36.29	37,137	33.01	14,359	12.76
1559	40,455	35.96	40,941	36.39	39,475	35.09	37,259	33.12	30,569	27.17	6,670	5.93
1569	39,633	35.23	40,213	35.75	38,442	34.17	35,705	31.74	27,579	24.52	3,508	3.12
1579	38,214	33.97	38,762	34.46	37,102	32.98	34,536	30.70	26,861	23.88	3,324	2.95
1589	38,976	34.65	39,625	35.22	37,676	33.49	34,757	30.90	26,464	23.52	2,662	2.37
1599	37,689	33.50	38,461	34.19	36,186	32.17	32,755	29.12	23,195	20.62	1,145	1.02
1609	38,113	33.88	39,061	34.72	36,274	32.24	32,148	28.58	21,354	18.98	618	0.55
1619	38,986	34.65	40,029	35.58	36,973	32.87	32,500	28.89	21,131	18.78	314	0.28

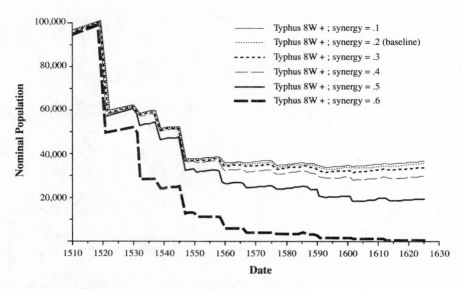

Figure 3.7 Agriculture-Epidemic Synergy Comparison

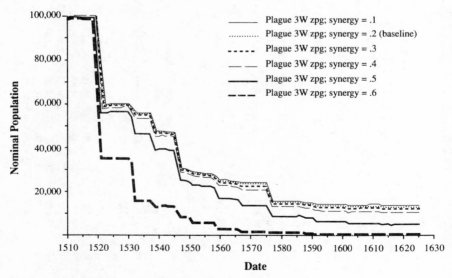

Figure 3.8 Agriculture-Epidemic Synergy Comparison

The surplus variable affects the scaling of the previously discussed factors since it sets the level of "crisis cushion" for MEXIPOP families. A relatively high cushion will virtually eliminate the excess mortality effects, at least for relatively small values of labor tribute. For example, a surplus goal of 10 percent of a PU's annual consumption demand (about 80 kg of maize) has the effect of virtually eliminating the excess mortality called forth by a 10 percent labor withdrawal (Figure 3.9). Similarly, a surplus "cushion" of 10 percent mitigates the effect of a severe (0.2) labor withdrawal as well (Figure 3.9). This "cushioning" effect does not extend to maize tribute withdrawal, however, since (unlike the situation for labor withdrawal) production units (PUs) plan for the maize tribute by increasing production so having a surplus in addition to the extra production planned for the tribute conveys no increased security (Figure 3.9).

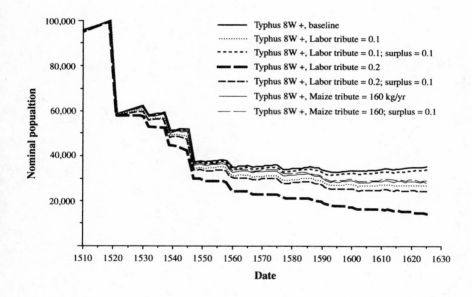

Figure 3.9 Withdrawal Variables-Surplus Comparison

The provision of surplus also mitigates the detrimental effects of agricultural production-epidemic synergy. This effect is variable, however, and is more effective for large values of synergy (Figure 3.10). This variability is to be expected since synergy only operates in epidemic crisis years and small values of synergy have little effect on the resulting population dynamics in any case.

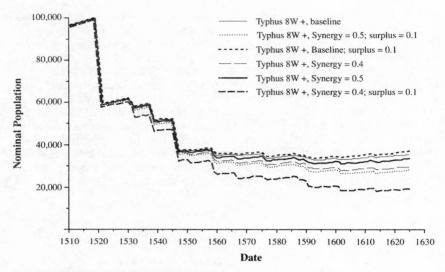

Figure 3.10 Synergy-Surplus Comparisons

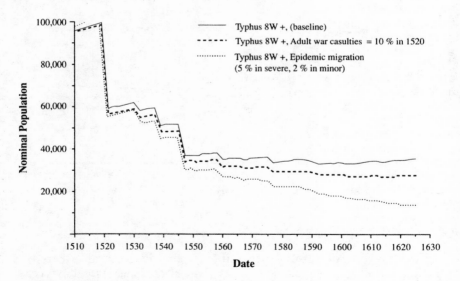

Figure 3.11 Migration and Homicide Effects

The surplus variable only acts as a mitigating variable, that is to say, changes in its value do not call forth any changes in population by itself—only relatively constant modifications in the action of another variables. In effect, it acts as a constant, the value of which is incorporated in the values assumed by the variables it modifies. For that reason, it is unnecessary to model changes in surplus independently of other variables.

The effects of migration and homicide are simple to envision, yet complex in their ultimate effect on population size. For example, examination of a simulation in which it is assumed that 10 percent of the adult (aged 15-60) population perished in the wars of conquest in 1520 (this is the only excess homicide mortality assumed in this run) shows that the immediate effect on population size is not profound, but the altered age structure of population that results has a surprisingly great impact on the subsequent trajectory of population as compared to the baseline (Figure 3.11). Even larger impacts on total population size is engendered if it is assumed that 5 percent of the population (all ages) emigrate in years of severe epidemic (1520, 1532, 1546, and 1576) and 2 percent emigrate in years of minor epidemics (1530, 1550, 1558, 1559, 1563, 1566, 1587, 1590, 1592, 1601, 1604, 1613, and 1615) (Figure 3.11). These simple examples show how important migration may have been in the Basin's population dynamics. There seems to be little attention to migration in the literature of the early colonial period and for that reason its scale and timing are conjectural. Kicza and Robinson argue that urbanward migration during crisis periods was likely.[50] If so, it is not unreasonable to posit higher morbidity rates for this migrant population since they would have been more likely to have contacted diseases in the confined cities. Since MEXIPOP does not address internal population distribution, however, this argument cannot be addressed here. It is reasonable to argue, however, that net emigration peaked in crisis times, although the values used in this example may be too large. Like the withdrawal variables, migration will be used to "fine tune" simulations to their corresponding historical reconstruction group.

In summary then, alterations to the level of labor tribute alters the population dynamics of non-crisis periods primarily. The maize tribute variable behaves in the same manner. This is in contrast to the effects obtained by alteration of the synergy level, where the population dynamics are changed primarily for the crisis years.[51] Level of surplus affects both labor tribute and synergy, but differently. Increased surplus attenuates the

---

[50] John E. Kicza, "Migration to Major Metropoles in Colonial Mexico," in David J. Robinson (ed.), *Migration in Colonial Spanish America*, Cambridge: Cambridge University Press, 1990, p. 193-211; Robinson, "Typology of Migration."

[51] Of course, the changes to the population dynamics engendered by these variables (labor tribute, maize tribute, and synergy) are not as simple as just portrayed. Any alteration in the population age structure will alter the subsequent dynamics of a population. Changes to any of these variables do alter the population age structure, however, the dominant effect on the overall trajectory of population is as noted.

deleterious effect of labor tribute at any level; while increased surplus is significantly more effective at damping the negative effects of synergy at high levels of synergy. Migration and homicide exert complex effects on the population trajectory depending on their scale, timing, and the age pattern of the migrating group. The alteration of these variables thus creates a powerful set of tools to "shape" a simulation resulting from one of the baseline assumptions.

MITIGATING OR ESCALATING VARIABLES SUB-MODEL

The complex discussion in the previous section helps to establish another set of variables (a "simplified"sub-model) to be paired with the original eight baseline simulations. The idea is to produce a reasonably sized set of simulations that encompass a wide range of assumptions and produce a wide range of possible population outcomes. Consideration of the calibration results discussed above leads to the definition of a third set of sub-models (the first 2 are the demographic and the epidemic), the "interactive," that will, when paired with the other sub-models, produce a wide range of possible results. The more benign interactive sub-model assumes the baseline model, including synergy level (= 0.2), while the more malignant sub-model utilizes a 0.5 synergy level along with the other baseline assumptions. Mating these 2 additional sub-models to the 8 introduced previously results in 16 "standard" models. The 8 standard models using the benign assumptions are, in fact, the 8 baseline sub-models introduced above, while the 8 severe ones are identical except in the synergy level assumption.

Simulation to Reconstruction-group Mating

BASIC METHODOLOGY

The goal here is to establish simulation runs that reasonably mimic the population dynamics described by the historical reconstruction groups. The first step is to establish one of the 16 "standard" simulation runs as that closest to the historical. Next, alterations to the surplus, migration, and withdrawal variables will be performed to allow a "fine-tuning" of the best-fitting standard simulation to produce a closer match with the historical reconstruction group. There are two methodological problems to consider in this process, that of scaling the nominal output of MEXIPOP to the specific population numbers in the historical groups and that of defining the criteria for establishing a good "fit" of a simulation to a historical group.

Depopulation Ratio Scaling

The simulations in MEXIPOP begin with an initial population of 100,000 in 1500. Any figure could be used, of course (providing it reflected the correct initial age structure), but it is convenient to start with this nominal population. The output runs of MEXIPOP must then be scaled so that they are directly comparable with the historical reconstruction groups. Since virtually all the population figures for the historical reconstructions are based on mid-century data, it is advisable to scale the MEXIPOP simulations so that a given simulation run matches the population figure for the mid-century, "datum" population in the historical reconstruction. Unfortunately these datum dates (and their accompanying population estimates) vary so that in a single historical group (e.g., the severe group) there is no single date or population figure that serves as the basis for all the estimates. This problem does not arise for the mild group since it consists only of Cook and Simpson's estimates, and these are predominantly based on the estimate for 1565. Thus, the population at 1565 serves as the datum for scaling for the mild group.

To overcome this problem for the other groups, a best-fit line (and accompanying best-fit points for each date) is defined for each group by joining a series of best-fit lines separately determined for each segment of the whole. This is accomplished by calculating a best-fit line for historical estimates at pairs of dates. For example, the best-fit line between the 1518-1519 estimates and the 1532 estimates for the severe group is determined by using the 1518 and 1532 estimates of Slicher van Bath, the 1519 estimate of Borah and Cook, and the 1532 estimate of Cook and Borah (see Figure 3.2). This process proceeds until all the estimates for the entire group are approximated by a series of best-fit segments (e.g., see the series of segments for the severe group in Figure 3.2). Table 3.4 details the best-fit values and individual historical values for each group. In addition, the depopulation ratio (i.e., the proportion of the initial population remaining) at each date is calculated for the fitted values.

The population value calculated for each group's fitted line at a specified, "datum," date is then used to scale the simulations for that group. In the moderate case, this datum date is 1569 when the implied population is 343,018 (Figure 3.2). Similarly, for the severe group the datum date is 1568 when the population is 321,591 (Figure 3.2). For example, to fit the "Typhus 8W + baseline" simulation run to the mild group necessitates determining the ratio of the mild group historical value for 1565, 517,461, to the nominal simulation output at this date, 39,957, a value equal to 12.95. Multiplying every value of the simulation output by 12.95 will produce a scaled simulation output comparable with the historical values.[52] Refer to Table 3.9 for a summary of the simulation fitting procedure.

Comparison Criteria

Scaling the simulation output allows comparison, but does not specify the precision to which simulations are to be mated with their matching historical group estimates. It is futile to attempt an optimal solution, that is, to create a simulation that exactly matches each historical group estimate at each date (i.e., that matches the best-fit estimates that result from the fitted line for each historical group). The best that can be accomplished is to

---

[52] In the analysis that follows, "actual" (i.e., scaled) population figures will be used to describe the simulation outputs—not the nominal figures used earlier in the chapter to describe the effects of various variables.

search for a "non-inferior" solution such that no other reasonable solution improves the fit of the simulation to the historical reconstruction.[53]

TABLE 3.9 SIMULATION FITTING PROCEDURE

(1) Calculate segmented best-fit line for each historical reconstruction group.

(2) Use mid-century datum date population value for each historical reconstruction group to scale simulation. Symbolically: Scaled Simulation Value $_{t\,=\,i}$ = {Historical Reconstruction Population Value datum / Simulation Value datum} * Simulation Value $_{t\,=\,i}$

(3) Calculate the sum of absolute deviations for each scaled simulation for each value in each historical group. Rank, according to their deviation, the scaled simulations for each historical group.

(4) Select the 6 standard scaled simulations with the smallest summed deviations to compare with +/- 25 % uncertainty bands around best-fit historical reconstruction values.

(5) Select the best simulation (as determined from steps 3 & 4) for each historical group.

(6) Fine tune resulting standard scaled simulations using differing assumptions regarding migration, synergy, casualty, and tribute values to obtain a better fit.

Fundamentally, measuring the fit of a simulation to the historical data involves ranking simulations using "metrics" that measure the "distance" of the simulation value to the historical reconstruction value at each relevant date. However, all such rankings involve tradeoffs. Ranking simulations using a single distance metric (e.g., by choosing the minimum of the sum of the absolute value of the deviations at each point) may give rise to a simulation with a good fit at most points, but a very poor fit at a single date of interest. Thus the "shape" of the simulation will not correspond well to that of the historical reconstruction. Conversely, using a criteria that rejects simulations that fall outside specified uncertainty bounds may give rise to a simulation that has a "good shape" but is not all that close a fit at any date. Further, such a criteria does not help in choosing among multiple simulations that satisfy the uncertainty bounds criteria. For these reasons, a dual criteria (using both methods) is employed here to judge the fit of a simulation to its historical reconstruction.

This dual approach necessitates choosing appropriate "distance" measurements. All methods that measure the distance of a proposed "solution" from the desired value weight the distances the deviations fall from the desired value. For example, a commonly used definition of distance (in this case a second-order metric) weights the deviations

---

[53] Jared L. Cohon, *Multiobjective Programming and Planning*, New York: Academic Press, 1978, p. 69.

according to the square of their distance from the desired point. Employing a criteria that rejects simulations if any of their points fall outside established uncertainty bounds, is equivalent to using a distance metric of an infinite order because values that fall outside the authorized range are given infinite weight.[54] Similarly, using a criteria that ranks simulations by the minimum of the sum of their absolute deviations[55] is equivalent to using a first-order distance metric since only the absolute values of the deviations are used (rather than using the squared values as in a second-order metric).[56] Since all distance measuring metrics fall between these extremes, this last pair (the first-order, sum of absolute values of deviations and, the infinite-order, absolute uncertainty bounds) are appropriate choices.[57]

In particular, the use of the sum of absolute values of deviations (hereafter, Σ abs dev) to measure the fit of a simulation (the first-order metric) is preferable to using higher order metrics since, in this case, the historical data consists of values that have declining values at subsequent dates. A second-order (or higher order) metric would emphasize the importance of fit at earlier dates verses later dates, since the target values at the earlier dates are larger.[58] This biasing is not entirely undesirable, however, since the values for the eve-of-the-conquest values are of more interest (and are more controversial) than the later values.

Zambardino's criticism of the "Berkeley school" estimates provides an initial set of guidelines to determine a reasonable figure for the confidence limits of the uncertainty bounds.[59] Essentially, he multiplies an assumed uncertainty for each step in the calculation of a population estimate to produce a total uncertainty for the resulting estimate.[60] Hence, estimates that involve more steps, usually those "farthest" from the datum, have the greatest uncertainty. He determines differing uncertainty ranges for the estimates at differing dates, ranging from +/- 15 percent to over +/- 80 percent.[61] These specific values only apply to Cook and Borah's method of estimation, however.[62] Taking Zambardino's figures as convenient extremes, uncertainty values of +/- 25 percent for each date are reasonable. Subsequent "fine-tuning" of the simulations may allow choosing simulations that simultaneously satisfy the +/- 25 percent criteria and

---

[54] Cohon, *Multiobjective Programming*, pp. 184-185.

[55] Symbolically, this is given by the expression: min { $\Sigma_{i=1}$ [|deviation$_i$|]}.

[56] Cohon, *Multiobjective Programming*, pp. 184-185.

[57] Cohon, *Multiobjective Programming*, p. 185.

[58] This point notwithstanding, a first order metric also biases the ranking in favor of larger (in this case earlier) values, although not as much.

[59] Zambardino, "Mexico's Population."

[60] See Whitmore and Turner, *Population Reconstruction of the Basin of Mexico*, pp. 24-25, for a fuller discussion.

[61] Zambardino, "Mexico's Population."

[62] Cook and Borah, *The Indian Population of Central Mexico*.

TABLE 3.10 STANDARD SIMULATIONS RANKED BY SUMS OF ABSOLUTE DEVIATIONS

Mild Group		Moderate Group		Severe Group	
T 8W+ Baseline	306,092	P 3W+ Baseline	389,844	P 3Wzpg syn = 0.5	1,523,848
T 8Wzpg Baseline	332,729	T 8W+ syn = 0.5	415,434	P 3W+ syn = 0.5	1,889,128
T 3W+ Baseline	364,116	P 3Wzpg Baseline	428,256	T 3Wzpg syn = 0.5	1,921,249
P 8W+ Baseline	574,727	P 8W+ syn = 0.5	460,376	T 3W+ syn = 0.5	2,231,780
T 3Wzpg Baseline	594,491	T 8Wzpg syn = 0.5	473,529	P 8Wzpg syn = 0.5	2,585,861
P 8Wzpg Baseline	692,547	P 8Wzpg Baseline	489,822	P 8W+ syn = 0.5	2,811,978
P 3W+ Baseline	801,459	P 8Wzpg syn = 0.5	544,121	T 8Wzpg syn = 0.5	2,916,564
T 8W+ syn = 0.5	832,677	T 3Wzpg Baseline	551,898	P 3Wzpg Baseline	3,034,302
T 8Wzpg syn = 0.5	992,132	P 8W+ Baseline	578,956	T 8W+ syn = 0.5	3,123,703
P 3Wzpg Baseline	1,131,452	T 3W+ Baseline	785,941	P 3W+ Baseline	3,282,266
P 8W+ syn = 0.5	1,213,959	T 3W+ syn = 0.5	793,772	P 8Wzpg Baseline	3,378,815
P 8Wzpg syn = 0.5	1,460,917	T 8Wzpg Baseline	852,014	T 3Wzpg Baseline	3,435,496
T 3W+ syn = 0.5	1,596,180	T 8W+ Baseline	923,831	P 8W+ Baseline	3,461,923
T 3Wzpg syn = 0.5	1,951,558	T 3Wzpg syn = 0.5	1,079,641	T 3W+ Baseline	3,652,069
P 3W+ syn = 0.5	2,068,437	P 3W+ syn = 0.5	1,125,104	T 8Wzpg Baseline	3,714,666
P 3Wzpg syn = 0.5	2,465,001	P 3Wzpg syn = 0.5	1,489,913	T 8W+ Baseline	3,780,851

KEY: (see text for more complete descriptions/definitions)

"T" => typhus epidemic sub-model

"P" => pneumonic plague sub-model

"8W zpg" => 8 west demographic sub-model, zero growth

"8W +" => 8 west demographic model, 0.1% growth

"3W zpg" => 3 west demographic sub-model, zero growth

"3W +" => 3 west demographic model, 0.1% growth

"Baseline"=> agricultural-epidemic synergy = 0.2

"Syn = 0.5" => agricultural-epidemic synergy = 0.5

minimize sum of absolute deviation from the historical groups. The basic procedure is summarized in Table 3.9.

MILD GROUP

Best Standard Fit
Table 3.10 shows the standard simulations scaled for the mild group, and arranged in rank order by the sum of their absolute deviations. Unfortunately, none of these produce estimates that fall within the +/- 25 percent bounds at all of the relevant mild group dates (Table 3.11). Even though it exceeds the target for 1597, the best of this group is the simulation, T 8W+ Baseline (Figure 3.12). [63]

TABLE 3.11 MILD GROUP SIMULATION ANALYSIS

	Percentage of Mild Group value at Date *				
SIMULATION MODEL	1519	1540	1565	1597	Σ ABS DEV
T 8W+ syn = 0.0 LT = 0.2**	111	98	100	115	203,872
T 8W + syn = 0.0	111	98	100	*141*	295,919
T 8W + syn = 0.1	112	98	100	*141*	299,796
T 8W + Baseline	113	99	100	*139*	306,092
T 8W + syn = 0 LT = .05	115	100	100	*138*	320,488
T 8W + syn = 0.3	115	101	100	*137*	336,075
T 8W + syn = 0 war =.05	119	101	100	*135*	373,184
T 8W + syn = 0 E migr =.02	120	101	100	*133*	377,232
T 8W+ syn = .2 War = .05	121	102	100	*134*	407,548
T 8W+ syn = .2 E migr = .02	122	103	100	*131*	411,918
T 8W+ syn = .2 LT = .1	*127*	107	100	*129*	505,400

* Italic type indicates a value outside +/- 25 % limits
** Labor tribute; initiated only after 1565

KEY: (see text for more complete descriptions/definitions)
    "T" => typhus epidemic sub-model
    "P" => pneumonic plague sub-model
    "8W zpg" => 8 west demographic sub-model, zero growth
    "8W +" => 8 west demographic model, 0.1% growth
    "3W zpg" => 3 west demographic sub-model, zero growth
    "3W +" => 3 west demographic model, 0.1% growth
    "Baseline" => agricultural-epidemic synergy = 0.2
    "Syn = 0.5" => agricultural-epidemic synergy = 0.5
    "E migr" => epidemic-induced migration rate.
    "LT => Labor tribute rate

---

[63] See above and Table 3.11 for a guide to the interpretation of this coding.

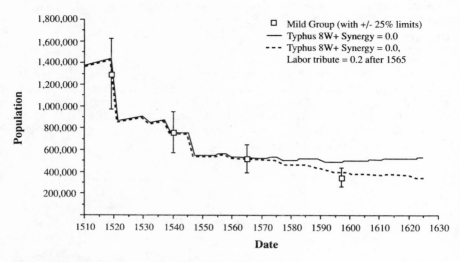

Figure 3.12 Mild Group and Candidate Simulations

Alterations to Best Standard Fit

Only modification of the best-fitting standard simulation will be undertaken in an attempt to improve the fit. There is a potential problem in this methodology, however, since it does not exhaust all the possible combinations that might produce acceptable results. To do so would demand alteration of all 16 standard simulations using each of the four basic types of modifications (i.e., changed synergy, labor tribute, war casualty, and epidemic emigration) for each historical group. A minimum of 384 additional runs (for all three historical groups) would be necessary in that case. This effort is surely futile for the vast majority of the possible combinations. Furthermore, an examination of Table 3.10 shows that the chance of producing an acceptable fit for most of the unused alternative standard runs is small since their closeness to the desired historical pattern is so poor (i.e., their Σ abs dev are so large so as to preclude success). Additionally, for the standard runs that are generally similar to the best fitting ones (i.e., ranked among the top in lowest Σ abs dev), the results of their modification is likely to be quite similar to the result of modifying the best choice. So while completeness argues for this expanded effort, reason suggests that very few—if any—possible solutions are discarded in using the less arduous procedure (i.e., modifying only the best standard simulation in an attempt to produce a better fit).

To attempt to produce a simulation that better mimics the historical data involves the systematic alteration of key variables one-at-a-time and comparing the resulting simulations with the historical data goal. This process will be most complete if, at first, each of the modifications is attempted on the base simulation (i.e., standard simulation that emerged best in the first round of comparisons). Subsequent rounds of experimentation using the best new (i.e., modified) simulations to emerge from the previous rounds of fine tuning will also be conducted. This multistage, "round robin" approach improves the possibility of obtaining the best quality fit.

It is reasonable to begin this process with the important agriculture-epidemic synergy variable (synergy). Since the best-fitting standard simulation assumes a synergy of 0.2, a trial with synergy = 0.3 is a good first choice. This simulation (T 8W+ syn = 0.3) also fails to meet the +/- 25 percent criteria for 1597 and has a higher sum of absolute deviations as well (Table 3.11). Changing the synergy value in the opposite direction, to synergy = 0.1, has the more positive effect of reducing the Σ abs dev, but the value for 1597 still exceeds the +/- 25 percent limit. Further reduction of synergy to 0.0 results in an even smaller Σ abs dev, but the end-of-century value is still stubbornly high (Table 3.11 and Figure 3.12). Since no further reduction in the synergy variable is possible, synergy = 0.0 is the best choice for this variable.

Again using the best fitting standard simulation, T 8W+ syn = 0.2, a better fit was attempted using a labor tribute of 0.1. The fit resulting from this simulation both worsened the +/- 25% fit (it exceeded the bounds at both 1519 and 1597) and increased the Σ abs dev so it was rejected (Table 3.11). The standard simulation, without this modification, is a better choice.

Using an assumption of war casualties equal to 5% in 1520 also failed to improve the fit of the standard simulation. The resulting plot did not improve the +/- 25% fit and worsened the Σ abs dev figure (Table 3.11). Thus, the standard simulation is a better choice than this modification.

Modifying the standard simulation by assuming that there was epidemic induced emigration of 2% in 1520, 1531, 1546, and 1576 also resulted in a poorer fit than the standard simulation. These trials indicate that no modification of the standard simulation, save that of synergy, results in a better fit. A further round of trials using the synergy = 0.0 version is now indicated.

Fine Tuning

It may be possible to achieve a better fit for the best-fitting simulation from above (T 8W+ syn = 0.0) if a labor tribute is assumed for the entire period. Utilizing an assumption of a 5 percent labor tribute does not significantly improve the fit at 1597, and results in a higher Σ abs dev (Table 3.11). Since additional labor tribute will not improve the fit, the best choice for this variable is zero.

Unlike the every-year effect of labor tribute, casualties in the war of conquest in 1520 will have a large initial effect and a small, but noticeable effect subsequently. Adding a 5 percent adult (aged 15-60) war casualty figure to the best-fitting simulation (T 8W+ syn = 0.0 war = 0.05) still does not resolve the problem of fit at 1597, and results in a higher $\sum$ abs dev. Since this alteration provides no improvement in fit, it is also rejected.

Another possible fine-tuning involves the use of migration. It is reasonable to postulate emigration occurring in the years of most severe epidemics (1520, 1531, 1546, and 1576). If an emigration of 2 percent of the entire population is assumed for these dates and combined with the best-fit simulation already determined, an even less satisfactory fit results (Table 3.11).

Since the simulation only fails to fit within the +/- 25 percent criteria at the last date, 1595, a modification that results in a reduced simulation population figures for the post-1565 period is indicated. Altering the labor tribute variable so that there is a 20 percent withdrawal of labor initiated *after* 1565, results in a simulation that does meet the +/- 25 percent criteria and also exhibits a minimum $\sum$ abs dev (Table 3.11 and Figure 3.12).

Figure 3.12 displays both the best fitting simulation, T 8W+ syn = 0.0 LT = 0.2 after 1565, and the initial, approximate, best fitting standard simulation, T 8W+ syn = 0.0, along with the mild group data.

This best-fitting simulation describes a situation in which the pre-conquest Basin is inhabited by a relatively healthy, growing population (the 8W + assumption). This population retains its propensity for growth in the years without severe crises as well. The crises that afflict this population, while severe by any measure, are essentially epidemic-only crises. This is because the agriculture-epidemic synergy level is set at 0.0. Each epidemic carries its own additional level of mortality, but there is no loss of agricultural production due to these epidemics so there is no accompanying famine mortality. Further, there is an imposition of crippling labor withdrawal after 1565 that depresses the agricultural productivity and, hence, population's growth.

MODERATE GROUP

Best Standard Fit

Unlike the situation obtaining for the mild group, two of the standard simulations, P 8W+ syn = 0.5 and T 8W zpg syn = 0.5, produced trajectories that fell within the +/- 25 % uncertainty bounds (Table 3.12 and Figure 3.13). While these runs are well ranked (fifth and sixth) according to the minimum of absolute deviations, they are not the top ranked ones (Table 3.10). Nevertheless, the criteria established above requires that to be selected, individual runs generate values that fall within the +/- 25 % limits. Since P 8W+ syn = 0.5 simulation run produced a somewhat smaller $\sum$ abs dev, it is preferred (Table 3.12).

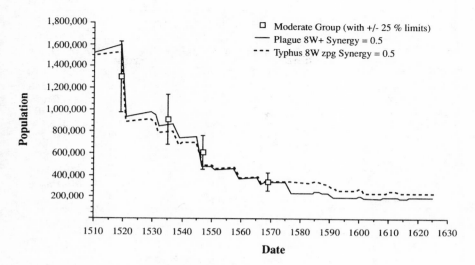

Figure 3.13 Moderate Group and Candidate Simulations

Alterations to Best Standard Fit

Beginning again with the synergy variable, the best standard run for the moderate group, P 8W+ syn = 0.5, utilizes a synergy value of 0.5. That a higher synergy value is inappropriate is demonstrated by the results of a trial in which synergy is set to 0.6 (Table 3.12). The very wide deviations generated by this run show that a synergy value of less than 0.6 is appropriate. Altering the synergy in the opposite direction, to syn = 0.4, also produces values that violate the +/- 25% limit (Table 3.12). Hence, the best value for synergy in this case is between 0.4 and 0.6, and a value of 0.5 will be utilized.

As in the mild case, increasing the labor tribute from its standard value of 0.0 to 0.1, produces simulation values that greatly exceed the +/- 25% limits as well (Table 3.12). This result implies that the standard value, 0.0, should be used.

A similar recalculation that sets initial (1520) adult war casualties at 5% produces simulation values that are much closer than those produced with the labor tribute variable, but overshoots the +25% bounds in 1519. Any larger assumption of war casualty will produce even larger deviations, so the standard assumption of 0.0 must be used.

The last relevant modification to the best standard run assumes epidemic induced emigration. Setting this value equal to 2% of the total population in 1520, 1531, 1546, and 1576 produces a run with values generally similar to that for the war casualty variable (Table 3.12). Unfortunately, this alteration fails to improve the fit of the standard

TABLE 3.12 MODERATE GROUP SIMULATION ANALYSIS

SIMULATION MODEL (KEY *)	Percentage of Moderate Group Value at Date*				
	1519	1535	1547	1569	Σ ABS DEV
P 8W + syn = 0.5	122	94	81	100	460,376
T 8W zpg syn = 0.5	118	88	79	100	473,529
P 8W + syn = 0.4	97	81	*70*	100	394,100
T 8W + syn = 0.5	107	82	*74*	100	415,434
P 8W + syn = 0.5 war = .05	*131*	97	82	100	536,729
P 8W + syn = 0.5 E migr = .02	*132*	97	82	100	545,483
T 8W zpg syn = 0.4	87	*71*	*60*	100	639,914
P 8W + syn = 0.5 LT = 0.1	*334*	*189*	*156*	100	4,205,211
P 8W+ syn = 0.6	*843*	*339*	*227*	100	12,647,459

* Italic type indicates a value outside +/- 25 % limits.

KEY: (see text for more complete descriptions/definitions)
    "T" => typhus epidemic sub-model
    "P" => pneumonic plague sub-model
    "8W zpg" => 8 west demographic sub-model, zero growth
    "8W +" => 8 west demographic model, 0.1% growth
    "3W zpg" => 3 west demographic sub-model, zero growth
    "3W +" => 3 west demographic model, 0.1% growth
    "Baseline"=> agricultural-epidemic synergy = 0.2
    "Syn = 0.5" => agricultural-epidemic synergy = 0.5
    LT => labor tribute
    E migr => epidemic induced migration

simulation also since it overshoots the +25% limit at 1519. Since none of the these alterations improved the fit of the best-fitting standard simulation, P 8W+ syn = .5, it is the best choice for this case. This simulation and the second best fitting simulation (T 8W zpg synergy = 0.5) are displayed in Figure 3.13.

Like the mild case above, this simulation presumes a moderately healthy, growing population, that tends to continue to grow in the absence of crises (the 8W + demographic sub-model). Unlike the mild case, this simulation assumes that pneumonic plague and not typhus was the pathogen responsible for the severe epidemics of the late 1540s and 1570s. Also unlike the mild case, this simulation assumes that epidemics significantly interfered with agricultural production, thus inducing additional mortality through famine. In each epidemic year 50 percent of the households who had adults who were taken ill failed to gain a harvest. This synergy is not as powerful as it may appear at first, since for most of the minor epidemic years, the epidemic morbidity is concentrated among the youth and, as such, has no effect on agricultural production (see Chapter 2 for a discussion of the assumptions of the epidemic sub-model and Chapter 4 for a discussion of the effects of particular epidemics on famine mortality). This famine effect is most important in years where the morbidity is universal, and that would be expected.

TABLE 3.13 SEVERE GROUP SIMULATION ANALYSIS

SIMULATION MODEL	Percentage of Severe Group value at Date *								Σ ABS DEV
	1519	1532	1548	1568	1580	1595	1607	1625	
P 3W zpg syn = 0.5; E migr = .04	98	71	50	100	77	82	81	143	1,140,579
P 3W zpg syn = 0.5; E migr = .06	104	73	51	100	75	79	77	136	1,153,736
P 3W zpg syn = 0.5; war = 0.1	96	69	50	100	80	86	85	151	1,208,537
P 3W zpg syn = 0.5; war = 0.2	107	72	52	100	79	83	81	144	1,243,477
P 3W zpg syn = 0.5; E migr = 0.2	92	69	50	100	79	85	84	150	1,339,849
P 3W zpg syn = 0.5; war = .05	91	68	50	100	81	87	86	154	1,373,017
P 3W zpg syn = 0.5	86	67	49	100	81	88	87	157	1,523,848
P 3W zpg syn = 0.4; war = 0.1	65	53	39	100	80	104	112	206	2,465,271
P 3Wz syn = 0.5; war = 0.1; Emigr = 0.02	60	50	36	100	77	106	118	218	2,680,921
P 3W zpg syn = 0.2; L T = 0.1	57	51	37	100	79	106	115	204	2,722,061
P 3W zpg syn = 0.4	57	51	38	100	81	107	117	216	2,736,218
P 3Wz syn = 0.5; E migr= 0.04; LT = 0.1	189	113	80	100	77	58	48	76	2,877,588
P 3Wzpg syn = 0.4; E migr = 0.04	54	47	35	100	79	108	119	228	2,896,674
P 3W zpg syn = 0.5; L T = 0.1	276	145	102	100	79	43	33	49	5,584,545
P 3Wz syn = 0.5; war = 0.1; LT = 0.1	289	146	101	100	78	42	32	47	5,931,815
P 3W zpg syn = 0.6	1124	298	214	100	77	15	6	2	32,614,384

* Italic type indicates a value outside +/- 25 % limits.

KEY: (see text for more complete descriptions/definitions)

"T" - typhus epidemic sub-model

"P" - pneumonic plague sub-model

"8W zpg" - 8 west demographic sub-model, zero growth

"8W +" - 8 west demographic model, 0.1% growth

"3W zpg" - 3 west demographic sub-model, zero growth

"3W +" - 3 west demographic model, 0.1% growth

"Baseline" - agricultural-epidemic synergy = 0.2

"LT = x" - labor tribute = (100*x) %

"Syn = x" - agricultural-epidemic synergy = x

"War = x" - adult war casulities (1520) = (100*x) % of adults

"E migr = x" - emmigration in severe epidemic years = (100*x) % of total population

SEVERE GROUP

Best Standard Fit

As with all the others in this case, the simulation run with the smallest Σ abs dev (P 3W zpg syn = .5) fails to generate values that fall within the +/- 25% bounds around the historical values (Tables 3.10 and 3.13). Indeed, this run generates values that fail this criteria at three dates, 1532, 1548, and 1625 (Table 3.13 and Figure 3.14). This points to the need to alter this, best fitting, simulation to attempt a better fit.

Alterations to Best Standard Fit

Since the best-fitting standard run generated values that were rather low for the initial years, the first choice in altering the synergy variable would be to increase it from 0.5 to 0.6 in an effort to raise the values. Examination of Table 3.13 indicates that this procedure raised the early-century values—but far more than desired. This alteration failed to bring values to within the +/- 25% limits and vastly increased the Σ abs dev values (Table 3.13). Similarly, altering the synergy level to 0.4 so reduced values that they also remained outside the +/- 25% range and increased the Σ abs dev over the standard value as well (Table 3.13). We are left with synergy = 0.5 as the best value.

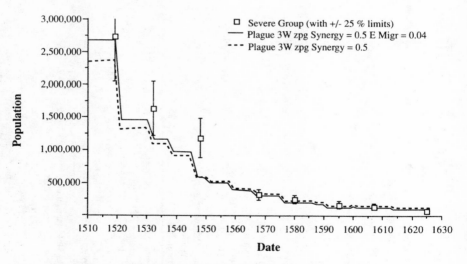

Figure 3.14 Severe Group and Candidate Simulations

Increasing the labor tribute variable from 0.0 to 0.1 also has the effect of increasing the Σ abs dev over the value produced by the standard simulation (P 3W zpg syn = .5), and failed to bring the simulation values to within the desired range. Thus, the standard value for labor tribute, 0.0 emerged as superior.

Altering the war casualty rate from 0.0 to 5% (in 1520) reversed the trend towards increasing Σ abs dev (Table 3.13). This change did not move more values to the +/- 25% limits, but it did reduce the Σ abs dev over the standard simulation (Table 3.13). Increasing the war casualty rate to 10% also improved the Σ abs dev fit, but failed to pull values to within the +/- 25% range (Table 3.13). A third trial in which war casualty was set equal to 20% resulted in an increased Σ abs dev from the previous trial (Table 3.13). This indicates that a value for war casualty of 10% is the best choice for this variable.

Modifying the best standard simulation (P 3W zpg syn = .5) so that epidemic emigration is raised from its 0.0 standard value to 2% resulted in a run in which the Σ abs dev was reduced, but the +/- 25% limit criteria was still not met (Table 3.13). Similarly, raising the emigration value to 4% also resulted in a decreased Σ abs dev (Table 3.13). Since a third trial using a value of 6% for emigration produced an increased Σ abs dev, the best value for this variable is 4% (Table 3.13).

Fine Tuning

Unlike the limited success enjoyed in the mild and moderate cases, initial alterations of the best standard fit in this case produced real gains in the quality of fit. Since none of these changes resulted in a simulation that satisfied the +/- 25% criteria (and for completeness), further trials using the standard simulation as modified by war casualty (P 3W zpg syn = 0.5 war = 0.1) are warranted. Beginning with the synergy variable, we can rule out any value greater than 0.5 since it was demonstrated above that such values drive the system to extremes (see the last entry in Table 3.13). A trial with synergy = 0.4 resulted in values that were a poorer fit than at synergy = 0.5 (Table 3.13). Hence, the standard synergy value is the best choice here.

Assuming a value of 10% for labor tribute, and again using the modified simulation, P 3W zpg syn = 0.5 war = 0.1, results in a run that greatly misses the +/- 25% limits and also has a higher Σ abs dev. The standard value for labor tribute, 0.0, it is preferred to this modification.

Again using the modified standard simulation, a run adding an epidemic induced emigration of 2% resulted in a higher Σ abs dev (Table 3.13). This indicates that no modification of the P 3W zpg syn = 0.5 war = 0.1 simulation resulted in an improvement in fit. There remains, however, the possibility that modifications to the simulation P 3W zpg syn = 0.5 E migr = 0.4 may result in an even better fit.

The first choice of modifications here is to the synergy variable. Assuming a synergy value of 0.4 (resulting in a simulation characterized as P 3W zpg syn = 0.4 E migr = 0.4) led to a run in which both goodness-of-fit criteria were worsened (Table 3.13). Hence, the 0.5 value is preferred.

The last possible modification of this, already modified standard simulation (P 3W zpg syn = 0.5 E migr = 0.4), is to assume a labor tribute was extracted. Using a labor tribute value of 0.1 resulted in values that increased the Σ abs dev, however.

150

To summarize this complex procedure; initial modifications to the best-fit standard simulation (P 3W zpg syn = 0.5) resulted in two modified simulations that improved on its fit, one utilizing epidemic migration (P 3W zpg syn = 0.5 E migr = 0.4) and another utilizing war casualties (P 3W zpg syn = 0.5 war = 0.1). Modifications to these "new standards" resulted in no improvement. Thus, the best fitting simulation found for this case is the P 3W zpg syn = 0.5 E migr = 0.4 simulation (see Table 3.13). This simulation and the initial, approximate, best fit simulation, P 3W zpg synergy = 0.5, are plotted in Figure 3.14.

This severe case shares little with its mild and moderate peers. The initial (pre-conquest) demographic assumption is of a population with a relatively high mortality and virtually no growth. Like the moderate simulation, the severe simulation assumes the plague epidemic sub-model and a 50 percent synergy rate. In addition, this simulation posits a emigration (or homicide) rate of 4 percent (across all ages of the population) in the severe epidemic years of 1520, 1531, 1546, and 1576.

Summary

The techniques detailed in this chapter form the essential bridge between the individual, historical population estimates that are to be examined and the MEXIPOP population simulations. These techniques consist of three relatively independent procedures. The first identifies and quantifies Basin population estimates. Using these estimates, the individual estimates are arranged into groups that reflect a similar set of assumptions about the sixteenth-century depopulation. These grouped estimates are then generalized by a single fitted line that closely captures the sense of the group. The result of this process is to create three cases ("mild, "moderate," and "severe"), reflecting differing levels of implied depopulation.

The second process necessitates creating a simulation run that can closely "mimic" the population dynamics of one of the grouped historical reconstructions. To reduce the possible number of simulation runs needed to produce a result close to an historical case, a group of assumptions that detail the "baseline" assumptions were developed. This simplification produced 16 "standard" simulation candidates. To allow for "fine tuning" of these 16, a group of "mitigating" or "escalating" variables were also identified.

The last process involves scaling the simulation runs and "fitting" them to historical reconstruction cases. Since the MEXIPOP simulations are all run with nominal 100,000 initial populations, it is necessary to scale the simulations to be directly comparable with the historical reconstruction groups. This is done using the mid-century (1560s) historical estimate for each case as the datum from which to scale the comparable simulation value at that date. Once scaled, simulation population trajectories are compared with each historical population trajectory. The criteria for choosing the best fitting simulation trajectories are two-fold: the minimum of the sum of the absolute deviations, provided that the simulation values were within a +/- 25 percent envelope bracketing the historical figures.

Applying this complex series of processes resulted in different simulations that satisfied both criteria for the "mild" and "moderate" historical cases. No simulation tested satisfied the +/- 25 percent criteria for the "severe" group, however.

Chapter 4

INTERPRETATIONS

In the previous chapter, MEXIPOP simulations were matched to corresponding historical population reconstruction groups. It is now possible to compare these simulations, to interpret the data implicit in them, and to choose among them. These exercises should illuminate the cultural ecological and demographic patterns of the sixteenth-century Basin and facilitate assessment of the relative accuracy of each simulation. To accomplish these ends, this chapter is organized in six parts. The first discusses general comparative data on population dynamics among the three cases. The second "goes behind" the population numbers and examines the role of different causal forces that shaped the pattern of overall population change. The third section uses the information developed in the previous two sections to choose one of the simulation cases as the most probable simulation of the sixteenth-century Basin Amerindian population trajectory. The fourth section examines temporal patterns of basic demographic measures and population composition implied by the simulations, and comments on the importance of these measures in understanding the demography and cultural ecology of the sixteenth-century Basin. The fifth section discusses some implications of the temporal patterns of population decline and other demographic measures for historical reconstructions, and the major findings are summarized in the last section.

Population Dynamics Compared

To compare the population dynamics among the historical groups it is first necessary to examine the implied scale of population loss implied by their matching simulations. Emphasis is given to the scales of depopulation between selected dates within the century, since it is for these decadal or "generational" periods that the true impact of the population loss is best understood. After each group's historical and simulation depopulation figures are examined, they will be compared against each other.

TABLE 4.1 SIMULATION–HISTORICAL COMPARISONS

	Mild Group				Moderate Group				Severe Group			
	HISTORICAL		SIMULATION		HISTORICAL		SIMULATION		HISTORICAL		SIMULATION	
Date	Fitted Line	% of initial (a)	Mild Simulation (b)	% of initial (a)	Fitted Line	% of initial (a)	Moderate Simulation (c)	% of initial (a)	Fitted Line	% of initial (a)	Severe Simulation (d)	% of initial (a)
1519	1,293,652	100.00	1,271,095	100.00	1,304,390	100.00	1,590,768	100.00	2,736,594	100.00	2,701,153	100.00
1532	—	—	—	—	—	—	—	—	1,639,557	59.91	1,161,054	42.98
1535	—	—	—	—	912,068	69.92	865,951	54.44	—	—	—	—
1540	755,493	58.40	738,397	58.09	—	—	—	—	—	—	—	—
1547	—	—	—	—	611,788	46.90	492,906	30.99	—	—	—	—
1548	—	—	533,092	41.94	—	—	—	—	1,191,634	43.54	597,795	22.13
1565	517,461	40.00	517,461	40.71	—	—	—	—	—	—	—	—
1568	—	—	—	—	343,018	26.30	—	—	321,591	11.75	321,951	11.92
1569	—	—	—	—	—	—	343,018	21.56	—	—	—	—
1580	—	—	455,457	35.83	—	—	230,630	14.50	252,962	9.24	193,932	7.18
1595	—	—	—	—	—	—	193,299	12.15	161,804	5.91	132,887	4.92
1597	346,698	26.80	397,455	31.27	—	—	—	—	—	—	—	—
1607	—	—	376,957	29.66	—	—	183,033	11.51	141,182	5.16	113,719	4.21
1625	—	—	337,739	26.57	—	—	195,618	12.30	73,314	2.68	104,715	3.88

(a) Percentage of initial population remaining at date
(b) Typhus, 8W+, synergy = 0.0, labor tribute = 0.2 after 1565
(c) Plague, 8w+, synergy = 0.5
(d) Plague, 3W zpg, synergy = 0.5, emigration = 0.04

MILD GROUP

As noted in Chapter 3, a good fit was obtained between the fitted line defining the mild group of historical estimates and the mild group simulation. Indeed, no simulation value differed from the corresponding mild group value by more than 15 percent (Table 3.11). This good fit is reflected in the figures showing a close congruence between the scale of depopulation implied by the mild group historical estimates (at the dates of historical estimation) and their matching simulation estimates (Table 4.1).[1]

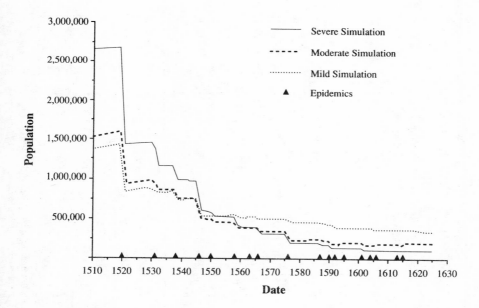

Figure 4.1 Simulations Compared

The "mild" label is a misnomer for the pattern of depopulation implied in this case (Figure 4.1). The total population calculated in the mild simulation for 1625, after the first 100 years of Spanish occupance in the Basin, totals about 25 percent of the pre-contact total (Tables 4.1 and 4.2), representing, at minimum, a loss of three persons in every household of four. But this statistic alone, grim as it is, obscures the more tragic experience of the Basin peoples.

---

[1] In Table 4.1 simulation estimates are displayed for dates in each of the general "decades" for which historical population estimates are made for the Basin (e.g., the dates 1532, 1535, 1540 all fall within a "decade" in this sense, as do the dates 1547 and 1548). This allows a better comparison between the historical groups since they differ in the range of their dates.

TABLE 4.2 RELATIVE LOSS RATES COMPARED

Mild Simulation

RELATIVE		AVERAGE	
Date	Population	% Loss (a)	Loss Rate (b)
1519	1,271,095	—	—
1540	738,397	41.91	2.59
1548	533,092	27.80	4.07
1565	517,461	2.93	0.18
1580	455,457	11.98	0.85
1597	397,455	12.73	0.80
1607	376,957	5.16	0.53
1625	337,739	10.40	0.61
1519	1,271,095	—	—
1625	337,739	73.43	1.25
1519	1,271,095	—	—
1565	517,461	59.29	1.95
1625	337,739	34.73	0.71

Moderate Simulation

RELATIVE		AVERAGE	
Date	Population	% Loss (a)	Loss Rate (b)
1519	1,590,768	—	—
1535	865,951	45.56	3.80
1547	492,906	43.08	4.70
1569	343,018	30.41	1.65
1580	230,630	32.76	3.61
1595	193,299	16.19	1.18
1607	183,033	5.31	0.45
1625	195,618	6.88	0.37
1519	1,590,768	—	—
1607	183,033	88.49	2.46
1519	1,590,768	—	—
1569	343,018	78.44	3.07
1607	183,033	46.64	1.65

Severe Simulation

RELATIVE		AVERAGE	
Date	Population	% Loss (a)	Loss Rate (b)
1519	2,673,062	—	—
1532	1,157,472	56.70	6.44
1548	596,673	48.45	4.14
1568	321,951	46.04	3.08
1580	194,214	39.68	4.21
1595	133,230	31.40	2.51
1607	114,104	14.36	1.29
1625	105,142	7.85	0.45
1519	2,673,062	—	—
1625	105,142	96.07	3.05
1519	2,673,062	—	—
1568	321,951	87.96	4.32
1625	105,142	67.34	1.96

(a) Relative % Loss = {1-(previous population/subsequent population)} * 100
(b) Average loss rate per year = [Ln (previous population/subsequent population)] / interval length; expressed as a percentage

In *each* of three periods in the sixteenth century (each more or less one generation in length, 1519-1540, 1540-1565, and 1565-1597), the Amerindian population of the Basin suffered proportional population losses approaching or exceeding the total proportional loss estimated for England in the "Black" fourteenth century. During the first of these periods, after the first two decades of Spanish occupation, the Basin's population was reduced to slightly less than 60 percent of its initial, 1.2 million level (Tables 4.1 and 4.2). This 40 percent loss is comparable to or larger than the loss rate experienced in a somewhat larger (4 to 6 million) English population during the "Black Death" bubonic plagues of the fourteenth century.[2] The mild case simulation indicates for the Basin that this loss was suffered in only 20 years, however.

A further 20 percent was lost in the second 25 year period from 1540 to 1565, so that only about 40 percent of the pre-conquest indigenous population total for the Basin would have been counted in the Spanish surveys of the 1560s (Tables 4.1 and 4.2). The loss in this period represents fully one-third of the 1540 population, however, and is thus comparable to England's entire fourteenth-century experience.

This pattern of "reduced" rates of population collapse was continued for the next 35 years, so that by the "turn of the century" (1597), the Amerindian population was reduced to about one-third of its pre-conquest total (Tables 4.1 and 4.2). While the population loss in this later period represented "only" about 10 percent of the 1519 total, it totaled about a 25 percent loss from 1565. The rate of loss for the next 30 years virtually stabilized, so that the 1625 total is scarcely different than the 1597 figure, indicating that the nadir of population probably occurred sometime after 1597—most likely in the early decades of the seventeenth century (Tables 4.1 and 4.2).

MODERATE GROUP

The best-fit moderate simulation matches the moderate case less closely than its counterpart does for the mild. Despite the fact that the moderate group historical estimates span only the first 50 years of Spanish occupance, the best fitting simulation generated values within 20 percent of the historical fitted line in only three of four dates, exceeding the 1519 value by 22 percent (Table 3.12). This less-precise fit explains the differences in the depopulation figures evident in Table 4.1 for the moderate group fitted line versus the moderate group simulation. Because of these differences, the discussion below notes both the historical reconstruction figures and the simulation results. Nevertheless, since the simulation satisfies the +/- 25 percent goodness-of-fit criteria established in Chapter 3 and since the same patterns of depopulation for the early century are evident in both cases (i.e., historical and simulation), the depopulation totals produced by this

---

2   McEvedy and Jones *Atlas*, p. 42; Russell, *British Medieval Population*, pp. 260-81; Slack, *Impact*, p. 15; and Hatcher, *Plague, Population and the English Economy*, p. 68.

simulation for dates later in the century are certainly reflective of the general pattern of depopulation established by the moderate group fitted line, and thus may be used confidently.

The total sixteenth-century depopulation calculated using the moderate simulation is greater than 85 percent: that is to say, the 1625 Basin Amerindian population was less than 15 percent of its 1519 total (Figure 4.1 and Tables 4.1 and 4.2). But even this figure pales if the rates of depopulation for decades within the century are considered. In this "moderate" case, the relative scale of depopulation in *each* of four periods (1519-1535, 1535-1547, 1547-1569, and 1569-1580—each less than 22 years in duration) exceeds 30 percent. Thus, in the first 60 years of Spanish colonial rule, the Basin experienced *four* traumatic depopulations, each roughly the scale of the total proportional loss in England's cataclysmic fourteenth century.[3]

The initial (1519-1535) depopulation implied by the historical fitted line, about 30 percent, is significantly smaller than that generated by the moderate simulation for the same period, about 45 percent (Table 4.1). These differences aside, these totals, spanning only 15 years, are comparable to the total proportional loss in fourteenth-century England.[4]

In the next decade or so (from 1535-1547), the Amerindian population suffered a similar proportional loss. The moderate simulation indicates that the Basin suffered a loss of about a 40 percent (relative to the 1535 figure) and an absolute loss to about 30 percent of the initial, 1519 total, while the historical fitted line indicates a smaller, 33 percent proportional loss to about 45 percent of the initial total (Tables 4.1 and 4.2).

Once again, in the years between 1547 and 1569 the simulation generates a population loss of about 30 percent relative to the 1547 total (to a total of only about 20 percent of the 1519 total), while the historical fitted line indicates an even larger proportional loss from 1547 of 44 percent (to a sum roughly equal to 25 percent of the 1519 sum) (Tables 4.1 and 4.2).

The simulation shows that a fourth loss, of about 33 percent (again similar in magnitude to that of fourteenth-century England's), occurred in the period from 1569 to 1580 (Tables 4.1 and 4.2). The rate of loss slowed in the next 27 years so that by 1607 the relative loss from 1580 was "only" 20 percent, although the total population was scarcely greater than 10 percent of the pre-Hispanic total (Tables 4.1 and 4.2). The last 20 years of the moderate simulation show slight population growth, indicating that the nadir of population was reached sometime between 1607 and 1625 (Tables 4.1 and 4.2).

---

[3] Hatcher, *Plague, Population and the English Economy*, p. 68; McEvedy and Jones, *Atlas*, p. 42; Russell, *British Medieval Populations*, pp. 260-81; and Slack, *Impact*, p. 15.

[4] Hatcher, *Plague, Population and the English Economy*, p. 68; McEvedy and Jones, *Atlas*, p. 42; Russell, *British Medieval Populations*, pp. 260-81; and Slack, *Impact*, p. 15.

SEVERE GROUP

The shape of the population trajectory implied by the severe group's fitted line is not a close fit with the severe simulation trajectory, especially for the first half of the century (Figure 3.14). Accordingly, the scale of depopulation, especially for the early part of the sixteenth century, implied by the severe historical fitted line and the severe simulation differ. Since, as is noted below and in Chapter 5, there is reason to doubt the early figures of this historical group, I will separate the discussion of depopulation implied by the historical date from that generated by the simulation.

The historical fitted line implies a quite severe overall depopulation of about 97 percent from 1519 to 1625 (Figure 4.1 and Table 4.1). Unlike the more uniform pattern noted above for the mild and moderate cases, the rates of population loss between dates are quite variable for the severe historical fitted line. In the 13 years between 1519 and 1532, a 40 percent loss, is indicated (Table 4.1). A much smaller loss of about 27 percent is implied for the next period from 1532 to 1548 (Table 4.1). This loss, nevertheless, leads to a population in 1548 that is only slightly above 40 percent of the 1519 total. The relatively small loss in the 1532-1548 period is followed by a profound collapse of 73 percent from 1548 to the datum date of 1568, where a scant 12 percent of the initial (1519) population total remains (Table 4.1). Relatively speaking, the population loss in the next period, 1568-1580, is again small, 21 percent, but implies that the population sank to a total of less than 10 percent of its pre-conquest high (Table 4.1). While the population totals are quite small proportionally (relative to the pre-conquest totals), the rate of loss in the next 15 years is again large, 36 percent (Table 4.1). Similarly, the loss in the last 30 years is proportionally large, 55 percent from 1595, but the totals are very small, reaching only about 3 percent of the 1519 total in 1625.

The severe simulation generates a more regular, if not less catastrophic, pattern of depopulation than does the severe historical fitted line. In *each* of the less than 20 year-long first four periods (i.e., 1519-1532, 1532-1548, 1548-1568, and 1568-1580) this simulation returns a depopulation of greater than 40 percent (compare with the 30 percent depopulation implied for each similar period in the moderate case noted above). For the initial 13 years, the population plummeted to a scant 43 percent of its initial total, a loss of greater than 56 percent (Tables 4.1 and 4.2). This catastrophic loss was almost matched in the next period, from 1532 to 1548, where the population fell to only 22 percent of its initial value, a relative loss of 49 percent from 1532 (Tables 4.1 and 4.2). Again, from 1548 to 1568 the simulated population declined by 46 percent to a total equal to only 12 percent of the large 1519 sum (Tables 4.1 and 4.2). A fourth loss of 40 percent for the 12 year period from 1568 to 1580 results in a 1580 total of less than 8 percent of the initial (Tables 4.1 and 4.2). The next 15 year period, 1580 to 1595, witnessed a loss of "only" 31 percent, reaching a total of less than 5 percent of the pre-conquest value (Tables 4.1 and 4.2). The rate of depopulation slowed, at last, for the final 30 years of this period to "only" 21 percent.

SIMULATIONS COMPARED

A plot of the simulation trajectories, while generally similar to a plot of historical fitted lines, shows a good deal more detailed variation (cf. Figure 4.1 and Figure 3.2). This variation, moreover, is relatively regular for the simulations, since they all are based on the same dates for epidemics and adverse agricultural conditions. The "stair-step" quality of depopulation common to each of the simulations is one of their few similarity, however.

Perhaps the most obvious difference among the simulations lies in their overall depopulation. The mild simulation returns an overall depopulation of nearly 75 percent (i.e., the nadir population is scarcely 25 percent of the 1519 zenith population total) (Table 4.2). This figure is large by any measure for such a large population—except in comparison with the moderate and severe cases. The moderate simulation produces an overall depopulation of nearly 90 percent at its 1607 nadir (Table 4.2). Even this is exceeded by the total depopulation for the severe case (reached at the 1625 nadir), which exceeds 95 percent (Table 4.2). By way of comparison, the total depopulation figures estimated for England in the fourteenth century ranged from 33 to 50 percent.[5]

Further, the severe case's *rate* of depopulation outstrips that of the mild and moderate cases. The total depopulation of the mild case, 75 percent, is reached by the severe case in less than 30 years (1519-1548), and the total depopulation of the moderate case, nearly 90 percent, is reached in only 49 years (1519-1568) in the severe scenario. The moderate case's rate also exceeds the mild case, since it returns a depopulation of roughly 75 percent in only 50 years (1519-1569) as compared to the 106 years (1519-1625) necessary for such a loss in the mild case.

If the Basin's simulated population losses are expressed as average annual decline rates, the comparison is even clearer. Using the most severe value in the range suggested for England, a 50 percent loss in 100 years, the average annual rate of decline equals only 0.7 percent.[6] For 106 years in the Basin (1519-1625) under the mild case, the average annual rate of population loss equals 1.25 percent, roughly double the rate of England's calamitous fourteenth century (Table 4.2). This rate is eclipsed by that for the moderate case. In this simulation, the nadir is reached in 1607 so the total interval is shorter, 88 years, and the average annual rate of loss is roughly double that of the mild case, 2.46 percent (Table 4.2). The 106 years (1519-1625) under the severe simulation assumption were witness to an even more rapid average annual population loss rate, 3.05 percent (Table 4.2).

---

5   Hatcher, *Plague, Population and the English Economy*, p. 68; McEvedy and Jones, *Atlas*, p. 42; Russell, *British Medieval Population*, pp. 260-81; and Slack, *Impact*, p. 15.

6   The average decline rate is computed using the standard equation for population change: Average annual rate = {Ln(initial pop/subsequent pop)}/number of years in the interval. The change is *not* uniform of course, but this average figure captures the general sense of the rapidity of change.

These differences notwithstanding, there are some similar patterns in the rates of change between the three simulations. The average annual rate of change from 1519 to the 1560s (roughly the mid-point of the 80 years of Spanish occupance in the sixteenth century) is roughly double that of the rate of change for the last half of the century (i.e., 1560s to 1607 or 1625) (Table 4.2). Accordingly, the total scale of depopulation for the first "half-century" (1519 to 1565 or 1569) is more-or-less double that for the last "half-century" in the mild and moderate cases (Table 4.2). The severe case indicates a more profound collapse in the last "half" of the century, over 75 percent of the value for the first "half-century" and close to double that of the mild and moderate cases (Table 4.2).

Causal Links

On the most basic level, all population change is due to changes in the primary demographic variables: fertility, mortality, and migration. One should note, however, that migration does not enter into the simulations that track the moderate and mild cases. For the severe case, migration is explicitly limited to emigration in the four most severe epidemic years. Thus, with the severe case exception noted, population change for the simulations results from changes in fertility and mortality. Short-term changes in fertility and mortality are due to the immediate effects produced by epidemics, famines, and Spanish actions; longer-term changes result from altered age distributions in the population (themselves a result of the short-term disruptions). The following sections discuss the relative contributions of these causal variables; a subsequent section explores the longer-term pattern of fertility and mortality.

EPIDEMICS

Examination of Figure 4.1 suggests that the dates of epidemics are closely linked to the dates of most rapid population change. Indeed, it is obvious that the periods of precipitous population collapse coincide with periods of epidemic illness (Figure 4.1). This is, of course, to be expected since MEXIPOP was constructed to track the effects of variables thatengender population change, especially epidemics. Epidemics produce population change three ways: they increase mortality rates while they are active; they decrease fertility rates while they are active; and they alter longer-term mortality and fertility rates as a result of changed population age structure—itself a result of the short-term periodic changes in mortality and fertility. (This last point is discussed in the "Longer-Term Demographic Patterns" section below.)

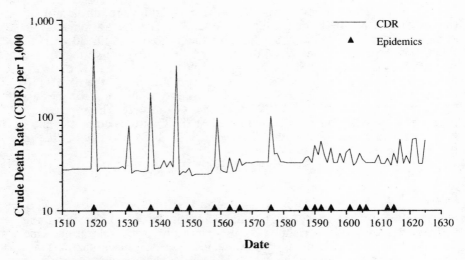

Figure 4.2 Crude Death Rate and Epidemics (mild case)

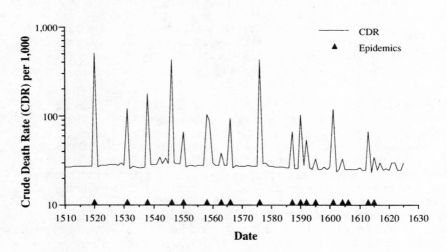

Figure 4.3 Crude Death Rate and Epidemics (moderate case)

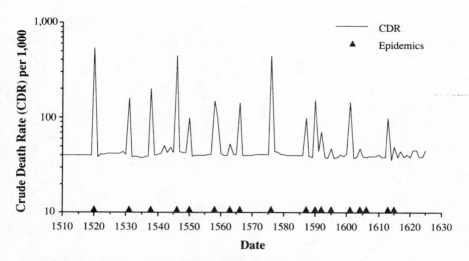

Figure 4.4 Crude Death Rate and Epidemics (severe case)

Mortality Effects

Plots of the approximate crude death rate (CDR or CDRs hereafter) for the period 1510-1625 allow examination of the way epidemics alter mortality. In all the cases, there is a pattern of very large increases in the death rate coincident with dates of epidemics (Figures 4.2, 4.3, and 4.4). The most severe epidemic years result in CDRs of over 500/1000, as compared with the "usual," non-crisis rates of approximately 30/1000 (40/1000 in the severe case)—an over 16-fold multiplication (over 12-fold in the severe case) (Figures 4.2, 4.3, and 4.4). There are three "over 400/1000 CDR" epidemic events (in 1520, 1546, and 1576) in the severe and moderate cases compared with one, in 1520, for the mild case, however (cf. Figures 4.2 and 4.3 and 4.4).

The most severe epidemic-induced increases in CDR, in 1520, 1531, 1538, 1546, 1558, and 1576, all lead to profound population drops in the severe and moderate cases (Figures 4.1, 4.2, 4.3, and 4.4). The mild case differs from the other two in that the population declines in 1558 and 1576 are not as severe since the epidemics for 1558 and 1576 are modeled as typhus (as opposed to pneumonic plague) for this case, hence their CDRs differ. (see Chapters 2 and 3 for details on how this epidemic modeling differs) (Figures 4.1 and 4.2).

Fertility Effects

The overall pattern of crude birth rates (CBR or CBRs hereafter) is similar to that for death rates except that the perturbations to the long-term pattern decrease the rate rather than increase it (Figures 4.5, 4.6, and 4.7). It is also clear that the most serious periods of diminishment of the crude birth rate are coincident with epidemic years (Figures 4.5, 4.6, and 4.7).

164

The scale of decrease for birth rates is less than that for death rates. This is because CDRs are only bounded by unity (i.e., 1.0, the logical limit, where everyone in the population dies), hence the range of increase is larger than for birth rates that are bounded to minimum values of roughly one-third the "usual" value (i.e., no matter the severity of the crisis, there is a minimum birth rate—the birth rate cannot reach its logical limit of 0.0) (see Chapter 2 for a discussion of the birth rate function). The most serious epidemics (in 1520, 1531, 1566, 1588, 1590, 1601, and 1603 for the moderate and severe cases; 1520, 1531, 1546, 1566, and 1590 for the moderate case) depress the CBRs to their minimum values of around 10/1000 (Figures 4.5, 4.6, and 4.7).

The general pattern of sporadic, epidemic-induced precipitous decrease in crude birth rates is similar among the cases. One exception, however, is the 1546 epidemic, which is modeled as typhus in the mild case and pneumonic plague in the moderate and severe cases; and typhus has a more profound effect on the childbearing age class. The severity of decline in CBR for the 1550, 1556, 1588, 1601, and 1613 epidemics is also somewhat less for the mild case than for the others. This is due to the differing age composition of the population, not to differences in the epidemic assumption.

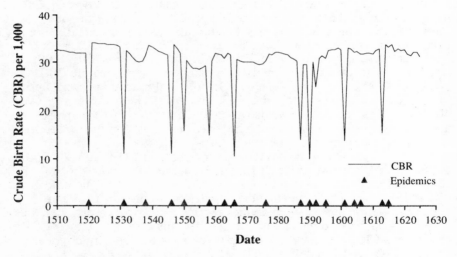

Figure 4.5 Crude Birth Rate and Epidemics (mild case)

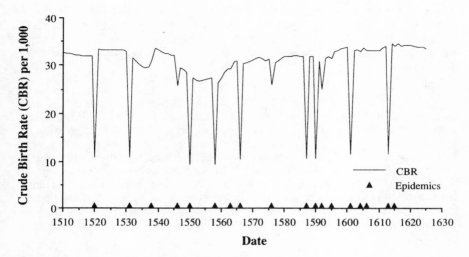

Figure 4.6 Crude Birth Rate and Epidemics (moderate case)

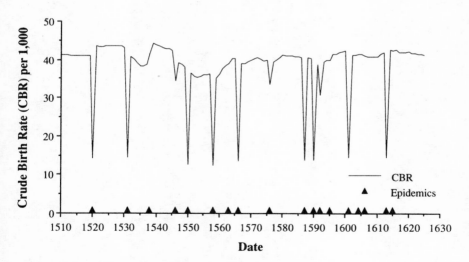

Figure 4.7 Crude Birth Rate and Epidemics (severe case)

It is important to separate the crisis-induced "spikes" from the secular trend of CBRs because the general pattern of crude birth rates is important in understanding the overall demographic history of the Basin. (These longer-term trends will be discussed in the "Long-Term Temporal Patterns" section below.)

EPIDEMIC INDUCED FAMINES

A rough measure of famine, "nutritional sufficiency," is plotted for the three cases in Figures 4.8, 4.9, and 4.10. In these, a value of 1.0 indicates a level of maize nutrition (i.e., energy and protein derived from maize) adequate to support the population at its customary nutritional level. Inspection of these graphs shows that the level of nutrition during the sixteenth century was anything but uniform, especially in the period from 1590-1625 (Figures 4.8, 4.9, and 4.10). Departures from the "sufficient" level are engendered by epidemics (in the case of the severe and moderate cases) and by adverse agricultural conditions (i.e., poor harvests). The dates of these perturbations are noted in the figures (Figures 4.8, 4.9, and 4.10).

TABLE 4.3 EPIDEMIC–FAMINE INTERACTIONS:
CRUDE DEATH RATES (SEVERE CASE)

DATE	CDR (/1000) SYNERGY = 0.0	CDR (/1000) SYNERGY = 0.5	Famine ADDITION (%)
1520	513	538	4.6
1531	86	160	46.1
1538	198	202	2.0
1546	444	449	1.1
1550	49	99	50.7
1558	51	150	66.3
1559	95	103	8.3
1563	53	53	0.2
1566	48	143	66.2
1576	446	452	1.3
1587	46	100	53.7
1590	56	152	63.0
1592	60	72	16.4
1595	48	48	-1.0
1601	48	147	67.4
1604	48	48	-0.2
1606	40	39	-2.8
1613	45	100	54.9
1615	49	50	0.8

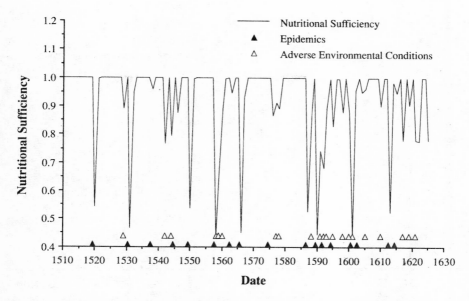

Figure 4.8 Nutritional Sufficiency, Epidemics, and Adverse Agricultural Conditions (severe case)

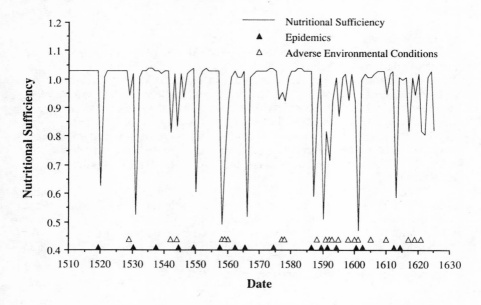

Figure 4.9 Nutritional Sufficiency, Epidemics, and Adverse Agricultural Conditions (moderate case)

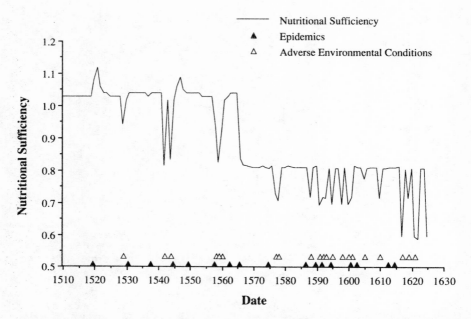

Figure 4.10 Nutritional Sufficiency, Epidemics and Adverse Agricultural Conditions (mild case)

Mortality Effects

As noted in Chapter 3, the best possible fit of a simulation to the historical data for the moderate and severe cases necessitated assuming that famine engendered a significant increase in mortality during epidemics. An opposite assumption obtains for the mild case, where it was assumed that there was *no* additional mortality due to agricultural losses in famine years. The scenario for the severe and mild cases was played-out by assuming that 50 percent of the households of adults who were stricken by a disease suffered loss of their harvests in the year they were stricken. While this assumption seems like a momentous one, its effect is surprisingly inconsistent.

This inconsistency is shown by examining Tables 4.3 and 4.4, which show the approximate crude death rates for epidemic years for the severe and moderate cases (see also Figures 4.11, 4.12, 4.13). The effect of famines in epidemic years may be examined by calculating the CDRs for epidemic years using both an assumption of 50 percent harvest loss and an assumption of zero loss (in Tables 4.3 and 4.4 these assumptions are labeled as "synergy = 0.5" and "synergy = 0.0").

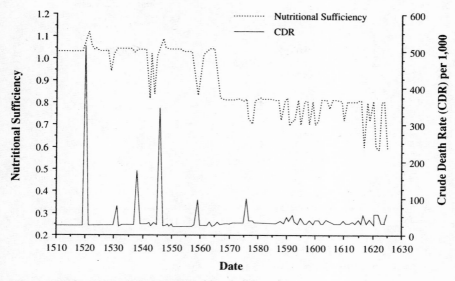

Figure 4.11 Crude Death Rate and Nutrition (mild case)

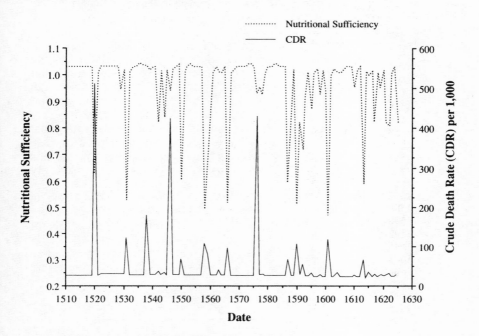

Figure 4.12 Crude Death Rate and Nutrition (moderate case)

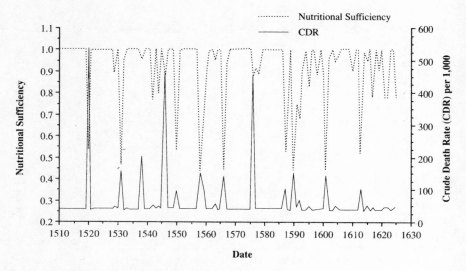

Figure 4.13 Crude Death Rate and Nutrition (severe case)

TABLE 4.4 EPIDEMIC–FAMINE INTERACTIONS: CRUDE DEATH RATES (MODERATE CASE)

DATE	CDR (/1000) SYNERGY = 0.0	CDR (/1000) SYNERGY = 0.5	Famine ADDITION (%)
1520	495	510	2.9
1531	77	122	36.6
1538	176	178	1.1
1546	423	426	0.7
1550	33	68	50.5
1558	34	105	67.4
1559	83	88	6.1
1563	39	39	-0.3
1566	33	94	64.9
1576	428	432	0.9
1587	30	66	54.3
1590	44	103	57.8
1592	47	54	14.0
1595	33	33	1.5
1601	31	118	74.0
1604	34	33	-0.9
1606	26	25	-2.4
1613	28	67	57.8
1615	35	35	0.3

Among the most severe epidemics (in 1520, 1531, 1546, and 1576) (see Figure 4.1) only the 1531 measles epidemic generates any significant additional famine mortality (Tables 4.3 and 4.4). This phenomenon may be explained by noting that the pneumonic plague epidemics in 1546 and 1576 were characterized by high case fatality, but relatively low morbidity (Table 2.6). This low morbidity generates relatively few households with production losses, hence famine effects in these years are minimized (Figs 4.2 and 4.3). For the 1520 epidemic, the epidemic induced increase in mortality was so great that the additional mortality contributed by famine was small (Figures 4.12 and 4.13). This is so because the total mortality for any age group is not a simple sum of epidemic mortality and background mortality (which includes famine mortality) because such a simple sum would overstate the mortality since some who would be expected to die from "background" causes (including famine) in the year in question will perish from epidemic illness in that year—and conversely. Instead, the total mortality rate is figured to be equal to the largest component (usually epidemic mortality) plus one-half of the smaller component (see the Health/Interaction Subsystem section of Chapter 2).

Low values of famine-induced addition to CDRs also are found in the measles epidemics of 1538, 1563, 1592, 1595, 1604, 1606, and 1615 (Figures 4.12 and 4.13 and Tables 4.3 and 4.4). Here the reason for the low famine addition to the CDRs is also low morbidity in the adult population (Table 2.6). This low morbidity is due to the immunity developed by the population that has been exposed previously to measles. The adults in the years in question suffer a low morbidity rate since many of their number contracted measles as children in previous epidemics and survived to be immune to the disease at later dates. The plague epidemic of 1559 is also characterized by low morbidity, not so much because of immune survivors (although that is part) but because of the nature of the disease (see discussion in the Epidemic Mortality section of Chapter 2).

High rates of epidemic-induced famine mortality occur in 1531, 1550, 1558, 1566, 1587, 1590, 1601, and 1613 (Figures 4.12 and 4.13 and Tables 4.3 and 4.4). All these dates are characterized by epidemics with relatively low case fatality and relatively high morbidity rates (Table 2.6). The low case fatality rates indicate that the resulting epidemic mortality rates are not so high as to "overpower" the background mortality rates, thus the modified sum (discussed above) of the two has a greater contribution by the famine component. Indeed, the background mortality (including famine) may be larger than the epidemic famine for many age groups in many of these cases, relegating the epidemic contribution to the lessor.

In two of these "high famine impact" epidemic years, 1558 and 1601, there is an additional factor that raises famine mortality—coincidental poor harvests due to adverse environmental conditions in the previous years (Table 2.15 and Figures 4.12 and 4.13). As will be noted below, this effect is small, but it is noticeable.

Fertility Effects

In addition to raising mortalities, epidemic-induced famine serves to depress fertility in the severe and moderate cases (Figures 4.14, 4.15, and 4.16 and Tables 4.5 and 4.6). This effect is not as profound as for mortalities, but epidemic-induced famines additionally depress crude birth rates in 1550, 1558, 1587, 1601, and 1613 (Figures 4.15 and 4.16 and Tables 4.5 and 4.6). There is not a significant famine effect in the serious epidemic years of 1520, 1531, 1546, and 1576, however (Tables 4.5 and 4.6). For the 1520 and 1531 epidemics the reason that there is only a small effect is that the CBR is close to the absolute minimum set in the fertility assumptions of MEXIPOP (see Births section in Chapter 2 and Tables 4.5 and 4.6). For 1546 and 1576, the relatively low adult epidemic morbidity combined with low famine-induced morbidity (a consequence of low epidemic morbidity) failed to depress the CBR significantly over the no famine situation (Tables 4.5 and 4.6). Indeed, the low epidemic morbidity in these years failed to reduce the CBR all that much over the "usual" rate (Figures 4.15 and 4.16). As is noted below, however, the fact that epidemic-induced famines did not alter the CBRs greatly from their epidemic-only values does not mean that the epidemic-induced reductions in CBRs did not have a very significant effect on the overall population dynamics of the Basin.

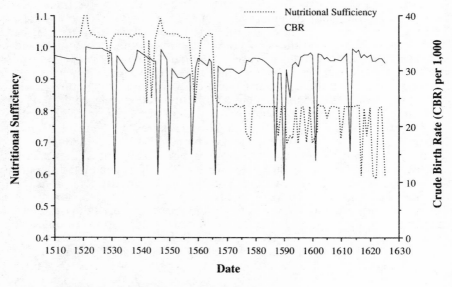

Figure 4.14 Crude Birth Rate and Nutrition (mild case)

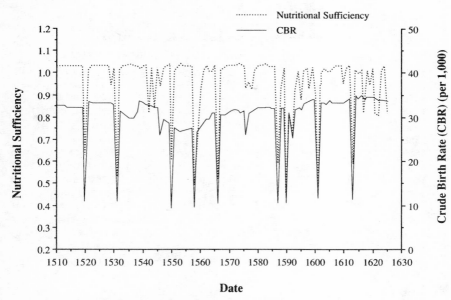

Figure 4.15 Crude Birth Rate and Nutrition (moderate case)

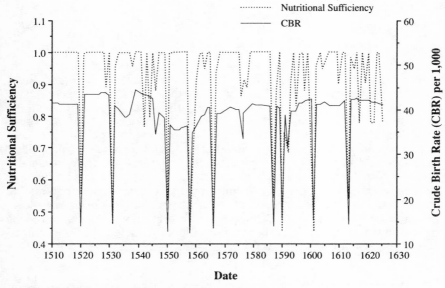

Figure 4.16 Crude Birth Rate and Nutrition (severe case)

TABLE 4.5 EPIDEMIC–FAMINE INTERACTIONS:
CRUDE BIRTH RATES (MILD CASE)

DATE	Synergy = 0.0 CBR (/1000)	Synergy = 0.5 CBR (/1000)	Famine SUBTRACTION (%)
1520	14.4	14.3	0.70
1531	14.4	14.5	-0.69
1538	41.6	41.4	0.48
1546	33.7	34.3	-1.75
1550	16.1	12.7	26.77
1558	15.5	12.4	25.00
1559	36.0	35.0	2.86
1563	38.6	38.9	-0.77
1566	13.5	13.6	-0.74
1576	32.9	33.4	-1.50
1587	17.5	13.8	26.81
1590	13.6	13.7	-0.73
1592	33.7	30.8	9.42
1595	40.7	40.0	1.75
1601	18.4	14.5	26.90
1604	41.9	41.5	0.96
1606	41.1	41.0	0.24
1613	18.4	14.4	27.78
1615	41.7	42.4	-1.65

FAMINES INDUCED BY ADVERSE AGRICULTURAL CONDITIONS

Examination of Figures 4.8, 4.9, and 4.10 show that decreases in nutritional sufficiency are associated with periods of adverse agricultural conditions (hereafter, agriculturally-induced famines). The decreases in nutritional sufficiency show up in the year following the year in which the harvest shortfall is noted (see Chapter 2 and Table 2.15). These agriculturally-induced famines are especially evident in Figure 4.10 since it lacks the epidemic-induced nutritional insufficiency "spikes." The scale of reduction in nutrition for the years following harvest shortfalls is usually less than for the years following epidemics. A typical year with adverse agricultural conditions generates a nutritional sufficiency level of about 0.8, that is to say, the maize nutritional level is 80 percent of its customary level (Figures 4.8, 4.9, and 4.10). This is a less profound shortfall than for the most severe epidemics that produce a nutritional sufficiency of less than 50 percent the usual value (Figures 4.8 and 4.9).

TABLE 4.6 EPIDEMIC–FAMINE INTERACTIONS:
CRUDE BIRTH RATES (MODERATE CASE)

DATE	Synergy = 0.5 CBR (/1000)	Synergy = 0.0 CBR (/1000)	Famine REDUCTION (%)
1520	10.9	11.0	0.91
1531	10.9	10.8	-0.93
1538	31.1	31.2	0.32
1546	25.8	25.5	-1.18
1550	9.42	13.9	32.23
1558	9.29	13.5	31.19
1559	26.4	26.9	1.86
1563	29.4	29.1	-1.03
1566	10.4	10.3	-0.97
1576	26.0	25.7	-1.17
1587	10.7	15.8	32.28
1590	10.7	10.6	-0.94
1592	25.2	26.6	5.26
1595	31.6	31.8	0.63
1601	11.5	16.7	31.14
1604	33.1	33.3	0.60
1606	33.3	33.3	0.00
1613	11.5	17.1	32.75
1615	34.2	33.6	-1.79

Mortality Effects

This less profound reduction in nutritional sufficiency is shown in the scale of reduction in CDRs engendered by agriculturally-induced famines. The effects of these famines on CDRs may be tracked by comparing simulations that include agro-environmental effects to the same simulations run without the agro-environmental effects (Table 4.8). These comparisons show that increases in CDRs attributable to agriculturally-induced famines range to over 50 percent (Table 4.8). More typical increases range from 10-30 percent, and in many years the effect is so small as to be negligible (since the CDRs measured in Tables 4.7 and 4.8 are approximate, small values, both positive and negative, must be ignored). It is enlightening to compare the effect of these famines with those induced by epidemics.

Epidemic-induced famines (only for the severe and moderate cases) often produce a greater multiplication of CDR than do agriculturally-induced famines (*cf*. Table 4.8 and Tables 4.3 and 4.4). This is evident since the epidemic-induced famines produce increases that typically range from 10-50 percent as opposed to the 10-30 percent increases for the agriculturally-induced ones. Thus, as modeled, agriculturally-induced famines are roughly half as "effective" in increasing CDRs than are epidemic-induced famines. This disparity is greater if agriculturally-induced famines are compared with epidemic-induced (as opposed to epidemic-induced famine)

TABLE 4.7 AGRICULTURAL FAMINE INTERACTIONS: CRUDE BIRTH RATES COMPARED

	Mild Case			Moderate Case			Severe Case		
Date	NO AGRICULTURAL PROBLEMS CBR (/1000)	AGRICULTURAL PROBLEMS CBR (/1000)	PERCENT Reduction	NO AGRICULTURAL PROBLEMS CBR (/1000)	AGRICULTURAL PROBLEMS CBR (/1000)	PERCENT Reduction	NO AGRICULTURAL PROBLEMS CBR (/1000)	AGRICULTURAL PROBLEMS CBR (/1000)	PERCENT Reduction
1529	33.6	33.6	0.00	33.3	33.2	0.30	43.7	43.6	0.23
1542	32.5	32.4	0.31	32.7	32.5	0.61	43.1	43.1	0.00
1544	32.0	31.8	0.63	32.3	32.2	0.31	42.7	42.8	-0.23
1558	15.0	13.3	11.33	9.3	9.29	-0.11	12.4	12.4	0.00
1560	32.0	32.1	-0.31	28.2	27.6	2.13	37.2	36.3	2.42
1577	31.9	31.8	0.31	30.5	30.7	-0.66	39.1	39.5	-1.02
1580	32.2	32.3	-0.31	31.8	32.0	-0.63	40.8	41.2	-0.98
1588	29.8	29.6	0.67	31.7	31.9	-0.63	40.2	40.5	-0.75
1591	30.3	29.8	1.65	31.3	31.0	0.96	38.9	38.7	0.51
1592	25.4	23.8	6.30	25.9	25.2	2.70	32.0	30.8	3.75
1593	31.0	30.7	0.97	31.7	31.6	0.32	39.7	39.5	0.50
1595	31.0	30.6	1.29	31.8	31.6	0.63	40.3	40.0	0.74
1598	32.8	32.7	0.30	33.6	33.5	0.30	42.1	41.9	0.48
1599	32.9	33.1	-0.61	33.8	33.8	0.00	42.3	42.2	0.24
1601	15.3	11.2	26.80	11.5	11.5	0.00	14.6	14.5	0.68
1605	32.1	32.4	-0.93	34.1	33.7	1.17	42.2	41.6	1.42
1610	31.8	32.0	-0.63	33.3	33.3	0.00	41.0	40.9	0.24
1617	33.0	32.6	1.21	34.1	34.1	0.00	41.7	42.0	-0.72

TABLE 4.8 AGRICULTURAL FAMINE INTERACTIONS: CRUDE DEATH RATES COMPARED

	Mild Case			Moderate Case			Severe Case		
	NO AGRICULTURAL PROBLEMS	AGRICULTURAL PROBLEMS	PERCENT	NO AGRICULTURAL PROBLEMS	AGRICULTURAL PROBLEMS	PERCENT	NO AGRICULTURAL PROBLEMS	AGRICULTURAL PROBLEMS	PERCENT
Date	CDR (/1000)	CDR (/1000)	Increase	CDR (/1000)	CDR (/1000)	Increase	CDR (/1000)	CDR (/1000)	Increase
1529	27.8	29.3	5.12	28.3	29.9	5.35	41.9	44.2	5.20
1542	28.6	34.3	16.62	29.0	34.8	16.67	42.9	50.6	15.22
1544	28.6	33.5	14.63	29.0	33.8	14.20	43.0	48.6	11.52
1558	27.8	37.5	25.87	68.3	105.0	34.95	101.0	150.0	32.67
1560	25.4	27.2	6.62	28.3	29.7	4.71	40.6	42.5	4.47
1577	33.1	39.1	15.35	28.6	29.5	3.05	42.1	43.7	3.66
1580	32.5	32.4	-0.31	27.6	27.5	-0.36	41.3	41.1	-0.49
1588	30.5	38.1	19.95	24.7	26.1	5.36	37.5	39.7	5.54
1591	29.9	41.6	28.13	24.3	28.4	14.44	37.7	44.4	15.09
1592	49.3	63.9	22.85	49.1	54.3	9.58	63.4	71.8	11.70
1593	31.4	38.6	18.65	25.2	26.3	4.18	37.6	39.0	3.59
1595	37.2	48.7	23.61	30.7	33.3	7.81	45.3	47.7	5.03
1598	31.9	40.4	21.04	25.3	26.8	5.60	39.1	41.3	5.33
1599	32.1	31.9	-0.63	25.4	25.3	-0.40	39.4	39.1	-0.77
1601	36.7	77.9	52.89	67.2	118.0	43.05	101.0	147.0	31.29
1605	32.2	34.4	6.40	25.3	25.1	-0.80	38.8	39.1	0.77
1610	31.9	38.4	16.93	25.1	26.2	4.20	39.3	41.0	4.15
1617	31.6	56.0	43.57	24.7	29.7	16.84	38.2	44.5	14.16

increases in CDRs. To produce the same multiplication in CDRs as epidemics, agriculturally-induced famine severities would have to be multiplied 6-7 times (Figs. 4.2, 4.3, and 4.4).

There is a similar pattern of agriculturally-induced famine-generated decreases in CDRs across the cases (Figures 4.11, 4.12, and 4.13). The mild case looks different due to the lack of epidemic-induced famines. Since there are no epidemic-induced famines, the population's age structure is different in this case—there are more youth and elderly proportionally in the mild case since their ranks were not winnowed by epidemic-induced famines; thus there is a larger proportion of the population at risk to agriculturally-induced famines. It should be noted, however, that the age structure for the each case is different because of the initial demographic assumptions. Also, there are no epidemic-induced famines to link with the agriculturally-induced ones in close succession (e.g., 1558-1560 and the 1590s) or to augment them (e.g., 1601) (Figures 4.11, 4.12, and 4.13).

Fertility Effects

Like the situation for epidemic-induced famines, agriculturally-induced famines are less effective in altering crude birth rates than they are in altering crude death rates. With only a very few exceptions, agriculturally-induced famines do not significantly alter CBRs (Table 4.7). The only significant effects are seen in the mild case, and there in only two years (Table 4.7). This is due to the altered age structure of the mild case (as opposed to the others that have epidemic-induced famines), where there is a population that is relatively "rich" in youth and elderly, the most affected age classes.

As compared to epidemic-induced famines, agriculturally-induced famines generally effect CBRs less, if only because the number of events with significant impact is much larger for the epidemic cases (Tables 4.5, 4.6, and 4.7). Similarly, the impact of severe epidemics on CBRs reduces them to one-third of their usual values while agriculturally-induced famines seldom have greater than a 10 percent effect (i.e., a fall to 90 percent of their usual values) (Figures 4.14, 4.15, 4.16).

OTHER CAUSES

Another cause of population decline, for the mild case only, is the assumed imposition of a 20 percent labor tribute in the period 1565 to 1625. This assumption results in a reduction of the agricultural product, lowering the nutritional sufficiency level to 80 percent (Figure 4.10). This new level of nutritional "insufficiency" results in a rise in the "non-crisis" CDR from the high 20s (per 1,000) to the low 30s (Figure 4.2). This pattern is in marked contrast to that exhibited by the moderate simulation, where the trend is towards decreasing CDRs for the same period, and to the severe simulation, where there is a pattern of steady CDRs for the same period (Figures 4.3 and 4.4).

There is no clear, long-term pattern of decreased CBRs due to this labor draft; in fact there is a rather unstable increasing trend from the nadir in the 1550s (Figure 4.14). Nevertheless, this semi-stagnation is in contrast to the relatively steady, gradual increase in CBRs shown by the severe and moderate cases over the same period (Figures 4.15 and 4.16). These longer-term trends will be discussed below, but it is clear that the decreased nutritional level due to the labor withdrawal contributes to the reluctance of the CBRs to rise after mid-century.

The net result of an increased base-level death rate and an only sporadically growing birth rate is a gradual decline in population in non-crisis years. This negative growth situation is in marked contrast to the pre-1565 situation, in which there is significant population growth in non-crisis years (Figure 4.1). Indeed, comparison of the two curves in Figure 3.12 graphically shows the depressing effect of the labor tribute on population growth.

While migration affects the population trend directly, it does not affect mortality and fertility if, as is assumed for the emigration in the severe simulation (4 percent emigration in each of the years 1520, 1531, 1546, and 1576), it involves all age groups equally.[7] So without affecting the mortality and fertility rates, this emigration partly accounts for the very large severe-case population losses at these dates. Emigration is a minor component in these losses, however, since it accounts for only about 10 percent of the population declines in 1520, 1546, and 1576, and about 20 percent of the decline in 1531.

Longer-term Demographic Patterns

There are two inter-linked patterns evident in the temporal plots of the basic demographic variables. The most obvious are the sharp, "spike" patterns of very rapid, but short-term, increase or decrease (e.g., see Figure 4.2). These almost-instantaneous changes show the immediate effects of epidemic or famine crises. The interconnection of these "spikes" with their causes has been discussed above. This section is devoted to the other, longer-term, patterns of more-gradual and smaller-amplitude changes (e.g., see Figure 4.2). Since MEXIPOP is designed to return constant levels of mortality and fertility in the absence of crises, these "non-crisis" changes are the result of changes in the underlying age composition of the population. By the same token, however, changes in the age structure of the population are the result of the previous experience of the population with situations that modify death and birth rates. For that reason, the longer-term patterns also result from the past epidemiological and nutritional experience of the population.

---

[7] During the crisis period of 1785-1786 in which harvest failures and disease caused substantial migration, there is evidence of wide-spread child abandonment and differential-age migration, see Robinson, "Typology of Migration." It is reasonable to argue that such was the case in the sixteenth century as well, but for simplicity, I assume equal migration of all age classes and sexes.

Concentrating on the longer-term patterns of fertility and mortality allows certain patterns of population change to be explained. For that reason, it is instructive to examine these longer-term patterns for the basic demographic variables; crude death rates and crude birth rates, and this is done immediately below. Following these, the temporal patterns of two derived demographic measures, dependency ratio and tributary ratio, also are discussed.

CRUDE BIRTH RATES

Crude birth rates (CBRs) are affected by the current state of health (i.e., the presence or absence of famine or epidemic illness) of reproducing-age adults and by the relative proportion of reproducing-age adults in the population. There is often a pattern of lagged effect, since a crisis typically affects youth more severely than the reproducing-age group. Hence, the crisis effects the reproducing-age group after a lag, when the affected age-group matures into the reproducing-age group.[8] The age-composition is a result of the population's previous health experience, and reflects previous changes in death rates and birth rates.

Severe and Moderate Cases

The overall pattern (i.e., without crisis spikes) for the severe and moderate simulations are remarkably similar, although they are both different from the mild case (Figures 4.5, 4.6, and 4.7). This similarity is evident despite the differences in the underlying demographic assumptions (see Chapters 2 and 3 for a discussion of the differences in these assumptions). The severe and moderate simulations share a common epidemic sub-model (the pneumonic plague version), however, and this suggests that the mortality and fertility effects engendered by this sub-model differ enough from those engendered by the typhus epidemic sub-model used in the mild case to produce the differing CBR pattern from the mild case (but see below for additional effects on the mild simulation's CBR by other factors). Hence, differences in the specification of only three epidemics (two of them severe, however) outweigh the differences in the assumed, underlying demographic patterns for the three cases. This may not be true, for very large differences in demographic assumptions, but it is suggested for the scale of difference between the differing demographic sub-models used in MEXIPOP.

Since the severe and moderate cases are quite similar, their temporal patterns are discussed together. The first important pattern is the "wave" of declining CBRs in the period from roughly 1529 to 1536 and the subsequent rising CBRs from 1536 to 1540 (Figures 4.6 and 4.7). This decline in CBRs is not profound, only from about 33 per 1,000 to about 29 per 1,000, but it is of interest because its cause illustrates a general pattern.

---

[8] For example, an epidemic that killed many children aged 0-15 would have negative consequences for the birth rate in subsequent years as the now-smaller-than-usual youthful cohorts mature to reproductive age, since there would be a relatively smaller proportion of reproducing adults in the population.

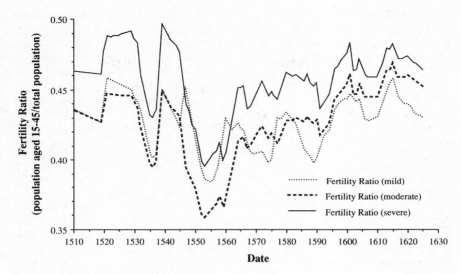

Figure 4.17 Simulated Fertility Ratios

That this fall is due to changing age structure and not to a pattern of illness or famine may be demonstrated by examination of Figures 4.15 and 4.17. Aside from the immediate effects during the epidemic of 1531 and the adverse agricultural conditions of 1528, there is no *trend* of nutritional insufficiency or epidemic illness that would serve to reduce the non-crisis birth rate.[9] Instead, the declining birth rate is a consequence of reduction in the proportion of young children due to the 1520 epidemic. The high rates of death among the 0-5 age group in the 1520 epidemic means that 10-15 years later the 15-45 age class (the reproductive age group) would be under-represented in the population, leading to reduced crude birth rates (Figure 4.17 and Table 2.6). The situation begins to turn in the late 1530s as this group is augmented by the maturation of children born after 1520. By 1540, "customary" CBRs are achieved (Figures 4.6, 4.7 and 4.17).

The upward swing of CBRs is abruptly terminated by 1540, and from then to the early 1550s CBRs decline again—this time to their lowest sixteenth-century values, around 27 per 1,000 in the early 1550s (Figures 4.6 and 4.7). This time the decline is due to two factors, however, poor harvests and epidemics. The food shortages that must have resulted from the poor harvests in 1528 increased the proportional loss of 0-5 year-old children (Table 2.15). The effects of this reduced group appear in decreased CBRs after 10-15 years, that is, 1538-1543 (Table 2.15 and Figures 4.15

---

9 In the "real world" this decline could also be the result of a pattern of reduced frequency of intercourse, reduced fecundity, or other factors. In the "simulation world" of MEXIPOP, however, such changes are not allowed. In the absence of famine or epidemic morbidity, the birth rate per age pp. 15-45 adult is constant.

children (Table 2.15). The effects of this reduced group appear in decreased CBRs after 10-15 years, that is, 1538-1543 (Table 2.15 and Figures 4.15 and 4.17). Adding to this are the poor harvests of 1541 and 1543. Like those before them, they depressed nutritional sufficiency and resulted in increased death rates for young children. Again, the effects of a reduced 15-45 age group is felt 10-15 years later, in the early 1550s.

After 1545, this gentle decline was further augmented by a decreased proportion of child-bearing-age adults due to the effects of the epidemics of 1531 (Figure 4.17). The epidemics of 1531 greatly impacted the infant age group and, after the 15 years they need to mature to the child-rearing ages, the proportion in the reproducing age group declined—forcing down the CBRs (Table 2.6 and Figs 4.6, 4.7, and 4.17). Similarly, the epidemic of 1538 greatly affected the 0-5 age group—forcing down the CBRs 10-15 years after, in 1548-1553 (Table 2.6, Figures 4.6, 4.7, and 4.17).

After 1555, CBRs again began to rise, a pattern of general increase that was to continue, with some minor set backs, until the first decade of the seventeenth century (Figures 4.6 and 4.7). The initial segment of this rise (from 1552-1560) reflects, in part, the maturing of the children that were the result of the increased CBRs in the 1540s (Figures 4.6, 4.7, and 4.17). In addition, the effects of the 1538 epidemic on the reproducing-age group were passing off by the early 1550s. Further, 10-15 years after the catastrophic epidemic of 1546, the 15-45 age group again began to increase its proportion. Indeed, the proportion of the population aged 15-45 reached its sixteenth-century ebb in the 1550s, and climbed rapidly to 1565, and more slowly and unevenly until 1590 (Figure 4.17).

In the decade of the 1590s CBRs rose again, mostly due to the rapid increase in the proportion of reproducing adults in that decade (Figures 4.6, 4.7, and 4.17). There was an increasing proportion of mating adults in the population because the decline in 0-15 year-olds engendered by the epidemics of 1576 was passing off by the 1590s. The "troubles" of the 1590s once again reduced the proportion of reproducing-age adults in the first decade of the 1600s and, consequently, slightly lowered the CBRs of that decade (Figures 4.6, 4.7, and 4.17).

Mild Case

The differences in CBR pattern between the mild case and the others are due to the differences in the epidemic model used (typhus instead of plague), the assumption of no epidemic-induced famine, and the assumed imposition of a labor tribute in the decades following 1565. The lack of epidemic-induced famines in the mild case results in a post-epidemic population with a slightly higher proportion of reproducing-age adults since the famines affect the youth proportionally more (Figure 4.17). The higher proportion of reproducing-age adults accounts for the slightly higher post-epidemic CBRs for mild case verses the moderate case (which has the same initial demographic sub-model assumptions) (Figure 4.17).

The second divergence is a result of the differing epidemic assumption for the mild case verses the severe and moderate cases. The typhus epidemics of 1546, 1558, and 1576 (the mild case assumption) did not reduce the 0-5 age class and 5-15 age class proportionally as much as the 15-45 age class (Table 2.6). This differential age-class mortality resulted in a CBR decline between 1540-1553 that was more muted in the mild case (Figures 4.5, 4.6, and 4.7). The pattern after the 1576 epidemic more closely resembles that in the moderate and severe cases since the age-class differential mortality for the epidemics for this date is broadly similar to that of the pneumonic plague epidemic sub-model used for the moderate and severe cases (Table 2.6).

There is a difference in mild case CBRs in the post-1565 period, however. The mild case has an assumed labor tribute that reduces nutritional sufficiency, and this, in turn, reduces CBRs over those of the moderate case, which shares demographic assumptions and epidemic assumptions save for that of 1576 (Figures 4.5, 4.6, 4.15, and 4.8).

CRUDE DEATH RATES

As with crude birth rates, crude death rates are determined both by immediate factors (e.g., famines or epidemics that add to the death rates) and by the relative proportions of different age groups in the population. The later is because different age groups have different mortality rates, so that when a population suffers a change in the relative proportions among age groups, its CDR changes. Because it is sensitive to the total population age distribution, explanation of changes in CDR due to changes in population age structure is a little more complex than for crude birth rates (see above). This is because the respective age-class-specific death rates differ as well as the proportions of the population in those age groups.[10] Of course, the relative proportions of different age groups in a population is a consequence of the past experience of that population with factors that alter the basic pattern of fertility and age-specific mortality. In the case of MEXIPOP these factors are associated with epidemics and famines.

Moderate and Severe Cases

The patterns of non-crisis CDRs for the moderate and severe cases are similar, differing mostly in that the severe case has higher CDRs at all points, ranging from 39-43 per 1,000 verses the 24-30 per 1,000 range for the moderate case (Figures 4.3 and 4.4).

The first important non-crisis CDR change to note is the abrupt decline of CDRs (to levels below their pre-conquest totals) immediately after the measles epidemic of 1531 (Figures 4.3 and 4.4). This drop is a consequence of both the 1520 and 1531 epidemics. The first epidemic produced a smaller-than-normal group of children, and when they matured to the lower age-specific death rate age groups, the overall CDR was

---

10 For example, it may be that one event that reduces the number of infants (who have a death rate greater than that for the population as a whole) decreases the CDR for the population as a whole. This reduction may be less than that due to a second event that reduces the number of elderly (who also have a greater than group-average death rate) because the elderly comprise a greater proportion in the population.

reduced. Since the measles epidemic of 1531 attacked the elderly and infant age groups most strongly (and these groups have the highest age-class mortalities) and the 5-45 ages least (and theses ages have the lowest age-specific mortalities), the resulting CDRs would be immediately decreased (Table 2.6). This is partly confirmed by examining Figure 4.17, which shows an increase in the 15-45 age group's proportion. This skewed age distribution is reduced over time and the CDRs rise from their 1532 low to a relative peak in the late 1540s (Figures 4.3, 4.4, and 4.17). This is because the relatively large "middle-age" (ages 5-45) population has moved into older age groups and thus suffers from higher rates of death.

A similar reduction in CBRs occurs after 1547, when CDRs fall to near their pre-conquest levels (Figures 4.3 and 4.4). This drop reflects the effect of the 1531 and 1538 epidemics since these epidemics greatly affected the 0-5 age groups, producing a smaller-than-normal youth group, which, 10-15 years later, results in a smaller-than-normal young adult group. Since the young adult age groups have the lowest age-specific death rates, reduction in their numbers reduces the CDR.

A third such reduction is seen in the period bounded by about 1577 and 1600, when CDRs again fall to levels slightly below their pre-conquest values (Figures 4.3 and 4.4). As in the previous cases, this fall is due to a complex interplay of immediate and lagged effects. Significant among these is the trend towards an increasing proportion of reproducing-age group population in this period (Figure 4.17). Since this group has a low death rate, increasing its proportion (over that of the initial population) will result in a decreased CDR (as compared with the initial population). From about 1600 onward, there are relatively stable non-crisis CDRs (Figures 4.3 and 4.4). This stability is at a level slightly lower than that obtaining before the conquest. This difference, however, is small, and the non-crisis CDRs of the early 1600s (about 25 per 1,000) are scarcely smaller than the approximately 27 per 1,000 immediate pre-conquest levels.

Mild Case

There are two reasons to expect a different pattern of non-epidemic CDRs for the mild case as opposed to the moderate and severe cases; there are no epidemic-induced famines in the mild case and it has a period of labor tribute-induced nutritional insufficiency after 1565. The lack of epidemic-induced famines results in a post-epidemic population that typically is not as devastated in the youth and elderly age groups since their death rates are more highly sensitive to nutritional levels than are the middle age groups'. This has the paradoxical effect of *reducing* CDRs to even lower levels in the period after 1520 (*cf*. Figs 4.2 and 4.3). These are reduced because the combined epidemic-plus-famine crises in the moderate and severe cases more closely mimic the "usual" pattern of CDR, while the mild case's epidemic-only mortality pattern affects the higher mortality age groups even more strongly.

The effect of the post 1565 labor tribute-induced nutritional insufficiency is immediate evident in Figure 4.2. This reduction in nutrition increases the non-crisis CDR (to about 32 per 1,000), resulting in a level that is greater than that of pre-conquest times (of about 28 per 1,000) (Figure 4.2). Hence, the mild case exhibits CDRs in the early 1600s that are a good deal higher than those exhibited by the moderate case, about 26 per 1,000 (Figures 4.2 and 4.3).

DEPENDENCY RATIOS

The dependency ratio is a derived demographic measure defined as the sum of the population in the 0-15 age group plus that in the 60-99 age group divided by the total in the 15-60 age groups.[11] It is important because it roughly measures the ratio of the non-productive (but consuming) proportion of a population to the productive portion. In other words, it is a crude measure of how hard each productive member of a population must work to support the non-productive members as well. It does not account for other demands placed on the productive proportion, however (e.g., support for a non-productive elite class).

Two patterns within the sixteenth-century dependency ratios are evident (Figure 4.18). First, this ratio is far from uniform, especially in the first forty years of Spanish occupancy. The deviations away from the pre-conquest level (about 0.7 to 0.75) in this period, both plus and minus, are significant in all cases. The second remarkable feature of this graph is the long period (approximately from 1545-1600) that dependency ratios were above their immediate pre-conquest values (the mild case is different as will

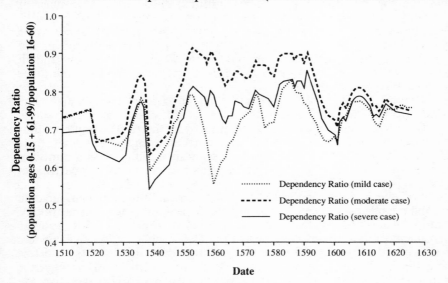

Figure 4.18 Dependency Ratios

---

[11] Symbolically, this is expressed as: $\{pop_{(0-15)} + pop_{(61-99)}\}/pop_{(16-60)}$.

be noted below) (Figure 4.18). This is important since dependency ratio is a crude measure of the difficulty a typical family has in providing support to all their members. In short, high dependency ratios signal a population at relatively high risk since each productive member has a relatively heavy burden of other individuals to support.

The temporal pattern of change in the dependency ratio reflects the current and past experience of a population exposed to forces that alter the relative population proportions. In general, the dependency ratio curve will "mirror" (i.e., invert) the pattern of the curve that plots the proportion of the population in the reproductive ages (15-45) (Figure 4.17) because this segment of the population is largest in size.

Moderate and Severe Cases

Beginning with the severe and moderate curves, since they exhibit a similar shape, the first pattern of note is the wave-like decline in the 1520s and subsequent increase in the late 1520s and early 1530s (Figure 4.18). This pattern of falling then ascending dependency ratios reflects the wave-like movement of an epidemic-diminished youthful cohort as it matures from a non-productive, dependent age class to a productive one (Figure 4.18). The abrupt drop in dependency ratio in the 1520s is due to the age-specific mortality pattern of the 1520 epidemic. It killed young and old in greater proportion than the middle age groups. That is to say, the increase in age-specific death rates for these targeted groups was greater than the increase for the more fortunate age groups, thus the usual pattern of mortality was skewed (Figure 4.18). This point is amplified in Figure 4.17 that shows the increase in the proportion of 15-45 year-olds at the same period. After the calamity of the initial epidemic and disruption, this period may have been one where the production of surplus by the Amerindian agricultural force was bountiful since the domestic demands were more easily met (Figure 4.18).

From the "valley" of the 1520s, dependency ratios increased in the late 1520s to a peak in the later 1530s. This increase is due to maturation of the (1520 epidemic) decimated youth-age groups into the 15-45 age group, thus reducing the proportion of 15-45 ages. Further, the gradual death of the 1520-epidemic-reduced elderly age classes resulted in the less-diminished middle-age groups taking their place, thus increasing the proportion of elderly (Figures 4.17 and 4.18).

Somewhat similar to the 1520 epidemic, but a little more complex, the second notable dependency ratio "regularity" is another wave-like cycle of decline, followed by increase (Figure 4.18). From its 1536 "peak," dependency ratios plummeted to a nadir in 1538, only to climb up again to a zenith in the early 1550s (Figure 4.18). This pattern also reflects the effect of a diminished youthful cohort as it matures from a non-productive, dependent age class to a productive one (Figure 4.18). Because the epidemics of 1531 and 1538 strongly affected youth, the proportion of youth was reduced, thus reducing the subsequent dependency ratio. As these reduced size groups matured and entered the productive-age groups,

10-15 years later, the dependency ratio was increased. This increase is due to the reduced proportion of the reproducing-age population that leads to higher dependency ratios by diminishing the denominator in the defining ratio. It is interesting to note that while dependency ratios increase (about 1538-1553), CBRs are in a declining phase (Figures 4.6, 4.7, and 4.18). This is to be expected since the reproducing-age portion of the population is smaller than "usual."

The first two "waves" of declining and falling dependency ratios were produced by the great epidemics of 1520, 1531 (also 1538) during which youth suffered a disproportionally high mortality. That the third pattern evident in the severe and moderate cases does not exactly mimic the first two is due to the different nature of the mortality pattern of the third great epidemic in the Basin, that of pneumonic plague, in 1546. The age-specific mortality pattern of this epidemic was not as biased against youth and, hence the "wave" of a reduced size cohort moving through subsequent age classes is less evident. Nevertheless, there is a moderate decline in dependency ratio from 1552 to 1560, followed by a more steep drop to a low in 1564, subsequently there is a slow, uneven increase to 1590 (Figure 4.18). This two-stage decline is the result of the immediate effects of the epidemics of 1550 and 1558, and the ragged rebound results from a similar "working through" of the reduced youth cohorts (Table 2.6). The relatively long period without significant swings in the rather high dependency ratios from about 1560 to 1590 reflects the nature of the epidemics of the period. Either they were severe, but without significant age-structure altering qualities such as that of 1576, or they were minor events that affected the ratio little.

The great decline in dependency ratios from 1590 to 1600, however, marks the effect that the epidemics of the troubled 1590s had on the youth population (Figure 4.18 and Table 2.6). This drop is, once again, followed by a small "rebound" effect in the period 1600-1608 (Figure 4.18). Lastly, there is a moderate drop late in the first decade of the 1600s due to the epidemics of 1604-1607 and 1613. After the prodigious decline of the 1590s, the dependency ratios in the early 1620s cluster near their initial, pre-conquest values.

Mild Case

The pattern for the mild case is substantially the same as for the moderate and severe ones with two exceptions. Since the epidemic sub-model for the mild case differs only for the 1546, 1558, and 1576 epidemics, differences in the dependency ratios only appear as a result of these different assumptions. Unlike the 1546 typhus epidemic, which was relatively age-neutral in its mortality pattern, the 1558 typhus epidemic more strongly increased mortalities for youth.[12] This is because the older age

---

12 By age-neutral, it is meant that the age-specific epidemic mortality pattern more closely follows the differences in age-specific mortality exhibited by the population in the absence of the epidemic.

188

groups had been previously exposed and were partially resistant, while the youth were not. This age bias in mortality is reflected in the (now typical) "wave" of decline (in the 1550s) and increase (in the 1560s) exhibited by the mild curve (Figure 4.18). A second, smaller such "wave" is evident as a result of the 1576 typhus epidemic, and is due to the same causes.

Since the mild simulation assumes that there was no epidemic-induced famines, each epidemic in the mild case is slightly less biased to attack the youth and elderly since famines affect these age groups more proportionally. This factor is illustrated in the dependency ratio curves as reduced amplitude of post-epidemic "waves" (Figure 4.18).

TRIBUTARY RATIOS

A second derived demographic measure of interest is tributary ratio (Figure 4.19). This is defined as the ratio of the total population divided by one-half of the 15-60 age-group population, and is an approximation of the ratio used by historians[13] to determine the total population from tributary counts.[14] The denominator used here (age 15-60 population/2), a figure roughly equal to the number of adult men, is *not* the same as the number of tributaries as computed by historical scholars, nevertheless it is valuable to examine the ratio of which this is a part.

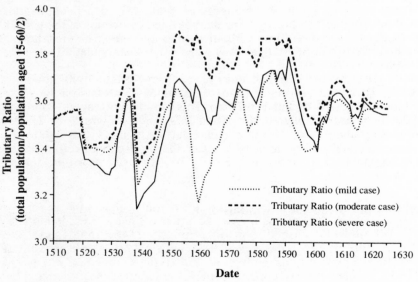

Figure 4.19 Tributary Ratios

---

[13] For example, see Cook and Simpson, *The Population of Central Mexico in the Sixteenth Century*; and Cook and Borah, *The Indian Population of Central Mexico*.

[14] Symbolically: tributary ratio = (total population)/{(population 15-60)/2}.

The values in Figure 4.19 are not directly comparable to those used by historical scholars because their numbers reflect differing proportions of the tribute exempt population and other factors; but they do fall into the general range of values used in the literature.[15] For example, Cook and Simpson assume a tributary multiplier of 4.0 in 1565 (as compared with the mild curve value at this date, about 3.4), Cook and Borah use a value of 3.3 for 1568 (as compared with a severe curve value of about 3.5 at this date), and Gibson uses a multiplier of 2.8 for the 1570s (as compared with a moderate curve value of about 3.7) (Figure 4.19).[16] The tributary ratio values plotted here are smaller than those used by these scholars, except for Cook and Simpson. Since the plotted values do not incorporate adjustments for the tribute exempt classes, widows, and so on, it would be expected that a tribute multiplier that incorporates these factors would be larger since the number of tribute payers is reduced—and this is what obtains in the Cook and Simpson figure. The fact that for Cook and Borah, and Gibson this relationship is reversed suggests that either their assumptions of population age-structure (used to determine their tributary ratios) are faulty or that the simulations produce faulty age-structures.

Not surprisingly, the basic shape (if not the amplitude) of the tributary ratio curve closely resembles the dependency ratio curve (*cf.* Figures 4.18 and 4.19). Thus, like the dependency ratio curve, its most obvious attribute is its non-uniformity, especially for the early part of the century (and throughout for the mild case) (Figure 4.19). The large range of values renders questionable simple calculations, such as those that assume a relatively constant tributary ratio at different dates. For example, a typical calculation used to establish the population at a date with less complete tributary data assumes that the ratio of tributaries to total population is constant. This method uses a ratio of the number of tributaries for a community at a well-documented date to the tributary number at the less well-documented date to establish a ratio that is subsequently used to project a population at the less well documented date. If there is a significant difference is the tributary ratios between the dates, the estimate projection will be unreliable.

Selection of "Best Fit" Simulations

A major goal of this work is to assess the historical statistics-derived population trajectories of the Basin of Mexico during sixteenth-century in a manner independent of the historical tributary data used to construct them. Before so doing, a review of the logic of simulation methodology as the

---

[15] See Whitmore and Turner, *Population Reconstruction of the Basin of Mexico*, for a brief discussion of these factors.

[16] Cook and Simpson, *The Population of Central Mexico in the Sixteenth Century*; Cook and Borah, *The Indian Population of Central Mexico*; and Gibson, *The Aztecs*.

means of assessment is warranted. It is argued that the various historical reconstructions are properly represented by their group's fitted lines, and further, that these groups' fitted lines are accurately represented by their matched simulations (where they do, in fact, match). Therefore, discrimination among the simulations is equivalent to discrimination among the matching historical reconstructions. To judge these surrogate simulations, I have developed variables other than population change *per se*. These variables help explain particularities of the population trajectory that would not be possible without their use, and they help in judging specific simulations against the criteria used to evaluate their likelihood (see below).

It must be noted, however, that even with the wealth of information available after such interpretation, it is not possible to reject outright any simulation. This is because none of the simulations as modeled are *prima facia* impossible. Since the simulation structure (i.e., the logical interconnections of causes and effects) are assumed to be possible (see Chapter 2) and the data used to inform each variable is also assumed to be possible, the population dynamics that result *must* be possible. Thus, logical validity alone is not a sufficient criteria for judging among the simulations. Nevertheless, it is possible to choose among the simulations by applying several criteria that help measure the probability of each simulation.

SELECTION CRITERIA

There are three criteria by which the simulations (and the historical data for which they are surrogates) are judged. The first compares the historical reconstruction population data against that developed by the most closely matching simulation (e.g., see Figures 3.12, 3.13, and 3.14). The historical reconstruction group is rejected (or seriously doubted) if it is impossible to fit (within reasonable uncertainty bounds) a credible simulation of it (e.g., see Figure 3.14). This criterion is a "test" of the historical population data (primarily based on manipulation of tribute counts) against the logical structure and causal relationships of the simulations (primarily based on epidemiological, demographic, and cultural data). Essentially, each simulation forms a "hypothesis" of a pattern of population collapse, against which the statistics-based historical reconstruction data are compared. Thus, the historical reconstruction is rejected if it fails to match any credible causal hypothesis.

The second, and perhaps most important, criterion judges a simulation's "fit" with other historical data. A simulation (and the historical group it represents) is doubted if it produces results that run contrary to independent historical data. Hence, a "possible" simulation (i.e., one that is logically consistent and informed with "possible" data) and the historical data it represents may be questioned if the simulation generates data that are in conflict with other historical facts. This is essentially a "reality" test, judging the consistency of the simulation results with other known, non-population number, data. This criterion is extended so that if the implications of data generated by a simulation are unlikely, based on the best evidence, the simulation is questioned as well.

The last criterion is more subjective. A simulation is doubted if it demands assumptions (to make it fit with the historical reconstruction group) that strain credulity. Essentially, this criterion is the requirement that to be true (as opposed to valid), a logical syllogism must be constructed with "true" data. In other words: if the logical, causal structure of the simulation model is valid, and the data inputs are true, then the simulation results are true. This criterion is subjective to the degree that the determination of what data inputs are "true" is subjective.

SELECTION AND JUSTIFICATION

Of the three cases examined here, the moderate case is selected as that most likely to have occurred. Since each simulation is judged to be possible *prima facia*, this selection is based on the agreement of the simulations with the choice criteria. It does not significantly violate any of the choice criteria set out above. Alone, this fact only consigns the moderate case to a group of potential choices, since others may have also satisfied the choice criteria. Indeed, the choice might have been more difficult if the mild or severe cases had only mildly violated one criterion. Nevertheless, the fact is that the mild and severe simulations each significantly violate two or more of these criteria, hence, the moderate one emerges as the only acceptable choice.

This, however, is not as negative a reason for its choice as it may appear to be at first sight. The moderate simulation closely matched the historical reconstruction data developed specifically for the Basin (thus errors of scaling did not cloud the issue). Hence, the moderate simulation represents a credible causal hypothesis for the historically-reconstructed population trajectory. This simulation produced no outcomes that strongly contradict independent (non-population number) historical data for the period, thus it fits within the more-or-less accepted vision of the Basin's history. Lastly, the assumptions used to create this simulation are not unreasonable. It must be noted, of course, that this choice is not entirely objective because the judgement criteria are not entirely objective, nor can they ever be. But, given the present state of knowledge it seems entirely reasonable.

Mild Group

The mild simulation violates the most important criteria, fit with other historical data, in three ways. First, the assumption of no epidemic-induced famines generates a nutritional-sufficiency pattern that is at odds with historical observations (see Figure 4.10). For example, in the first forty years of Hispanic occupance, Gibson notes periods of increasing maize prices and famines in several years following epidemics (e.g., 1547-1551, 1551, and 1564, all following years without reported agricultural problems).[17] This strongly suggests that epidemic-induced agricultural shortfalls were among the causes of the famines and price inflation. The

---

[17] Gibson, *The Aztecs*, pp. 452-453.

mild simulation fails to produce these famine conditions (i.e., the nutritional sufficiency measure generated in the mild simulation is not reduced in the periods in question) (Figure 4.10).

The generation of a famine by the mild simulation, when there was little evidence for it in the historical record, is the second "reality test" failure for the mild simulation. This is a result of an attempt to model adequately the mild group's depopulation pattern after 1565 (Figures 3.12 and 4.1). To sufficiently reduce the non-crisis population growth rate, the mild simulation utilized a 20 percent labor tribute to reduce the agricultural yield (and thus increase the mortality rate and decrease the fertility rate) (Figures 4.11 and 4.14). While there are scattered references to famine and higher grain prices for the latter half of the century, there is no evidence for the continuous and severe food shortfall implied in the simulation.[18] Of course, it is not necessary to assume the labor tribute, and for the same simulation without this factor this argument does not apply. Nevertheless, the "sans-tribute" simulation badly fails to meet the fit criteria for 1597 (see Figure 3.12), and thus violates the first choice criterion.

The third problem with the mild simulation concerns the epidemic(s) of 1576-1581. Many scholars list this "Great *cocoliztli*" as one of the most severe in central Mexico (see also Chapter 2).[19] But because of the way it must be modeled in the mild case, its effect is almost negligible (Chapter 2 and Figure 4.1). The mild simulation returns a 1575 population of 498,068 and a post-epidemic, 1577, population of 461,874, a difference of 36,194 or a 7 percent loss. This serious loss is quite mild as compared with the other severe epidemics in the Basin, however (e.g., the mild simulation generates a 35 percent loss for the 1546 epidemic—one that is described as of similar intensity). Since the mild simulation clearly fails to reproduce the severity of the 1576 event, it must be questioned.

Two assumptions of the mild simulation (both clearly linked to the "reality test" problems noted above), that of no epidemic-induced food production shortfalls and that of a 20 percent labor withdrawal in the period 1565-1625, strain credibility. To posit that there were *no* food production losses due to *any* epidemic in the Basin, requires that each epidemic affected every community in a non-crucial period of the agricultural calender. Given the spatial and temporal wave-like pattern that epidemics usually follow,[20] this timing assumption seems unlikely. Further, it is hard to imagine that an agricultural community, suffering a virgin soil epidemic (in which virtually the entire population is affected, and a large proportion of the population perishes), would emerge with no production (i.e., as measured against needs) shortfall even if the epidemic attacked in a relatively slack season in the agricultural year.

---

18 See Gibson, *The Aztecs*, p. 453.

19 See Gerhard, *Historical Geography of New Spain*, pp. 23-24; Gibson, *The Aztecs*, p. 449; and Hassig, *Trade, Tribute, and Transportation*, p. 156.

20 Cliff *et al.*, *Spatial Aspects of Influenza Epidemics*.

The assumption of a 20 percent labor tribute seems equally unlikely. This assumption indicates a 20 percent agricultural production drop due to labor shortage. This is a large shortfall, and it must imply a very large and inopportune labor draft. Such a policy would be counterproductive for the Spanish since it would lead to increased Amerindian mortality at a time when labor was in short supply due to the effects of the early-century epidemics. Clearly, the Spanish did not always act in their own enlightened self-interest, but such a massive labor withdrawal also seems unlikely.

Severe Group

Examination of Figure 3.14 suggests that the severe simulation violates the first of the acceptance criteria, since it fails to match the historical reconstruction values at two dates, 1532 and 1548. *No manipulation of the simulation improved this fit, and it is judged quite unlikely that any alteration could make the simulation conform to the historical values* (see Chapter 3). This failure, by itself, is strong indictment of the historical data, and is amplified by examination (below) of the assumption necessary to bring the simulation curve as close as it comes to a fit.

There is an important caveat to keep in mind when examining this issue, however. The dates assigned to the Hispanic counts are by no means precise. For example, population figures that are assigned to 1532, may reflect the actual "on the ground" situation in 1530, 1531, or even earlier, or may reflect a count that extended over several years so as to include pre-epidemic and post-epidemic populations from different areas. This is crucial because if the population data refer to a date before the epidemic of 1531, the high population numbers would be much more probable (see Figure 3.14). Indeed, if the 1532 figure actually referred to 1530, the simulation would make a good fit at this date. The same situation obtains for the population estimate recorded for 1548. If it reflects the pre-epidemic population before 1546, it would be more probable and would fall within the 25 percent uncertainty bound for the estimate at that date (Figure 3.14).[21]

These arguments notwithstanding, the severe simulation presumes such a large 1519 population, that supporting it from within the Basin seems improbable, thus violating the "reasonable implications" criterion. The productivity assumptions used in the construction of MEXIPOP (see Chapter 2) were set at what may be termed the "high end" of reasonable estimates. The severe simulation would require that the Basin's pre-Hispanic agricultural productivity be nearly double that needed in the mild and moderate cases (to support about 2.7 million instead of about 1.5 million). This may not be impossible, but it strains the imagination. Further, as Hassig argues, it is not likely that high bulk, high weight

---

21 Of course, the same argument applies for estimates at other dates and for the other simulations. For the moderate simulation, such considerations would not alter the quality of fit of the simulation. In fact, for the 1535 and 1548 estimates in the moderate case, the quality of fit would be improved if the historical estimate actually referred to pre-epidemic populations (Fig. 3.13).

products such as grain staples were imported in great quantity, from any great distance, into the Basin.[22] This is because only human porters were available and the costs (in lost grain to feed the porters and their families) of transport would have matched or exceeded the value of the transported grain.[23]

Even if we relax the 25 percent uncertainty restrictions, and accept the simulation values for 1532 and 1548, the assumption needed to reach these values is questionable. In Chapter 3 it was demonstrated that a 4 percent emigration in each of the epidemic years of 1520, 1531, 1546, and 1576 is necessary to approximate a satisfactory simulation fit. Examination of this assumption shows that the migration numbers implicit in the seemingly low migration rate are large (e.g., in 1520, a 4 percent emigration generates over 80,000 migrants, in 1531 nearly 55,000, in 1546 over 30,000 and in 1576 about 10,000). The problem is, where would such a large number of migrants, especially for the early dates, go? It is by no means certain that it would be easy for over 20,000 families (in 1520) to relocate and find agricultural lands or other employment, and if so large a movement had been triggered, why is there no mention of it in contemporary documentation of surrounding regions? Tribal animosities and land tenure systems may have precluded such a migration. This point is by no means certain, however, and migration may have been important—but the numbers generated by this simulation are large.

Another possibility is that instead of emigration, this population perished in these epidemics (or famines) or at the hands of the Spanish (especially in 1520). Eighty thousand is not an impossible-to-believe number for war casualties in 1520, but it is significant, and homicide will not explain the large figures for the other dates. For the later dates we must presume that if there were no emigration the "extra" population loss was due to increases in the mortality of the diseases or famine. This is not impossible either, but it does indicate that the mortality was fully 10 percent greater than that originally assumed. Indeed, for the high morbidity epidemics of 1520 and 1531 the "care factor" variable (see Chapter 2) comes into play to increase the mortality over the assumed value, making this 10 percent addition even less likely. Aside from trying to fit this simulation, there is no compelling reason to presume this additional mortality.

---

22 Hassig, *Trade, Tribute, and Transportation*, Chapter 2.

23 While the Spanish introduced carts and beasts of burden relatively early in the sixteenth century, the use of Amerindian porters did not vanish because until mid-century livestock numbers and production were low, see Hassig, *Trade, Tribute, and Transportation*, p. 187.

Implications for Reconstruction

The analyses in this chapter point to several issues concerning the dates and nature of the historical reconstruction counts. The most important general observation is that the sixteenth century was a period of very unstable demography in the Basin. Unlike the view implicit in most of the literature, the population change trajectory was not a "smooth" function; rather, it resembled a sort of punctuated equilibrium in which periods of relative stability were interrupted by crises that greatly altered the immediate pre-existing conditions and lead to altered subsequent conditions. This point is important in assessing the general Amerindian cultural environment and its "evolution." In particular, it is important in understanding the conditions under which the Hispanic counts of tributaries were made, since the nature of the "demographic environment" certainly affected the accuracy of the counts. For that reason, examination of the conditions around the dates of the counts is illuminating.

The first issue concerns the dating of Hispanic counts with respect to the dates of epidemics and coincident population declines. Neither the dates for counts nor the dates for epidemics are absolutely fixed in time, indeed, they cannot be since both the process of traveling around central Mexico performing counts and the spatial diffusion processes of epidemics required significant time. The applicable time constants for these two are not known in all cases, and in some cases may well not be recoverable. For that reason, it is useful to compare the purported "census" dates to the recorded periods of epidemics.

Ignoring the estimates for 1519, the first "census" period in question encompasses the dates of 1532-1540 (see Table 3.4). There was an epidemic recorded in 1531, and if the counts attributed to 1532 and 1535 (for the moderate and severe cases) actually reflected the situation before or during this event, the counts would be quite skewed compared to the figures obtained after the epidemic (Figures 3.13 and 3.14). Further, any counts that spanned or immediately followed the epidemic would be suspect because of the degree of disruption engendered by the epidemic.

A further problem to accurate counting at this date, even if the epidemic period itself was avoided, is that the basic demographic measures were instable and not at their "traditional" values. CBR and CDR were both declining and below "traditional" values (Figures 4.2-4.7). Conversely, the dependency ratio was rapidly increasing from a low level (Figure 4.18). This is a problem if one imagines how such "counts" may have been accomplished. It seems reasonable to posit that village elders, upon questioning from Spanish officers or clerics, might have done a simple (mental) household count, then multiplying this by a "traditional" estimate of family size and composition, to obtain a total figure. If this is so, a skewed result is obtained in times of rapidly changing household composition (i.e., changing CBR, CDR and dependency ratio).

A similar situation obtains for the counts dated 1540 and 1548, they presumably record the situation following the serious epidemics in 1538 and 1546, but the timing is uncertain in both. And for 1546, the span of the epidemic is recorded from 1545 to 1548.[24] Similar to the situation in 1531, the demographic measures at these dates also were unstable (Figures 4.2-4.7, and 4.18). These uncertainties make the counts at these dates relatively shakey foundations upon which to rest a depopulation pattern.

Fortunately, the situation in the late 1565s is less disturbed. The epidemics of the previous 5 years were less severe, making the timing issue less salient. Further, the effects of the severe epidemics of the early part of the century had "worked through" to some extent, and the other demographic measures were less erratic as well (Figures 4.2-4.7, and 4.18). Perhaps it is no coincidence that the data obtained for these dates are regarded as the earliest reliable data—it may have been the earliest date at which the demographic base was steady enough to permit a reasonably competent count.

The "great cocoliztili"[25] of 1576-1581 spanned or immediately preceded the count dated at 1580. The same objections that applied to the early counts apply here, except that the basic demographic rates are not all that disturbed in this period (Figures 4.2-4.7, and 4.18).

The counts dated to the late 1590s do not immediately follow a period of extreme mortality, but the period around 1590 was clearly an unsettled one so that the timing issue may have been important. The 1590s were a period of dramatically changing dependency (and tributary) ratios, however, and this factor may have affected the validity of the counts since the previous generation of high dependency ratios were falling to pre-conquest levels (Figure 4.18 and 4.19).

The late 1600s followed a serious mortality disruption in 1601, so that the issue of timing may have been important (Figures 4.2-4.4). It *may* be reasonable to assume, however, that as the century progressed and there were more Spanish in New Spain and the bureaucracy was established, that the dating of events was more reliable. Contrary to the case of the 1590s, the dependency and tribute ratios of the 1600s were climbing, but the CBR and CDRs were reasonably stable (Figures 4.18 and 4.19).

By 1625 the demographic situation (aside from population numbers, of course) more closely matched the immediate pre-conquest situation than at any time in the sixteenth century (Figs 4.2-4.7 and 4.18). This similarity may be misleading, however, since the numbers on which it is based are generated by simulations that do not presume that the population's primary behaviors have changed. By 1625, a century of Hispanic acculturation may have changed the Amerindian society's basic values and this change may have been reflected in their demographic behavior.

---

[24] Gibson, *The Aztecs*, p. 448.

[25] Gibson, *The Aztecs*, p. 449.

Summary of Major Findings

The major findings discussed in this chapter may be conveniently grouped under three headings: the nature of population change itself; the dynamics of other demographic measures of interest; and the causal linkages that are associated with these dynamics. Taken together these findings address the major research questions posed in Chapter 1 and illuminate other topics in the sixteenth-century demographic history of the Basin.

POPULATION DYNAMICS

A major research question motivating this study concerned whether the very large depopulations noted in the historical scholarship on the sixteenth-century Basin of Mexico were *possible*, given reasonable assumptions as to cause. Examination of the causal simulations performed here indicates that large depopulation was possible, indeed likely, given the probable causes illuminated here. As noted above, not all scales of depopulation are equally likely, but even the most severe is *possible* in the strict sense, if less probable.

Of the three examined here (and they encompass the full range of credible historical estimates of depopulation) the *moderate* case simulation is the one most likely to capture the actual sixteenth-century population dynamics of the Basin. This simulation generates an eve-of-conquest (1519) total population of 1.59 million for the Basin. This total was reduced in the course of the sixteenth century to a nadir population of 183,000 in 1607. The scale of this depopulation is remarkable, since this nadir population represents only 11.5 percent of the 1519 total.

Even more remarkable is the scale of population collapse in the early part of the century. By 1535 the Amerindian population had declined to only 54 percent of its total only 16 years earlier (to 866,000 from 1.59 million). This decline continued at an even more rapid rate to 1547 when the remaining population (493,000) totaled a mear 31 percent of its pre-conquest figure. Shortly after the mid-point of Spanish sixteenth-century occupancy in the Basin (1569), the Amerindian population total (343,000) only represented 21.5 percent of its zenith in 1519. The pace of collapse slowed in the later half of the century, so that the 1607 nadir (183,000) represented greater than 53 percent of the 1569 total.

This remarkable scale of depopulation was achieved in an equally exceptional way. The temporal pattern of depopulation was very irregular. Instead of a more-or-less uniform fall, the bulk of the Basin's Amerindian population decline occurred in a series of step-like catastrophes. Immediately following each severe epidemic, especially those in 1520, 1531, 1538, and 1546, the population total plunged to a lower level. Small population growth ensued for many of the periods between these epidemic-induced collapses.

OTHER DEMOGRAPHIC DYNAMICS

Like the pattern for population size, the temporal dynamics of the basic demographic variables (i.e., mortality and fertility) are quite unstable. They exhibit two inter-linked patterns. The most prominent are the notable "spikes" of increased mortality and decreased fertility associated with the epidemic periods. These "spikes" are not of long duration, typically one or two years, but they are of great magnitude. The serious epidemics (mostly in the first 40 years of Spanish occupance) increased the Amerindian crude death rates from their "usual" values of about 30 per 1,000 to over 500 per 1,000, a 16 -fold increase. Similarly, these epidemic events decreased the crude birth rates from the "usual" values of about 30 per 1,000 to scarcely 10 per 1,000, a drop of two-thirds.

In addition to, and indeed because of, these dramatic disruptions, the long-term (decadal) patterns of non-crisis (i.e., the rates in times without the crisis "spikes") crude death and birth rates were also unstable in the sixteenth century. The amplitude of these longer-term swings was far less than for the "spikes," however. Following the initial epidemics, crude birth rates declined about 10 percent in the early 1530s, briefly recovered, and subsequently plunged to their sixteenth-century minima (of about 80-85 percent of the "usual" level) in the early 1550s. From this nadir, the non-crisis crude birth rates gradually increased for most of the rest of the century, reaching values approximating those of 1519 in the early 1600s.

A similar, but reversed pattern obtains for non-crisis crude death rates. Initially, they increased about 10 percent from 1519 to the mid-1540s. From this sixteenth-century high, the non-crisis crude death rates followed a pattern of gradual decline throughout the century. By the 1610s the crude death rates were nearly 10 percent lower than their pre-conquest levels.

Because of these short-term and long-term fluctuations in the fundamental demographic measures, the long-term patterns in derived demographic measures were volatile as well. In the first 20 years of Spanish occupance, the dependency ratio traced a wave-like pattern of decline, rapid increase, and rapid decrease. So by the 1540s, the dependency ratio reached its sixteenth-century low (at about 85 percent of its 1519 level). A rapid and sustained increase in the dependency ratio followed, and from roughly 1550 through 1590 the dependency ratio hovered at levels approximately 30 percent higher than the pre-conquest level. A post-1590 decline brought the levels down to ones roughly similar to those at the time of conquest.

Tributary ratios (i.e., a rough measure of the multiplier needed to convert tribute counts to total population counts) parallel the dynamic pattern of dependency ratios. The value of this measure for the 1560s, about 3.7, is smaller than that used by Cook and Simpson (4.0), but larger than both those used by Cook and Borah (3.3) and Gibson (2.8).[26]

---

[26] Cook and Simpson, *The Population of Central Mexico in the Sixteenth Century*; Cook and Borah, *The Indian Population of Central Mexico*; and Gibson, *The Aztecs*.

CAUSAL LINKAGES

The catastrophic decline in the Basin's Amerindian population is due to the combined effect of a series of crises, each of which reduced the population significantly. It is this concatenation of calamity, rather than a single massive event, that produced such devastation.

By far the most important factor in these crises were the "virgin soil" epidemics. These epidemics produced profound short-term increases in mortality that profoundly reduced population totals. While fertility was significantly reduced at the same time and this effect cannot be neglected, it is not surprising that epidemic mortality emerges as the single most important cause of depopulation in the sixteenth-century Basin. It is this extra mortality that produces the "steps" of population collapse noted above.

A longer-term consequence of these epidemics was an increasing non-crisis death rate along with a decreasing non-crisis birth rate for the first 30-40 years after contact. This, in turn, led to decreasing rates of growth (indeed, to negative rates of growth) in the non-crisis intervals in this period. This trend reversed about mid-century and the disparity of the high secular death rates and the low secular birth rates was reduced, thus gradually increasing the non-crisis growth rates to their (low) pre-conquest values by the end of the century. While this pattern is noticeable, it is insignificant as an explanation for the bulk of the sixteenth-century collapse.

Epidemic illness did not work alone to winnow the Amerindian population, famine mortality was also a significant agent. Famines induced by both adverse environmental conditions for agriculture and by epidemic-induced labor shortage increased mortality and decreased fertility. Of these, epidemic-induced famines were the more significant. Indeed, epidemic-induced famines probably accounted for about 10 percent of the total depopulation. Neither type of famine altered the birth rates significantly, so it is famine mortality that accounts for its contribution to the depopulation.

Another factor that may have contributed to famine, labor withdrawals that led to production shortfalls, was judged to be unimportant for the accepted population decline scenario. Similarly, large-scale emigration or homicide need not have been important to generate the most reasonable population simulation.

Chapter 5

CALIBRATING POPULATION DECLINE:
MEASURING A CENTURY OF POPULATION CATASTROPHE

To this point, the simulation approach to the Basin's Amerindian depopulation has been technical, if not tedious. The reward of such an exercise, however, is the possibility of assessing various facets of the major debate over Central Mexican depopulation that is relatively independent of interpretations grounded in issues of documentary validity and that is more objective than personal observations or opinion. Here, then, the major findings of the present analysis are reviewed, conclusions and implications drawn, and its overall significance discussed.

The Scale of Population Decline

THE BASIN

Despite its power and sophistication as an analytical tool, *the simulation methodology developed here cannot absolutely eliminate any of the established reconstructions of the sixteenth century population dynamics of the Basin.* This is an important point that should not be lost for it counters the observations of those critics who contend that reconstructions positing large-scale depopulation are unrealistic, based on flawed data, or are reflective of biases on the part of the reconstructor.[1] To eliminate any group of historical reconstructions would require the failure to fit a credible simulation to that group, and that is not the case here. The historical values examined here are all within a general "envelope" of possibility.

Nevertheless, the severe and mild cases much more closely approach the boundaries of possibility than does the moderate case. A second major conclusion, then, is *that the extreme positions of relatively small collapse on the one hand, or very profound collapse on the other, are less likely to have taken place, and the moderate group is more likely to have occurred.*

---

[1]   For example, see Petersen, "A Demographers View"; and Petersen, *Population.*

It must be remembered, however, that the moderate case interpretation of the Basin's population trajectory represents an unparalleled depopulation in terms of the scale of decline for the size of population involved.[2] This conclusion, reached through simulation analysis, constitutes an "independent" evaluation since it does not rely in any important way on the possibly flawed data used in the historical reconstructions.

The simulation demonstrates that by the turn of the seventeenth century, the Amerindian population of the Basin had probably been reduced to a total scarcely more than 10 percent of the 1519 total: about 1.6 million was reduced to roughly 180,000 by 1607. To put the eve-of-the-conquest population figure in perspective, it is useful to compare it to other population figures for the same date. McEvedy and Jones estimate the 1500 population of *all* of Spain as 6.5 million (an overall population density of about 13 per km[2]), and that of England and Wales at 3.75 million (an overall population density of about 12 per km[2]).[3] Thus, the Basin's pre-Hispanic zenith population, 1.6 million, represented a large fraction of the total populations of two of Europe's major powers. Further, since the Basin is much smaller in area, about 7,000 km[2], its population density, of 230 per km[2], was far higher.

While the Basin's zenith population was comparable to that of selected European national populations, the sixteenth-century population collapse in Mexico was incomparable to any experienced in Europe. In each of four periods (each less than 25 years in length), the Basin's Amerindian population declined more than 30 percent from the previous level (Figure 5.1a). By way of comparison, estimates for the fourteenth-century European population holocaust resulting from the Black Death range from a loss of one-third from A.D. 1300-1400[4] to a 40-50 percent loss for the same period.[5] Thus, the sixteenth-century Mexican population catastrophe virtually equals *four Black Death equivalents in the span of a single lifetime.* As dramatic as these depopulation figures are, however, it is only through an examination of the population decline by on a more personal level that its impact as a human event can be truly gauged.

Imagine a young adult (say 20 years of age on the eve of the conquest) living in a village with a population of 100. If she survived to her thirty-fifth birthday (1535), she would have witnessed her village reduced to only 70 persons. By the time she reached middle age in 1547, a further 30 percent of the now diminished total would have perished, leaving only 49. Had she lived to full maturity at age 69, yet another 30 percent would have

---

2   Please refer to Figure 5.1 for a summary of the most probable population trajectory; crude death rate pattern; crude birth rate pattern; and pattern of nutritional sufficiency.

3   McEvedy and Jones, *Atlas*, p. 41, 101.

4   McEvedy and Jones, *Atlas*, p. 42; and Slack, *Impact*, p. 15;

5   Russell, *British Medieval Population*, pp. 260-281; and Hatcher, *Plague, Population and the English Economy* p. 68.

been winnowed from the "middle age" total, leaving only 34. And if she attained great age (80), a fourth 30 percent would have been lost, leaving only 24.

Since the simulations utilized here were constructed independently of the historical tributary count data used to produce the historical estimates, agreement of historical estimates with the simulation constitutes relatively independent support of these historical reconstructions. Conversely, failure to agree constitutes relatively independent refutation of the historical values. Hence, the simulation results strongly support the early century population totals and the 1519 to 1570 depopulation ratio argued by Gibson and Sanders, whose estimates were incorporated in the moderate case (see Chapter 3).[6] In contrast, because Cook and Simpson's estimates (used to construct the mild case) for this period imply a rate of depopulation that is scarcely less than one-half that obtained here, they are, at least partly, refuted. At the other end of the spectrum of depopulation ratios, Borah and Cook's population sums for this period (used as the basis for the severe case) call for a depopulation ratio roughly double that argued here. This seems even more unlikely.[7]

An important conclusion following from these results concerns the path of depopulation in this first 50 years of Spanish occupance. Since the tributary (and other) data for this period is less extensive and of lower quality than that for later dates, population estimates constructed using these data are more speculative and less well-supported. Hence, because of the paucity of data, even the more moderate historical reconstructions[8] may be questioned. Since the simulation population estimates developed here support these moderate values well, *the catastrophic nature of the initial phase of the population collapse is bolstered and is plausible given the circumstances* (Figure 5.1a).

Unfortunately, by concentrating on specific dates (or rather, the population estimates for these dates) and depopulation ratios there may be a tendency to presume that the population change between these dates was a relatively uniform phenomena. The simulations show that this is not the case, however. Rather, *the trajectory of population in the sixteenth century resembles a stair-step, where the "steps" represent relatively crisis-free periods, with only moderate population change (up or down), while the "risers" denote periods of catastrophic population decline* (Figure 5.1a). It is important to keep this pattern in mind when interpreting any phenomena in the sixteenth century Basin of Mexico.

Because of the instability of this trajectory, the timing of events is important in their interpretation. Nowhere is this more clear than for the

---

6 Gibson, *The Aztecs*; and Sanders, "The Population of the Central Mexican Symbiotic Region."

7 Borah and Cook, *The Population of Central Mexico*; and Borah and Cook, *Aboriginal Population of Central Mexico*.

8 For example, that of Gibson, *The Aztecs*.

dates of the Hispanic counts as compared to the dates of epidemics. Since the population data for the early part of the century are sparse, the counts usually dated to the mid 1530s and late 1545s are of particular importance. Unfortunately, the dates for these counts are not known with great precision, and significantly, neither are the dates of the important epidemics (usually dated to 1531 and 1545-1548) that are presumed to precede them (see Figure 5.1). There is a possibility that the counts reflect the population situation during or before the epidemics, rather than after. Since the population changed significantly during these events, this relative timing issue is important in interpreting the population trajectory.

This conclusion is significant for further research in this area. Particular attention should be given to the timing of events when examining new situations. It would also be valuable to undertake new research to clarify, as much as possible, the timing of events for the period and locale discussed in this work as well.

HEMISPHERIC DEPOPULATION: THE WIDER SCENE

While it is not valid to argue that Mexico's or the entire hemisphere's experience precisely mirrored the Basin's, the simulation results developed here are suggestive for other Amerindian cases.[9] Speculation on a larger scale is facilitated by concentrating on the proportions of collapse rather than the absolute scale of the decline. Examining the "conservative" position of McEvedy and Jones illustrates the argument .[10] They assume a small, only 14 million, population for the entire hemisphere in 1492, declining to 11.5 million by 1600.[11] The analyses performed here (for the Basin only, of course) suggest that it is extremely unlikely that any credible epidemic simulation would generate a total population collapse of only 20 percent

---

[9] Very large, presumably epidemic caused, population losses are reported for Polynesia and other places in Oceania in the eighteenth and nineteenth centuries (e.g., see B. G. Corney, "The Behavior or Certain Epidemic Diseases in Natives of Polynesia with Especial Reference to the Fiji Islands," *Transactions of the Epidemiological Society of London New Series* 3 (1884), pp. 76-95; Judd, "Depopulation in Polynesia"; and R. Lang, "Plagues and Pestilence in Polynesia: The Nineteenth-Century Cook Islands Experience," *Bulletin of the History of Medicine* 58 (1984), pp. 325-346). While the simulation results developed for the Basin will not be used to speculate on their validity, large-scale depopulation on the scale noted in the Basin does lend credibility to the similarly large-scale losses in Oceania.

[10] McEvedy and Jones' argument is based on the use of very conservative "eve-of-the-conquest" estimates for the Americas. For example, compare their estimates (McEvedy and Jones, *Atlas*, pp. 271-317 with Denevan's (*The Native Population of the Americas in 1492*, p. 291) "middle-of-the-road" estimates and with the earlier estimates of Kroeber, Rosenblat, and Steward (reprinted in Denevan, *The Native Population of the Americas in 1492*, p. 3.

[11] McEvedy and Jones, *Atlas*, p. 270.

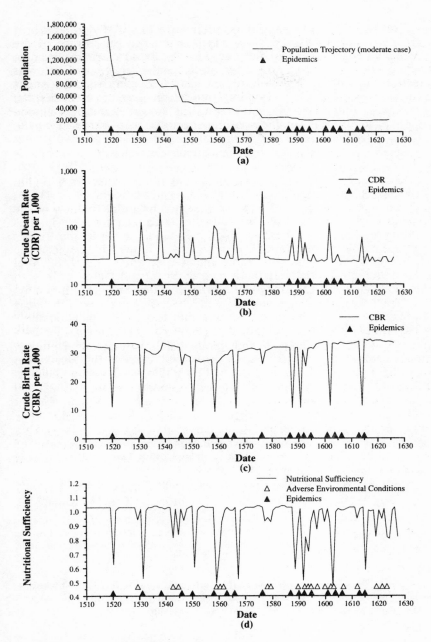

Figure 5.1 Most Probable Simulations

from 1500 to 1600 as is implied by their estimates.[12] To do so would require two unlikely assumptions: (1) that a large proportion of the population was not reached by the concatenation of Old World diseases, an unlikely event since a large proportion of the hemisphere's population was concentrated in the two "high culture" areas of Mesoamerica and the Andes and these areas were relatively completely Hispanicized; or (2) that the diseases were much less virulent among the Amerindians than among Europeans and others in similar, non-immune conditions—this seems to be an equally untenable position.

Similarly, although at the opposite extreme, estimates of a hemispheric population collapse of 95 percent in the sixteenth century[13] are also unlikely. To support such a position would require that each region experience a depopulation equivalent to the Basin's "severe" case. This is less extreme, but unlikely, if only because a substantial fraction of the hemispheric population was much less concentrated than in the Basin, thus enfeebling the epidemiological assumptions used to construct the Basin's severe case mortality functions. Further, regardless of the 1492 hemispheric total, it seems very likely that more than 5 percent of the 1492 total population remained relatively untouched by Spanish disease—at least in the sixteenth century. They may have perished at the same rate ultimately, but by then the Amerindian population was rebounding in many of the areas first affected, thus reducing the overall sixteenth century depopulation rate.

The simulation results obtained here are roughly comparable with Denevan's moderate Mexican and hemispheric estimates.[14] Denevan produces a Mexico estimate of 21.4 million by considering Borah and Cook's 25.2 million estimate and one of 11.4 million scaled from Sanders' Basin total.[15] Using a similar scaling for the moderate simulation 1519 population obtained here (about 1.6 million) gives a Mexico total of about 16 million. This total is about 75 percent of Denevan's Mexico total.[16] Thus a new, but rather speculative, hemispheric total may be computed by taking 75 percent of Denevan's hemispheric total. This calculation yields a total of about 43 million. This figure just barely nests within Denevan's proposed hemispheric total error range of 43-72 million.[17]

To put this figure into perspective, the 1500 European population is estimated by McEvedy and Jones to be 81 million.[18] They[19] estimate the

12 McEvedy and Jones, *Atlas*, p. 270.

13 See Dobyns, "Estimating," p. 415, for such a figure.

14 Denevan, *The Native Population of the Americas in 1492*, p. 291.

15 Denevan, *The Native Population of the Americas in 1492*, p. 291; and Sanders, "The Population of the Central Mexican Symbiotic Region," p. 130.

16 Denevan, *The Native Population of the Americas in 1492*, p. 291.

17 Ibid.

18 McEvedy and Jones, *Atlas*, p. 18.

19 McEvedy and Jones, *Atlas*, p. 349.

world total for 1500 at 425 million.[20] Based on McEvedy and Jones's conservative reckoning of the 1500 New World population (14 million), it's population represented only about 3 percent of humanity in 1500.[21] Assuming a more reasonable (and conservative) New World population of 50 million, and a world total of 461 million (425 plus the 36 million difference between 14 and 50), the Amerindian proportion of humanity in 1500 soars to about 10 percent. This estimate is more reasonable, and it is supported by the majority of historical demographic work in the Western Hemisphere.

Causes of Population Decline

The methodology used in this study is explicitly based on simulating the demographic responses of a population in the face of conditions that affect them. For that reason, it ties the statistics of population decline to their causes, both proximate and secondary. The proximate causes of population change are changes in fertility, mortality, and migration of the population. These changes are induced by secondary causes such as epidemics, famines, and so on. The simulation methodology developed here allows for the assessment of the importance of both the secondary and proximate causes of population change.

ROLE OF EPIDEMICS

So important are epidemics in understanding the Amerindian population collapse that, in essence, the simulation methodology developed here is a methodology of epidemic simulation. Unlike the famous epidemic periods in Europe where a single pathogen dominated, the sixteenth century Amerindian population was exposed to a series of invasions of different pathogens. It is the concatenation of the periods of extra mortality due to each new infectious agent that gives the Amerindian population collapse its unique scale (see Figure 5.1b). The effect in New Spain was of a series of "Black Death-scale" population collapses, with a new one following shortly on the heels of the previous. This realization is important because it points to an "easy" explanation of the much larger Amerindian depopulation. Further, the impact of epidemics demonstrated here serves to point to the

---

20   It must be noted that McEvedy and Jones may not be the best choice for European or world population estimates since there is good reason to question their New World figures as well as others (e.g., for Egypt see Douglas L. Johnson, and Thomas M. Whitmore, *Population Reconstruction of the Egyptian Nile Valley: 4000 B.C. to Present*, Millennial Long Waves in Human Occupance Project: Technical Paper #3, Clark University, 1987). Nevertheless, the *Atlas* is a good choice for this comparison since it is widely cited and represents an attempt to deal with all regions of the globe.

21   McEvedy and Jones, *Atlas*, pp. 270, 349.

importance of McNeill's much more general arguments about the importance of "micro-parasites" in the history of the world.[22]

It is not surprising then, that the data resulting from these simulations demonstrate that it is virtually certain that epidemics were responsible for the bulk of Amerindian population decline in the sixteenth century. Since epidemics can account for virtually all of the extra mortality in the sixteenth century, the principle of Occam's razor suggests that it is not necessary to assume that there were other important causes of death (but see famine below). Thus, no reliance on the "Black Legend" of Spanish homicide and cruelty is necessary to explain the observed population collapse. Cruelty and homicide were certainly present, however, and may have been important causes of depopulation for specific times and places. This general assertion may not be applicable to all areas of the New World, however, since the specific epidemiological and other variables are not consistent in all areas. Nevertheless, the presumption of disease mortality as the overwhelming cause of Amerindian population decline throughout the New World seems virtually irrefutable.

In addition to, and indeed as a result of, their primacy as catastrophic disruptions, epidemic diseases also produced important long-term demographic changes. The massive epidemics engendered very large increases in the crude death rates and similar decreases in the crude birth rates, but only for relatively brief periods (see Figures 5.1b and 5.1c). More pervasive were the secular changes to the CDRs and CBRs as a result of the changes in population age composition as a result of the epidemic crises (Figures 5.1b and 5.1c). The succession of "virgin soil" epidemics in the early part of the century gave rise to a half-century-long "trough" (extending roughly from 1540 to 1600) in the crude birth rates. This is primarily due to the maturation of epidemic mortality-reduced-size cohorts into the reproducing ages, thus reducing the number of reproducing couples in the population. This depression in CBRs is easily seen in the population trajectory for the non-crisis years after the 1531 epidemic. Instead of the vigorously increasing trend of population shown between the first epidemic crises, population change was virtually stagnant between epidemics in the later half of the century (Figure 5.1a).

This alteration affected the population in other ways as well. After an initial "wave" of decline, recovery, and decline from 1520 to 1540, the dependency ratios rose to high levels, that persisted for the rest of the century (roughly 1550 to 1590) (see Figure 4.18). As Hassig correctly notes, it is this extra burden on the productive portion of the population (and the reduction in the proportion of the productive portion) as much as the population decline *per se* that led to labor shortage and impoverishment.[23]

---

22 McNeill, *Plagues and Peoples*.
23 Hassig, *Trade, Tribute, and Transportation*, pp. 181-184.

Despite their importance in the causes and the virtually unprecedented scale of the collapse, the epidemic virulence assumptions used in MEXIPOP are "conservative" in the sense that they do not assume that the Amerindian population was genetically less able to resist successfully the diseases they encountered. The case fatality rate (i.e., the rate of death among those infected) applied to the Amerindian population in the MEXIPOP epidemics was, for the most part, developed from European data for these diseases.[24] The assumption is that the resistance to disease (i.e., the ability of the individual to fight off the disease successfully) was the same for all previously uninfected individuals (of the same age). Thus, the high mortalities experienced in the Basin of Mexico were not because the victims were a *particularly* defenseless population with low resistance to the imported diseases.

The high mortalities that resulted from these European diseases is the result of very high morbidity rates (i.e., the rate of infection in the total population) suffered by the non-immune Amerindian population.[25] The differences in morbidity rates between the European and Amerindian populations are a result of the immunizing effect possessed by most of the epidemic diseases considered here. Most infections trigger alterations in the immune system to produce infection-specific antibodies. A "pattern" for these specific antibodies is retained in survivors of a particular disease so that they are usually immune to further infections of the same disease because the immune system rapidly recognizes the specific infectious agent and produces the antibodies necessary to destroy the infectious agent. Previously uninfected individuals' immune systems lack these rapid recognition and destruction capabilities. The usual situation in the Old World limited the community mortality for each disease since the number of susceptible individuals (i.e., individuals with no previous infection—and no resulting immunity) was limited. This is because these diseases were relatively common (i.e., endemic) and a relatively small proportion of the population was infected in each outbreak. This is in contrast to the non-immune situation obtained when each disease first entered the Amerindian population. Since no one had previous exposure to the disease (thus no one had immunities as a result of surviving a previous exposure), the number of susceptible individuals was virtually the same as the total population.

---

24 In cases where the morbidity was extremely high, a compensating term in MEXIPOP, the care factor, gradually escalated the epidemic mortality to 1.25x its usual value when morbidity reached 90 percent. This term accounts for the fact that even rudimentary care reduces the case fatality rate—even for serious contagious diseases. The data from which the case fatality structure were drawn are mostly for circumstances in which such care was present. In situations where virtually the entire community (or family) suffers simultaneously, care for the ill is neglected and the case fatality rate rises. See Chapter 2 for a fuller discussion.

25 Symbolically the relationship is displayed:
Mortality = Morbidity * Case Fatality
(deaths/total pop) = (infections/total pop) * (deaths/infection)

These principles of epidemiology also explain the decline in epidemic mortality as the century progressed. Since the number of types of new pathogens (i.e., those capable of causing a "virgin soil" epidemic) that could be transported to the New World was limited, each new "virgin soil" epidemic reduced the number of possible "virgin soil" epidemics subsequently. Hence, there were fewer as the century advanced. Further, after the initial invasion of each new pathogen (resulting in a new "virgin soil" epidemic), subsequent outbreaks of the same pathogen produced community mortalities similar to those they produced in Europe, since the susceptible population was no longer so large a proportion of the total. Therefore, it is not necessary to argue that the gradual intermingling of Spanish and Amerindian blood produced a population with European resistance characteristics—the immunological experience of the Amerindian population was sufficient alone. Indeed, resistance to particular diseases is not heritable in that direct sense (i.e., offspring of Europeans would be as susceptible to European diseases with which they had no experience). Of course, the offspring of survivors of particular diseases may have inherited their parents' better-than-average immune systems and may be at less risk to those particular pathogens.[26]

ROLE OF DEMOGRAPHIC STRUCTURE

The demographic structure of a population is not, of course, strictly speaking, a cause of depopulation. This topic is properly examined here, however, because demographic structure does alter the effects of other mortality-causing factors. One advantage of the simulation method is that it allows examination of the effect changes in different aspects of the cultural-ecological situation, such as the demographic structure, have on the resulting population trajectory.

This advantage is clearly seen when the effects of changed demographic assumptions are weighed against changes in the epidemic pattern. At least for the range of demographic assumptions used here, changes in the specification of the epidemic sub-model (i.e., changes in the identification of three epidemics from typhus to pneumonic plague) produce more profound changes in the resulting population trajectory than do changes in the demographic sub-model, *ceteris paribus* (see Chapter 3). For situations with less virulent epidemics (i.e., non-virgin soil conditions) age structure may well be more important in determining the scale of population change in the face of disease. Of course, these results do not diminish the importance of detailed demographic data. Without such data or assumptions, the epidemic effects would be far less well-modeled.

Given the importance of epidemic disease in the demographic history of the New World, further research to more completely identify the specific pathogens responsible for epidemics is vital. Indeed, advances in the

---

26 The parents' immune systems may have been better-than-average since they survived infection with the particular pathogens. Pathogen-specific resistance is not usually thought of as inheritable, however.

accuracy of this simulation methodology rely on such advances in epidemiological history.

ROLE OF FAMINES

The impact of two types of famine is evident in the Basin. The first results from disruption during an epidemic, while the second is attributable to relatively independent harvest failures caused by adverse agricultural conditions (see Figure 5.1d). While famines are less important than epidemics in shaping the overall population history of the Basin, they do figure significantly, and it is not possible to have an accurate or complete view of the Basin's population without considering them. The role of famine is largely under-appreciated in studies of Amerindian depopulation and more research on topics germane to famines would certainly pay dividends in greater accuracy and understanding.

Epidemic-Induced Famines

While epidemic-induced agricultural shortages were a feature of all the epidemics modeled here, the demographic effects of these crisis famines varied considerably. For the most virulent, major epidemics, famines added little to the increase in CDRs or the decrease in CBRs, mostly because the epidemics themselves so altered the CBRs and CDRs that little additional change was possible. An exception to this pattern is the measles epidemic in 1531, where famine contributed significantly to the population decline that resulted. Many more minor epidemics triggered significant famine losses, however, increasing their impact on the overall population decline (see Figure 5.1d).

While it is clear that their role is significant, it is difficult to gauge the exact contribution of epidemic-induced famines to the Amerindian depopulation. Nevertheless, the overall depopulation probably would have been about 10 percent less profound if there had been no epidemic-induced famines (i.e., the total depopulation ratio would have been about 80 percent with no epidemic famines, as opposed to 89 percent with these famines) (see Chapter 3). This fact points to their importance. To produce an equal scale of depopulation without famines, epidemics would have had to have been 15-20 percent more potent. This is by no means impossible, but it seems unrealistic to posit even more virulent epidemics without accompanying agricultural disruption and famines. At the other end of the scale, the degree of epidemic disruption to agriculture is set in MEXIPOP at a maximum credible level, so that it is not reasonable to presume that epidemic-induced famines played a much greater role than is argued here. For other regions in the New World, epidemic-induced famines may have been more profound, however. The Basin possessed a particularly diverse and productive agricultural system(s) that may have been more robust in the face of epidemic disruption.

Despite their secondary importance as sources of crisis mortality, epidemic-induced famines served to alter the age-specific pattern of mortality in such crises. Generally, famines affected the aged and youth disproportionally more than did many epidemics. For this reason, famines were important in generating the altered age structure that was noted above.

Agricultural Failure-induced Famines

As modeled in MEXIPOP, famines resulting from environmentally-triggered agricultural failures played a minor role in the Amerindian population collapse (see Figure 5.1d). The modeling of these shortfalls is admittedly subjective and unsupported, and open to question for that reason. Nevertheless, the range of assumed shortfalls, from 5 to 20 percent seems quite within reason. Lesser values would eliminate these as factors, yet there are recorded shortages, price rises, and famines associated with poor agricultural years, and this implies that there were demographic effects as a result.[27] Greater shortfalls are probably not justified given the diversity of the Basin's agricultural regime.

Minor as they may have been, these famines certainly had the effect of helping reduce the rate of population growth is specific periods, especially when the bad years clustered, such as in the 1590s and late 1610s. Further, adverse agricultural conditions were coincident with epidemics in the late 1550s and in the 1590s, and in these times the demographic effects were additive and, thus, more significant.

Famines Due To Other Causes

Agricultural shortfalls may also be produced by labor shortages engendered by Spanish corvée drafts. The simulation calibrations show that in order for the demographic effects of such drafts to be significant, their magnitude must be relatively large (see Chapter 3). For example, an uncompensated labor withdrawal (each year from 1520 to 1625) that results in a 10 percent agricultural shortfall each year will depress growth rates enough to result in a roughly 25 percent smaller total population over 100 years. It is not necessary to presume such withdrawals, however, and they are not a feature of the best simulation developed here.

THE ROLE OF MIGRATION AND HOMICIDE

The best fitting simulation does not assume that there was any homicide or migration in the sixteenth century. Clearly this understates the actual situation. Nevertheless, this simulation methodology indicates that it is possible to produce a catastrophic collapse in the Basin's Amerindian population *without* assuming large levels of homicide or emigration. Calibration of the simulations, however, show that war casualties (assumed for 1520) of 10 percent of the adult population can have a much more profound effect on the total depopulation than their relatively small number indicates (see Fig. 3.11). Similarly, small emigration percentages, if repeated in each epidemic period, for example, can also have profound effects on the population trajectory (Fig. 3.11). It would be a mistake to fail to consider these in the Basin's population decline, yet their role may have been small since the most successful simulation fit best without them.

---

[27] See Gibson, *The Aztecs*, Appendix V.

Summary

Because of their number and complexity, the major findings of this work are summarized below. These findings address the major research questions posed in Chapter 1 and illuminate other topics in the sixteenth century demographic history of the Basin.

POPULATION DYNAMICS

- The very large depopulations noted in the historical scholarship of the sixteenth-century Basin were *possible*, given reasonable assumptions as to cause. This conclusion contradicts those critics who assert that such depopulations were unlikely.
- Of the three groups of simulations examined here, the moderate case most likely captures the actual sixteenth-century population dynamics of the Basin. This simulation generates an eve-of-conquest (1519) total population of 1.59 million for the Basin that generally supports moderate historical estimates such as those by Gibson and Sanders.[28] This total is generally consistent with Denevan's moderate 1492 Mexican and hemispheric estimates.[29]
- This total of 1.59 million was reduced in the course of the sixteenth century to a nadir population of 183,000 in 1607. The scale of this depopulation is remarkable, since this nadir population represents only 11.5 percent of the 1519 total—a scale of losses that may be unmatched for the size of the population involved outside the Americas.
- The scale of population collapse in the early part of the century was profound. By 1569, the Amerindian population total (343,000) represented only 21.5 percent of its zenith in 1519. This important result generally supports historically generated estimates for the period, despite their somewhat insecure foundation.
- The temporal pattern of depopulation was very irregular. Instead of a more-or-less uniform fall, the bulk of the Basin's Amerindian population decline occurred in a series of step-like phased catastrophes. This fact serves to emphasize the care in the dating of events necessary to obtain a clear picture in such unstable circumstances.

OTHER DEMOGRAPHIC DYNAMICS

- The temporal dynamics of the basic demographic variables (i.e., mortality and fertility) were quite unstable in the sixteenth century Basin. They exhibit two patterns.
- The most prominent are the notable "spikes" of increased mortality and decreased fertility associated with the epidemic periods.

---

28 Gibson, *The Aztecs*; and Sanders, "The population of the Central Mexican Symbiotic Region."

29 Denevan, *The Native Population of the Americas in 1492*.

- In addition to, and indeed because of, these dramatic disruptions, the long-term (decadal) patterns of non-crisis crude death and birth rates were also unstable. The amplitude of these longer-term swings was far less than for the "spikes," however.
- Because of these short-term and long-term fluctuations in the fundamental demographic measures, the long-term patterns in derived demographic measures such as the dependency ratio and the tributary ratio were also volatile. Volatility notwithstanding, the dependency ratio remained at high levels for most of the later half of the sixteenth century.

CAUSAL LINKAGES

- The catastrophic decline in the Basin's Amerindian population was due to the combined effect of a series of epidemic crises, each of which reduced the population significantly.
- By far the most important factor in these crises were the profound short-term increases in mortality engendered by the "virgin soil" epidemics. No reliance need be made on the so-called "Leyenda negra" of Spanish cruelty to explain the holocaust.
- Despite their devastation, the assumptions of epidemic virulence used here do not presume an Amerindian population genetically less able to successfully resist disease. No such presumption is needed.
- A longer-term consequence of these epidemics was an increasing non-crisis death rate along with a decreasing non-crisis birth rate for the first 30-40 years after contact. While this pattern is noticeable, it is insignificant as an explanation for the bulk of the sixteenth century collapse.
- Famine mortality, especially that engendered by epidemic disease, was also a significant agent in reducing the Amerindian population.
- Other factors that may have contributed to famine, such as labor withdrawals, were judged to be less important.
- Differing assumptions about the underlying demographic structure do not alter these results significantly.
- Large-scale emigration or homicide need not have been important to generate the most reasonable population simulation.

Methodological Significance

In addition to the contribution this study makes to the study of sixteenth-century Amerindian populations, the methodology developed in this study has wider significance for population studies in particular and for cultural-ecological studies in general. Foremost, this study places the study of population change within a more general cultural-ecological framework. Since human populations do not exist in isolation from their environment, a more complete understanding of population necessitates a broader approach that incorporates a population's cultural ecological *milieux*. This methodology is, therefore, an important advance because it allows the examination and weighing of the myriad of influences that affect populations. Advance may not be the proper term to use here, however, since this re-uniting of population change studies with their broader cultural-ecological surroundings represents a return to the geographies of old in which place and populace were treated together.[30]

There are several ways in which the technique introduced in this study is of benefit. First, simulation modeling connects change in population numbers with the causes purported to have changed them.[31] This characteristic is important because such connections allows for possibility or probability "testing." Aside from the most obviously impossible situations, population reconstructions that consist of a series of population numbers alone cannot be tested to ascertain if they are possible or probable given the conditions of the time. Only by linking *process* (those factors that influence population change) to *result* (the population change itself) is this testing possible—and that is precisely what systems dynamics simulation methodology accomplishes. Further, the population numbers themselves may be examined by a method that does not rely on the same data set used to generate the population estimates in the first place. This allows for relatively independent verification of the totals.

Second, this simulation methodology represents a move to a more "theory-based" approach to historical demographic studies since it generates findings as a result of explicit hypotheses of cause. These "hypotheses of cause" reflect generalizations (demi-theories) from other studies and situations that are applied anew, using study-specific data, to a particular problem. Thus, it is more firmly rooted in the general scientific method. Indeed, the simulation methodology is really no different than any general scientific method and may be applied in either a deductive mode (using "theories" developed in other situations to explain a given problem) or an inductive mode (using data from a given problem to calibrate a causal simulation model that represents a generalization or "theory" developed from that data). Unlike some scientific approaches, however, the simulation technique demonstrated here uses a complex structure, including multiple causal linkages and important internal feedbacks, to elicit understanding, avoiding simplistic and mono-causal approaches. Further, since it requires explicit specification of linkages, variable values, and feedbacks, this simulation methodology illuminates the underlying assumptions. This methodological step facilitates criticism (and, indeed, falsification) of the

---

[30] For example, see Sauer's *Early Spanish Main*.

[31] This then is a special case of geographic cultural ecology since cultural ecology "...has sought understanding primarily through systemic analyses and empirical examinations of problems and themes that link human activity and the physical environment," Turner, "The Specialist-Synthesis Approach," p. 92.

results as compared to less well specified "thought models" sometimes used in explanation.

Related to this synthetic approach is the value of addressing complex problems in a broader context that utilizes specialized knowledge from a multiplicity of disciplines. This study is an example of how such integration may be used within a systems simulation methodology. A multidisciplinary simulation approach is also of value in that it may uncover relationships and data that would not be evident if the problem were attacked in a more traditional or parochial fashion.

Third, simulation modeling allows for "what if...?" assessments. This is useful in discriminating among contradictory data. Performing a simulation using each contested data set may allow for the rejection of one or more alternatives, or, at least, it will show the ramifications of using each data set.

Fourth, this methodology is truly dynamic in the sense that subsequent conditions are a result of previously adopted assumptions or factors. This quality is superior to methodologies that generate population data for multiple dates, but fail to do so in a way that demonstrates the *dependence* of the data for later dates on prior conditions. This dependence is important for population studies since population numbers are an auto-correlated time series and later values are *not* independent of previous ones. This approach should not be confused with studies that only incorporate "time depth," however. Analyses that consist of systemic ecological descriptions at multiple dates without explicit causal mechanisms that demonstrate how the subsequent configurations are the result of the previous ones are not truly dynamic studies in the sense used here.

Lastly, appropriate simulations allow for the discovery of new data not possible in the traditional, accounting, approach. For example, even the best population reconstructions that generate accurate populations for a series of dates cannot capture the detailed trajectory possible in a simulation approach, and these data may be important in understanding the overall trend. Data emerging from simulations might allow one to identify time-period-specific conditions that could be investigated using more conventional archival/historical methods. Similarly, the dynamics of population composition and other demographic variables of interest are relatively easy to generate in simulations. Further, the simulation methodology can suggest the relative importance of different causes of population change.

As with all methods, the systems dynamics methodology has shortcomings, and these are expressed at three levels of specificity for the problem and model. In common with most cultural-ecological approaches, it is not guided explicitly by a "macro-theory" of the nature of society-environment interaction. This lack is expressed two ways in simulation modeling. First, the boundaries of analysis are not defined except by reference to relatively imprecise conceptions of which sub-systems to include in the analysis. This is an important shortcoming, since the failure to consider adequately an important causal factor(s) might lead to distorted interpretations of the importance of various actors within the model. Nevertheless, this approach does not differ from others since all techniques that attempt to explain must simplify reality, for that is the goal of explanation, and without adequate grand or "macro-theory" this simplification is not without problems.

A related second liability is that there is no basis for choice among the secondary-level theories that guide the specification of the interactive linkages within the simulation model. There are, perhaps, fewer controversies at this level, but careful assessment of the universe of possibilities is necessary regardless.

Further problems face the systems analyst at the "micro" level, where the explicit assumptions used to operationalize the systemic interactions may be challenged.[32] Of course, this is common to other methods as well, but the nature of this method highlights them. This is really not a deficit in the usual sense, however, since the explicit specification of assumptions is a hallmark of good science. These shortcomings notwithstanding, part of this methodology's value lies in the fact that virtually any question that requires understanding of process and change through time may be addressed using its broad methodological framework.

Finally, as in all science, this work should be seen as preliminary rather than definitive. It demands more detailed research to verify and "fine-tune" its variable data and logical structure. The structure of MEXIPOP demands data for a number of variables and interactions that have not been readily available in usual sources. Further research that uncovers more detailed and reliable data for these variables would improve the accuracy of the simulation. While it is problematic that the simulation demands these novel data, these new research leads may generate important reassessments of the primary data, and suggest new potential historical sources.

Similarly, the implications and conclusions that result from this analysis need verification. The relatively rich output of the simulation provides many potential points where historical data can verify or refute. Since the simulation generates data for a variety of phenomena that have not been usually tracked, searches for relevant historical data may uncover potentially valuable new lines of research.

Furthermore, this methodology suggests additional research avenues. Formost among these are comparative studies. The basic simulation structure can be used, with appropriate modification, to examine the sixteenth-century depopulation in other areas of the New World. The scale, timing, and rate of depopulation can be compared among case studies. Further, interesting aspects of the cases' differing spatial and ecological endowments can be compared with regard to the depopulation pattern.

---

[32] Challenges may be made to specific data values used to inform the simulation, e.g., the age-specific case fatalities for smallpox. Further, the nature of the structural linkages in the model may be questioned, e.g., the linkage that alters the proportion of available labor as a function of adult epidemic morbidity.

Appropriate choices for such comparative case studies include the northern Yucatan, highland Guatemala, and the Peruvian Andes.

It is hoped that this work is of value both as an advance in the study of historical population change, and as an introduction to a powerful conceptual tool. Specifically, I hope that this work helps understand the most tragic demographic event in human history, the Amerindian population holocaust.

Appendix

MEXIPOP DEFINING EQUATIONS

The simulations in this study were performed using STELLA (version 2.10), a systems dynamics modelling program for an Apple Macintosh microcomputer.[1] For a model "SE" Macintosh, each complete simulation run required approximately 15 minutes of computer time—exclusive of the time needed to set-up each run and to save the results. Including these, each complete simulation run took about an hour to complete.

This section is devoted to displaying the defining equations and graphs of the MEXIPOP simulation model. Reference to Chapter 2, particularly to Figures 2.3, 2.4, & 2.7, and to Figures A.1-A.3 in this section will be helpful in interpreting these equations.

These equations are denoted with a • and displayed in sections according to their STELLA type (i.e., stocks, convertors and flows, and graphical convertors). The variable names follow the same convention in these equations as in the figures (i.e., spaces between sections of a variable name are represented by _), but, unlike their representation in the text of the chapters, the variable names in this section are *not* displayed in italic type. There are a few additional conventions that apply in this chapter.

The numerical symbols are conventional, thus:

- * represents multiplication,

- / represents division,

- [ ] encompass the arguments in logical operators (see below), and

- { } and ( ) are used in their usual algebraic way.

---

[1] STELLA 2.10 requires a 512KE Macintosh or higher and utilizes 204 k of memory. STELLA is a registered trademark of High Performance Systems, 13 Dartmouth College Highway, Lyme, NH 03768.

The stock equations are displayed using a standard integral notation:

- Stock = $_{1500}\int^{1625}$ Flow * dt.

where 1500 is the starting time for the integration (and for the simulation) and 1625 is the ending time. "Flow" is the change in the variable "Stock" over each time interval, "dt." The initial value for each stock is displayed below the defining equation.

There are, in addition, a few logical operators used in the defining equations:

- MIN [,] returns the minimum value of the two arguments separated by the comma,

- MAX [,] returns the maximum value of the two arguments separated by the comma,

- DELAY [, c] returns the value of the first argument within the bracket at c time units earlier,

- The logical chain; IF [ ] OR [ ] THEN [ ] ELSE [ ], returns the value of the argument within THEN [ ] if the value of the arguments within IF [ ] or   OR [ ] are true. It returns the value of the argument within ELSE [ ] if they are false.

Stocks

- pop_0_1 = $_{1500}\int^{1625}$ (-dpa_0_1 + bpa - mpa_0_1 - mat_1) * dt
  Initial value = 0.0275 * 100000

- pop_15_45 = $_{1500}\int^{1625}$ (mat_15 - mat_45 - dpa_15_45 - mpa_15_45) * dt
  Initial value = 0.4583 * 100000

- pop_1_5 = $_{1500}\int^{1625}$ (mat_1 - mat_5 - mpa_1_5 - dpa_1_5) * dt
  Initial value = 0.0909*100000

- pop_45_60 = $_{1500}\int^{1625}$ (mat_45 - dpa_45_60 - mpa_45_60 - mat_60) * dt
  Initial value = 0.1390 * 100000

- pop_5_15 = $_{1500}\int^{1625}$ (-mat_15 - dpa_5_15 - mpa_5_15 + mat_5) * dt
  Initial value = 0.2017 * 100000

- pop_60_99 = $_{1500}\int^{1625}$ (-mpa_60_99 + mat_60 - dpa_60_99) * dt
  Initial value = 100000*0.0828

- storage = $_{1500}\int^{1625}$ (-add_cons_flow - storage_loss_flow + storage_flow - cons_flow) * dt
  Initial value = 0

- surplus_D_per_PU = $_{1500}\int^{1625}$(surp_D_incr) * dt
  Initial value = 0

- total_deaths = $_{1500}\int^{1625}$(total_dpa) * dt
  Initial value = 0.0

- total_labor = $_{1500}\int^{1625}$(ttl_labor_incr) * dt
  Initial value = pop_15_45 + pop_45_60

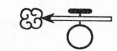

Converters and Flows

- add_cons_flow = MIN (storage, extra_cons + emerg_cons)

- Bkgd_morb = {(pop_0_1*B_morb_0_1) + (pop_1_5*B_morb_1_5) + (pop_5_15*B_morb_5_15) + (pop_15_45*B_morb_15_45) + (pop_45_60*B_morb_45_60) +(pop_60_99*B_morb_60_99)}/(pop_5_15+pop_15_45+pop_45_60 +pop_60_99+pop_1_5+pop_0_1)

- BM_0_1 = B_CF_0_1*care_factor*B_morb_0_1

- BM_15_45 = B_morb_15_45*care_factor*B_CF_15_45

- BM_1_5 = B_morb_1_5*care_factor*B_CF_1_5

- BM_45_60 = B_morb_45_60*B_CF_45_60*care_factor

- BM_5_15 = B_morb_5_15*B_CF_5_15*care_factor

- BM_60_99 = B_morb_60_99*B_CF_60_99*care_factor

- bpa = pop_15_45 * births_per_15_45

- bpa_lag_1 = DELAY [bpa,1]

- CBR = (bpa/total_pop)*1000

- CDR = (total_dpa/total_pop)*1000

- CH_env_loss_mult = CH_env_loss_fract*1

- CH_harvest = (1-CH_env_loss_mult)*CH_proj_yield

- CH_non_ag_extra_D = per_PU_demand*non_ag_PU_supp_by_C

- CH_plot_size_D = IF [CH_ttl_per_PU_D/CH_productivity $\geq$ 1]
  THEN [1]
  ELSE [CH_ttl_per_PU_D/CH_productivity]

- CH_productivity = 3000

- CH_proj_yield = CH_ttl_Yield_D*labor_avail_fract

- CH_ttl_area_D = net_CH_plot_size*no_CH_PUs

- CH_ttl_per_PU_D = per_PU_demand+extra_D_per_CH_PU

- CH_ttl_Yield_D = CH_productivity*CH_ttl_area_D

- cons_D_per_PU =total_cons_demand/number_PU

- cons_flow = MIN [total_cons_demand, storage_flow]

- cons_shortfall = total_cons_demand - cons_flow

- date = TIME

- dependency_ratio = (pop_0_1+pop_5_15+pop_1_5+pop_60_99)
  /(pop_45_60+pop_15_45)

- dpa_0_1 = IF [pop_0_1 $\leq$ 0]
  THEN [0]
  ELSE [pop_0_1*mort_0_1]

- dpa_15_45 = pop_15_45 * mort_15_45

- dpa_1_5 = mort_1_5*pop_1_5

- dpa_45_60 = pop_45_60 * mort_45_60

- dpa_5_15 = pop_5_15 * mort_5_15

- dpa_60_99 = pop_60_99*mort_60_99

- emerg_cons = MIN [cons_shortfall, storage]

- extra_cons = IF [storage - emerg_cons > 0]
  AND [storage - emerg_cons > ttl_surp_goal]
  THEN [storage - emerg_cons - ttl_surp_goal]
  ELSE [0]

- extra_D_per_CH_PU = CH_non_ag_extra_D/no_CH_PUs

- extra_D_per_IR_PU = IR_non_ag_extra_D/no_IR_PUs

- extra_D_per_TP_PU = Tp_non_ag_D/no_TP_PUs

- E_morb = {(pop_0_1*E_morb_0_1) + (pop_1_5*E_morb_1_5) + (pop_5_15*E_morb_5_15) + (pop_15_45*E_morb_15_45) + (pop_45_60*E_morb_45_60) + (pop_60_99*E_morb_60_99)}/total_pop

- E_mort_0_1 = E_morb_0_1*E_CF_0_1*1

- E_mort_15_45 = E_morb_15_45*E_CF_15_45*1

- E_mort_1_5 = E_CF_1_5*E_morb_1_5*1

- E_mort_45_60 = E_morb_45_60*E_CF_45_60*1

- E_mort_5_15 = E_morb_5_15*E_CF_5_15*1

- E_mort_60_99 = E_CF_60_99*E_morb_60_99*1

- IR_env_loss_mult = IR_env_loss_fract*1

- IR_harvest = IR_proj_yield*(1-IR_env_loss_mult)

- IR_non_ag_extra_D = non_ag_PU_supp_by_I*per_PU_demand

- IR_plot_size_D = IF [(IR_ttl_per_PU_D/IR_productivity) ≥ 2] THEN [2] ELSE [IR_ttl_per_PU_D/IR_productivity]

- IR_productivity = 1100

- IR_proj_yield = IR_ttl_yield_D*labor_avail_fract

- IR_ttl_area_D = net_IR_plot_size*no_IR_PUs

- IR_ttl_per_PU_D = extra_D_per_IR_PU+per_PU_demand

- IR_ttl_yield_D = IR_ttl_area_D*IR_productivity

- labor_availab = total_labor*trib_labor_fract

- labor_avail_fract = labor_availab/(pop_45_60+pop_15_45)

- matur_1 = bpa_lag_1*survivors_0_1

- matur_15 = matur_5_lag_10 * surv_5_2 * s_5_15_lag_10 * s_5_15_lag_18 * s_5_15_lag_17 * s_5_15_lag_11 *s_5_15_lag_12 * s_5_15_lag_16 * s_5_15_lag_15*s_5_15_lag_14 * s_ 5_15_lag_13

- matur_15_lag_30 = DELAY [matur_15, 30]

- matur_45 = matur_45b*matur_45a

- matur_45a = s_15_45_lag_53 * s_15_45_lag_42 * s_15_45_lag_46 * lag_15_45 * s_15_45_lag_30 * s_15_45_lag_41 * s_15_45_lag_52 * s_15_45_lag_43 * s_15_45_lag_44 * s_15_45_lag_45 * s_15_45_lag_47 * s_15_45_lag_49 * s_15_45_lag_51 * s_15_lag_30 * s_15_45_lag_50 * s_15_45_lag_48

- matur_45b = s_15_45_lag_54 * s_15_45_lag_40 * s_15_45_lag_58 * s_15_45_lag_36 * s_15_45_lag_55 * s_15_45_lag_56 * s_15_45_lag_57 * s_15_45_lag_31 * s_15_45_lag_32 * s_15_45_lag_33 * s_15_45_lag_34 * s_15_45_lag_35 * s_15_45_lag_37 * s_15_45_lag_38 * s_15_45_lag_39

- matur_45_lag_15 = DELAY [matur_45, 15]

- matur_5 = survivors_1_5 * s_1_5_lag_4 * s_1_5_lag_5 * s_1_5_lag_6 * mat_1_lag_5

- matur_5_lag_10 = DELAY [matur_5,10]

- matur_60 =s_45_60_lag_24 * s_45_60_lag_19 * s_45_60_lag_27 * s_45_60 * matur_45_lag_15 * s_45_60_lag_20 * s_45_60_lag_25 * s_45_60_lag_26 * s_45_60_lag_23 * s_45_60_lag_22 * s_45_60_lag_21 * s_45_60_lag_15 * s_45_60_lag_28 * s_45_60_lag_16 * s_45_60_lag_17 * s_45_60_lag_18

- mat_1 = matur_1

- mat_15 = matur_15

- mat_1_lag_5 = DELAY [mat_1, 4]

- mat_45 =matur_45

- mat_5 = matur_5

- mat_60 = matur_60

- morb_sum = E_morb + Bkgd_morb

- morb_ttl_15_45 = E_morb_15_45 + B_morb_15_45

- mort_0_1 = IF [ttl_EM_0_1+BM_0_1 - (MIN [ttl_EM_0_1, BM_0_1]/2) > 1]
  THEN [1]
  ELSE [ttl_EM_0_1+BM_0_1 - (MIN [ttl_EM_0_1, BM_0_1]/2)]

- mort_15_45 = IF [ttl_EM_15_45+BM_15_45 - (MIN [ttl_EM_15_45, BM_15_45]/2) >1]
  THEN [1]
  ELSE [ttl_EM_15_45+BM_15_45 - (MIN [ttl_EM_15_45, BM_15_45]/2)]

- mort_1_5 = IF [BM_1_5+ttl_EM_1_5 - (MIN [BM_1_5, ttl_EM_1_5]/2) > 1]
  THEN [1]
  ELSE [BM_1_5+ttl_EM_1_5 - (MIN [BM_1_5, ttl_EM_1_5]/2)]

- mort_45_60 = IF [ttl_EM_45_60+BM_45_60 - (MIN [ttl_EM_45_60, BM_45_60]/2) >1]
  THEN [1]
  ELSE [ttl_EM_45_60+BM_45_60 - (MIN [ttl_EM_45_60, BM_45_60]/2)]

- mort_5_15 = IF [ttl_EM_5_15+BM_5_15 - (MIN [ttl_EM_5_15, BM_5_15]/2) >1]
  THEN [1]
  ELSE [ttl_EM_5_15+BM_5_15 - (MIN[ttl_EM_5_15, BM_5_15]/2)]

- mort_60_99 = IF [ttl_EM_60_99+BM_60_99 - (MIN [ttl_EM_60_99, BM_60_99]/2) > 1]
  THEN [1]
  ELSE [ttl_EM_60_99+BM_60_99 - (MIN [ttl_EM_60_99, BM_60_99]/2)] mpa_0_1 =pop_0_1*mig_0_1

- mpa_15_45 = pop_15_45*mig_15_45

- mpa_1_5 = pop_1_5*mig_1_5

- mpa_45_60 = pop_45_60*mig_45_60

- mpa_5_15 = pop_5_15*mig_5_15

- mpa_60_99 = pop_60_99*mig_60_99

- net_CH_plot_size = MIN [CH_plot_size_D, 0.544]

- net_harvest = CH_harvest + IR_harvest + TP_harvest - net_tribute_loss

- net_IR_plot_size = MIN [IR_plot_size_D, 1.18]

- net_TP_plot_size = MIN [TP_plot_size_D, 2.71]

- net_tribute_loss = tribute_D_per_PU*number_PU

- non_ag_PU_supp_by_C = number_non_ag_PU*prop_supp_by_CH

- non_ag_PU_supp_by_I = number_non_ag_PU*prop_supp_by_IR

- non_ag_PU_sup_by_TP = number_non_ag_PU*prop_supp_by_TP

- no_CH_PUs = number_PU*prop_PU_in_CH

- no_IR_PUs = number_PU*prop_PU_in_IR

- no_TP_PUs = number_PU*prop_PU_in_TP

- number_non_ag_PU = number_PU*prop_non_ag_PU

- number_PU = {(pop_45_60 + pop_15_45)/4.075}

- nutr_disc = (ttl_cons/total_cons_demand)

- per_PU_demand = (tribute_D_per_PU
  +cons_D_per_PU+surplus_D_per_PU) prop_non_ag_PU = 0.298

- prop_PU_in_CH = 0.1169

- prop_PU_in_IR =0 .4995

- prop_PU_in_TP = 0.0856

- prop_supp_by_CH = 0.28

- prop_supp_by_IR = 0.72

- prop_supp_by_TP = 0.0

- PU_surplus = storage/number_PU

- PU_surplus_goal =cons_D_per_PU*0

- storage_flow = net_harvest

- storage_loss_flow = storage*0.15

- surp_D_incr = IF [PU_surplus ≥ PU_surplus_goal]
  OR [PU_surplus_goal = 0]
  THEN [-surplus_D_per_PU]
  ELSE [PU_surplus_goal - PU_surplus-surplus_D_per_PU]

- survivors_0_1 = 1-mort_0_1

- survivors_15_45 = 1-mort_15_45

- survivors_1_5 = 1-mort_1_5

- survivors_45_60 = 1-mort_45_60

- surv_5_2 = 1-mort_5_15

- s_15_45_lag_30 = DELAY [survivors_15_45, 1]

- s_15_45_lag_31 = DELAY [s_15_45_lag_58, 1]

- s_15_45_lag_32 = DELAY [s_15_45_lag_31, 1]

- s_15_45_lag_33 = DELAY [s_15_45_lag_32, 1]

- s_15_45_lag_34 = DELAY [s_15_45_lag_33, 1]

- s_15_45_lag_35 = DELAY [s_15_45_lag_34, 1]
- s_15_45_lag_36 = DELAY [s_15_45_lag_35, 1]
- s_15_45_lag_37 = DELAY [s_15_45_lag_36, 1]
- s_15_45_lag_38 = DELAY [s_15_45_lag_37, 1]
- s_15_45_lag_39 = DELAY [s_15_45_lag_38, 1]
- s_15_45_lag_40 = DELAY [s_15_45_lag_39, 1]
- s_15_45_lag_41 = DELAY [s_15_45_lag_30, 1]
- s_15_45_lag_42 = DELAY [s_15_45_lag_40, 1]
- s_15_45_lag_43 = DELAY [s_15_45_lag_42, 1]
- s_15_45_lag_44 = DELAY [s_15_45_lag_43, 1]
- s_15_45_lag_45 = DELAY [s_15_45_lag_44, 1]
- s_15_45_lag_46 = DELAY [s_15_45_lag_45, 1]
- s_15_45_lag_47 = DELAY [s_15_45_lag_46, 1]
- s_15_45_lag_48 = DELAY [s_15_45_lag_47, 1]
- s_15_45_lag_49 = DELAY [s_15_45_lag_48, 1]
- s_15_45_lag_50 = DELAY [s_15_45_lag_49, 1]
- s_15_45_lag_51 = DELAY [s_15_45_lag_50, 1]
- s_15_45_lag_52 = DELAY [s_15_45_lag_41, 1]
- s_15_45_lag_53 = DELAY [s_15_45_lag_52, 1]
- s_15_45_lag_54 = DELAY [s_15_45_lag_53, 1]
- s_15_45_lag_55 = DELAY [s_15_45_lag_54, 1]
- s_15_45_lag_56 = DELAY [s_15_45_lag_55, 1]
- s_15_45_lag_57 = DELAY [s_15_45_lag_56, 1]
- s_15_45_lag_58 = DELAY [s_15_45_lag_57, 1]
- s_1_5_lag_4 = DELAY [survivors_1_5, 1]
- s_1_5_lag_5 = DELAY [s_1_5_lag_4, 1]
- s_1_5_lag_6 = DELAY [s_1_5_lag_5, 1]
- s_45_60_lag_15 = DELAY [survivors_45_60, 1]

- s_45_60_lag_16 = DELAY [s_45_60_lag_28, 1]

- s_45_60_lag_17 = DELAY [s_45_60_lag_16, 1]

- s_45_60_lag_18 = DELAY [s_45_60_lag_17, 1]

- s_45_60_lag_19 = DELAY [s_45_60_lag_18, 1]

- s_45_60_lag_20 = DELAY [s_45_60_lag_19, 1]

- s_45_60_lag_21 = DELAY [s_45_60_lag_15, 1]

- s_45_60_lag_22 = DELAY [s_45_60_lag_21, 1]

- s_45_60_lag_23 = DELAY [s_45_60_lag_22, 1]

- s_45_60_lag_24 = DELAY [s_45_60_lag_23, 1]

- _45_60_lag_25 = DELAY [s_45_60_lag_24, 1]

- s_45_60_lag_26 = DELAY [s_45_60_lag_25, 1]

- s_45_60_lag_27 = DELAY [s_45_60_lag_26, 1]

- s_45_60_lag_28 = DELAY [s_45_60_lag_27, 1]

- s_5_15_lag_10 = DELAY [surv_5_2, 1]

- s_5_15_lag_11 = DELAY [s_5_15_lag_10, 1]

- s_5_15_lag_12 = DELAY [s_5_15_lag_11, 1]

- s_5_15_lag_13 = DELAY [s_5_15_lag_12, 1]

- s_5_15_lag_14 = DELAY [s_5_15_lag_13, 1]

- s_5_15_lag_15 = DELAY [s_5_15_lag_14, 1]

- s_5_15_lag_16 = DELAY [s_5_15_lag_15, 1]

- s_5_15_lag_17 = DELAY [s_5_15_lag_16, 1]

- s_5_15_lag_18 = DELAY [s_5_15_lag_17, 1]

- total_cons_demand = (70.6*pop_1_5 + 132.8*pop_5_15 + 128.6*pop_15_45 + 111.6*pop_45_60 + 111.6*pop_60_99)

- total_dpa = dpa_0_1+dpa_60_99+dpa_45_60+ dpa_1_5+dpa_5_15+dpa_15_45

- total_pop = pop_0_1 + pop_1_5 + pop_5_15 + pop_15_45 + pop_45_60 + pop_60_99

- TP_env_loss_mult = TP_env_loss_fract*1

- TP_harvest = (1-TP_env_loss_mult)*TP_proj_yield

- Tp_non_ag_D = non_ag_PU_sup_by_TP*per_PU_demand

- TP_plot_size_D = IF [TP_ttl_per_PU_D/TP_productivity ≥ 3]
  THEN [3]
  ELSE [TP_ttl_per_PU_D/TP_productivity]

- P_productivity = 350

- TP_proj_yield = TP_ttl_yield_D*labor_avail_fract

- TP_ttl_area_D = no_TP_PUs*net_TP_plot_size

- TP_ttl_per_PU_D = extra_D_per_TP_PU + per_PU_demand

- TP_ttl_yield_D = TP_productivity*TP_ttl_area_D

- trib_ratio = total_pop/(number_PU*2)

- ttl_cons = add_cons_flow + cons_flow

- ttl_EM_0_1 = E_mort_0_1*care_factor

- ttl_EM_15_45 = E_mort_15_45*care_factor

- ttl_EM_1_5 = E_mort_1_5*care_factor

- ttl_EM_45_60 = E_mort_45_60*care_factor

- ttl_EM_5_15 = E_mort_5_15*care_factor

- ttl_EM_60_99 = E_mort_60_99*care_factor

- ttl_labor_incr = (well_labor - total_labor)/DT

- ttl_surp_goal = PU_surplus_goal*number_PU

- well_labor = {1- (E_morb_45_60*0.5 + B_morb_45_60 -
  0.198)}*pop_45_60 + {1 - (E_morb_15_45*0.5 + B_morb_15_45 -
  0.14)}*pop_15_45

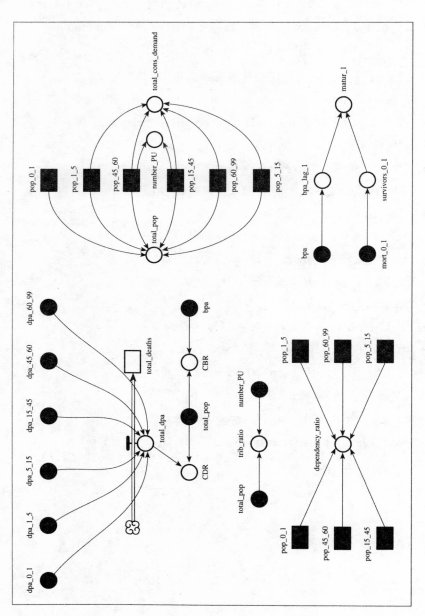

A.1 Various Counting Registers

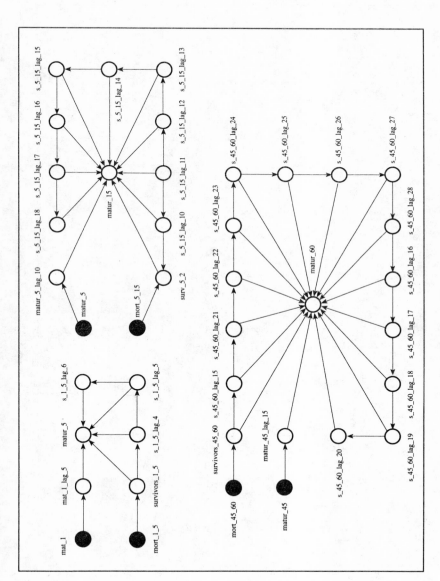

A.2 Maturity Calculations 5, 15, and 60

232

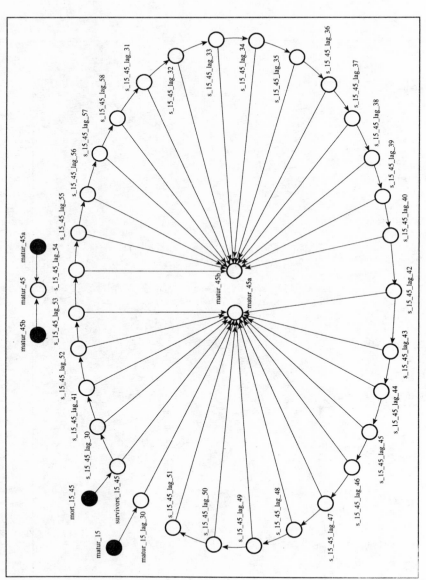

A.3 Maturity 45 Calculations

Graphical Convertors

A number of MEXIPOP variables are not defined by equations *per se*, rather, they are defined as graphical functions of other variables. The many variables that are functions of date are not displayed here. Examples of these variables include the epidemic case fatalities and morbidities (e.g., E_CF_0_1 and E_morb_0_1 in Figure 2.7) (they are zero except at the dates of the epidemics). These epidemiological relationships are not displayed here since doing so does not add to the information available in Table 2.6. Indeed, for all the date-dependent variables, the graphs are exceedingly simple since the values are zero for the vast majority of the time. Similarly, the values for the environmental losses (e.g., IR_env_loss_fract in Figure 2.11) are date dependent. These are not displayed here either, since the same information is available in Table 2.15. Further, migration (e.g., mig_0_1 in Figure 2.3), which is also modeled as a function of date, is not plotted here since migration information is available in Chapter 3. Tribute demand (see tribute_D_per_PU in Figure 2.11) also is modeled as a function of date and is not displayed here since the relevant information for this variable is found in Chapter 3. Lastly, labor tribute (see trib_labor_fract in Figure 2.7) is assumed to be a function of the date as well. This relationship is discussed in Chapter 3 as well.

There are several non-date-dependent graphically defined variables, however. The most numerous of these are the background case fatalities and background morbidities (see for example, B_CF_0_1 and B_morb_0_1 in Figure 2.4). These variables are functions of the nutritional level (see nutr_disc in Figure 2.4). I have grouped these 6 individual graphical relationships in two graphs for simplicity, Figures A.4 and A.5.

The care_factor variable (see Figure 2.4) is defined as a graphical function of the total morbidity (morb_sum) and is displayed in Figure A.6. The last of the graphically defined variables, the birth rate (see births_per_15_45 in Figure 2.3) is a function of the morbidity of the 15-45 year-old population (morb_ttl_15_45), and is displayed in Figure A.7.

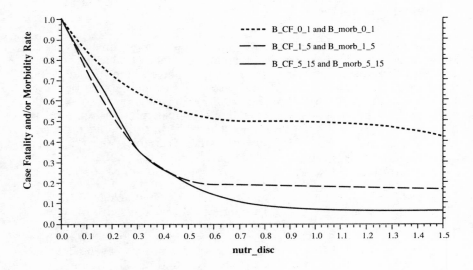

Figure A.4 Background Case Fatality and Morbidity Rates, Ages: 0-1, 1-5, 5-15

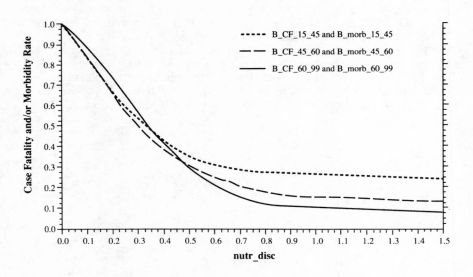

Figure A.5 Background Case Fatality and Morbidity Rates, Ages: 15-45, 45-60, 60-99

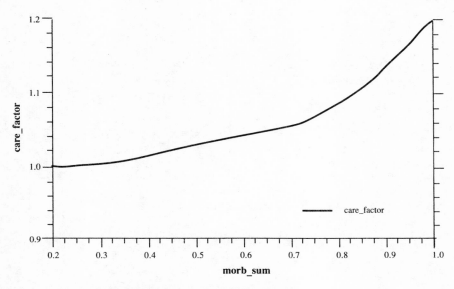

Figure A.6 Care Factor as Function of Morbidity Total

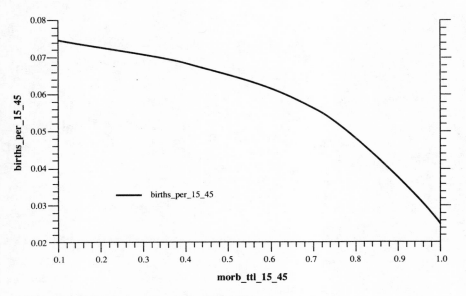

Figure A.7 Birth Rate as Function of Morbidity

Bibliography

Adams, R. E. W., "Settlement Patterns of the Central Yucatan and Southern Campeche Regions," in W. Ashmore (ed.), *Lowland Maya Settlement Patterns*, Albuquerque: University of New Mexico Press, 1981, 211-257.

Allison, M. J., A. Pezzia, and E. Gerszten, "Infectious Diseases in Precolombian Inhabitants of Peru," *American Journal of Physical Anthropology* 41 (1974), 468.

Anderson, Edgar, and R. H. Barlow, "The Maize Tribute of Moctezuma's Empire," *Annals of the Missouri Botanical Gardens* 30 (1943), 413-418.

Anderson, R. K., J. Calvo, G. Serrano, and G. C. Payne. "A Study of the Nutritional Status and Food Habits of Otomi Indians in the Mezquital Valley of Mexico," *American Journal of Public Health* 36 (1946), 883-903.

Armillas, Pedro, "Gardens on Swamps," *Science* 174 (1971), 653-661.

Aschmann, H., *The Central Desert of Baja California: Demography and Ecology*, Ibero-Americana 42, Berkeley: University of California Press, 1959.

Ashburn, P. M., *The Ranks of Death: A Medical History of the Conquest of America*, Frank D. Ashburn (ed.). New York: Coward-McCann, Inc., 1947.

Bang, F. B., "Famine Symposium—The Role of Disease in the Ecology of Famine," *Ecology of Food and Nutrition* 7 (1978), 1-15.

Barlow, R. H., *The Extent of the Empire of the Culhua Mexica*, Ibero-Americana 28, Berkeley: University of California Press, 1949.

Beisel, W. R., "Synergism and Antagonism of Parasitic Diseases and Malnutrition," *Reviews of Infectious Diseases* 4 (1982), 746-750.

Bell, J. A., and J. F. Bell, "System Dynamics and Scientific Method," in J. Randers (ed.), *Elements of the System Dynamics Method*, Cambridge, MA: M.I.T. Press., 1980, 3-22.

Benenson, A. S., "Smallpox," in A. S. Evans (ed.) *Viral Infections of Humans*, New York and London: Plenum Medical Book Company, 429-455.

238

Berdan, F. F., "A Comparative Analysis of Aztec Tribute Documents," *Actas XLI Congreso Internacional de Americanistas, 1974 Vol. 2* (1976).

Bergmann, G., *Philosophy of Science*, Madison, WI: University of Wisconsin Press, 1966.

Beveridge, William Ian, *Influenza: The Last Great Plague*, New York: Prodist, 1978.

Black, F.L., "Measles," in A.S. Evans (ed.), *Viral Infections of Humans*, New York and London: Plenum Medical Book Company, 1976, 297-316.

Blaikie, P., and H. Brookfield, "Defining and Debating the Problem," in P. Blakie and H. Brookfield (eds.), *Land Degradation and Society*, London: Methuen, 1987, 1-26

Blanton, R. E., *Monte Albán: Settlement Patterns at the Ancient Zapotec Capital*, New York: Academic Press, 1978.

Board on Science and Technology for International Development, Commission on International Relations, and The National Research Council, *Post Harvest Food Losses in Developing Countries*, Washington, DC: National Academy of Sciences, 1978.

Bongaarts, J., "Does Malnutrition Affect Fertility? A Summary of Evidence," *Science* 208 (1980), 564-569.

Borah, Woodrow, "Historical Demography of Aboriginal and Colonial America: An Attempt at Perspective," in W.M. Denevan (ed.), *The Native Population of the Americas in 1492*, Madison, WI: University of Wisconsin Press, 1976, 13-34

——————— "The Historical Demography of Latin America: Sources, Techniques, Controversies, Yields," in Paul Deprez (ed.), *Population and Economics: Procedings of Section V of the Fourth Congress of the International Economic History Association*, Winnipeg: University of Manitoba Press, 1970, 173-205.

——————— "América Como Modelo? El Impacto Demográfico de la Expansión Europea Sobre el Mundo no Europeo," *Cuadernos Americanos* 6 (1962), 176-185.

——————— *Early Colonial Trade and Navigation between Mexico and Peru*, Ibero-Americana 38, Berkeley: University of California Press, 1954.

——————— *New Spain's Century of Depression*, Ibero-Americana 35, Berkeley: University of California Press, 1951.

Borah, Woodrow, and Sherburne F. Cook. *The Aboriginal Population of Central Mexico on the Eve of the Spanish Conquest*, Ibero-America 45, Berkeley: University of California Press, 1963.

——————— "La Despoblación del México Central en el Siglo XVI," *Historia Mexicana* 12 (1962), 1-12.

——————— *The Population of Central Mexico in 1548*, Ibero-America 43, Berkeley: University of California Press, 1960.

——————— *Price Trends of Some Basic Commodities in Central Mexico, 1531-1570*, Ibero-Americana 40, Berkeley: University of California Press, 1958.

Boserup, Ester, *The Conditions of Agricultural Growth*, Chicago: Aldine, 1966.

Boyle, P. P., and C. O'Gráda, "Fertility Trends, Excess Mortality, and the Great Irish Famine," *Demography* 23 (1986), 543-562.

Bridges, E. L., *The Uttermost Part of the Earth*, New York: Dutton, 1949.

Brookfield, Harold C., "Intensification and Disintensification in Pacific Agriculture: A Theoretical Approach," *Pacific Viewpoint* 13 (1972), 30-48.

Brown, P., D. C. Gajdusek, and J. A. Morris, "Epidemic A2 Influenza in Isolated Pacific Island Populations Without Pre-Epidemic Antibody to Influenza Types A and B, and the Discovery of Other Still Unexposed Populations," *American Journal of Epidemiology* 83 (1966), 176-188.

Calneck, Edward E., "Settlement Patterns and Chinampan Agriculture at Tenochtitlan," *American Antiquity* 37 (1972), 104-115.

——————— "The Internal Structure of Tenochtitlan," in E. R. Wolf (ed.), *The Valley of Mexico, Studies in Pre-Hispanic Ecology and Society*, Albuquerque: The University of New Mexico Press, 1976.

Carrasco, Pedro, "The Joint Family in Ancient Mexico: The Case of Molotla," in Hugo G. Nutini, Pedro Carrasco and James M. Taggert (eds.), *Essays on Mexican Kinship*, London: The University of Pittsburgh Press, 1976, 45-64.

——————— "Social Organization of Ancient Mexico," in R. Wauchope (ed.), *Handbook of Middle American Indians*, Austin: University of Texas Press, 1971, Vol. 10, 349-357.

Centerwall, W. R., "A Recent Experience with Measles in a 'Virgin Soil' Population," In *Pan American Health Organization Scientific Publication #165, Biomedical Challenges Presented by the American Indian*, Washington, DC: Pan American Health Organization, 1968, 77-81.

Chevalier, F., *Land and Society in Colonial America*, L.B. Simpson (ed.). Berkeley: University of California Press, 1963.

Chayanov, A. V., "Peasant Farm Organization," in D. Thorner, B. Kerblay and R.E.F. Smith (ed.), *A.V. Chayanov on the Theory of Peasant Economy*, Homewood, IL: R.D. Irwin, 1966, 29-269.

Christensen, P. E., H. Schmidt, H. O. Bang, V. Andersen, B. Jordal, and O. Jensen, "An Epidemic of Measles in Southern Greenland, 1951," *Acta Medica Scandinavica* 144 (1953), 430-449.

Clark, W. A. V., and K. L. Avery, "The Effects of Data Aggregation in Statistical Analysis," *Geographical Analysis* 8 (1976), 428-438.

Clavijero, F. J., *Historia Antigua de Mexico*, Mexico City: Editorial Porrúa, 1964.

Cliff, Andrew D., Peter Haggett, and J. Keith Ord, *Spatial Aspects of Influenza Epidemics*, London: Pion Limited, 1986.

Cline, H. F., "Civil Congregations of the Indians in New Spain, 1598-1606," *Hispanic American Historical Review* 29 (1949), 349-369.

Coale, A. J., and P. Demeny, *Regional Model Life Tables and Stable Populations*, Princeton: Princeton University Press, 1966.

Cockburn, T. A., *The Evolution and Eradication of Infectious Diseases*, Baltimore: The Johns Hopkins University Press, 1963.

Coe, M. D., "The Chinampas of Mexico," *Scientific American* 211 (1964), 90-98.

Cohon, Jared L., *Multiobjective Programming and Planning*, New York: Academic Press, 1978.

Colson, E., "In Good Years and in Bad: Food Strategies of Self-Reliant Societies," *Journal of Anthropological Research* 35 (1979), 18-29.

Confrees Bellagio Confrence, "The Relationship of Nutrition, Disease, and Social Conditions: a Graphical Presentation," in R. I. Rotberg and T. K. Rabb (eds.), *Hunger and History, The Impact of Changing Food Production and Consumption Patterns on Society*, Cambridge: Cambridge University Press, 1983, 305-308.

Cook, Noble David, *Demographic Collapse: Indian Peru, 1520-1620*, New York: Cambridge University Press, 1981.

Cook, Sherburne F., *Santa María Ixcatlán: Habitat, Population, Subsistance*, Ibero-Americana 41, Berkeley: University of California Press, 1958.

——————— "The Aborginal Population of Alemeda and Contra Costa Counties, California," *Anthropological Records*, Berkeley: University of California Press, 1957, Vol. 16, 131-154.

——————— "The Aboriginal Population of the North Coast of California," *Anthropological Records*, Berkeley: University of California Press, 1956. Vol. 16, 81-129.

——————— "The Aboriginal Population of the San Joaquin Valley, California," *Anthropological Records*, Berkeley: University of California Press, 1955, Vol. 16, 31-78.

——————— *The Historical Demography and Ecology of the Teotlapan*, Ibero-Americana 33, Berkeley: University of California Press, 1949.

——————— *Soil Erosion and Population in Central Mexico*, Ibero-Americana 34, Berkeley: University of California Press, 1949.

——————— "The Incidence and Significance of Disease Among the Aztecs and Related Tribes," *Hispanic American Historical Review* 26 (1946), 320-335.

——————— *Population Trends Among the California Mission Indians*, Ibero-Americana 17, Berkeley: University of California Press, 1940.

——————— "Smallpox in Spanish and Mexican California, 1770-1845," *Bulletin of the History of Medicine* 7 (1939), 153-191.

——————— *The Extent and Significance of Disease Among the Indians of Baja California, 1697-1773*, Ibero-Americana 12, Berkeley: University of California Press, 1937.

Cook, Sherburne F., and Woodrow Borah, *Essays in Population History*, Vol. 3. Berkeley: University of California Press, 1979.

——————— *Essays in Population History*, Vol. 2. Berkeley: University of California Press, 1974.

——————— *Essays in Population History*, Vol. 1. Berkeley: University of California Press, 1971.

——————— *The Population of the Mixteca Alta*, Ibero-Americana 50, Berkeley: University of California Press, 1968.

——————— "On the Credibility of Contemporary Testimony on the Population of Mexico in the Sixteenth Century," *Suma Antropología en Homenaje a Roberto J. Weitlaner*, Mexico City: Instituto Nacional de Antropología e Historia, 1966.

——————— *The Indian Population of Central Mexico, 1531-1610*, Ibero-Americana 44, Berkeley: University of California Press, 1960.

——————— "The Rate of Population Change in Central Mexico," *Hispanic American Historical Review* 37 (1957), 463-470.

Cook, Sherburne F., and Lesley Bird Simpson, *The Population of Central Mexico in the Sixteenth Century*, Ibero-Americana 31, Berkeley: University of California Press, 1948.

Corney, B. G., "The Behavior or Certain Epidemic Diseases in Natives of Polynesia with Especial Reference to the Fiji Islands," *Transactions of the Epidemiological Society of London New Series* 3 (1884), 76-95.

Crosby, Alfred W., "The Influenza Pandemic of 1918," in June E. Osborn (ed.), *Influenza in America 1918-1976*, New York: Prodist, 1977, 5-13.

——————— "Virgin Soil Epidemics as a Factor in the Aboriginal Depopulation in America," *William and Mary Quarterly* 33 (1976), 289-299.

——————— *The Colombian Exchange: Biological and Cultural Consequences of 1492*, Westport, CN: Greenwood Press, 1972.

——————— "Conquistador y Pestilencia: The First New World Pandemic and the Fall of the Great Indian Empires," *Hispanic American Historical Review* 47 (1967), 321-337.

Curry, L., "A Note on Spatial Association," *The Professional Geographer* 18 (1966), 97-99.

Davenport, F. M., "Influenza Viruses," in A. S. Evans (ed.), *Viral Infections of Humans*, New York and London: Plenum Medical Book Company, 1976, 273-296.

de Oviedo y Valdés, Gonzalo Fernández, *Historial General y Natural de las Indias*, Vol. 4. Juan Pérez de Tudela (ed.), Madrid: Ediciones Atlas, 1959.

Denevan, William M., "Carl Sauer and Native Population Size in the New World," Paper presented at the annual meetings of the Association of American Geographers, Baltimore, MD. 1989.

——————— (ed.), *The Native Population of the Americas in 1492*, Madison, WI: University of Wisconsin Press, 1976.

————————*The Aboriginal Cultural Ecology of the Llanos de Mojos of Bolivia*, Ibero-Americana 48, Berkeley: University of California Press, 1966.

Díaz del Castillo, B., *Historia Verdadera de la Conquista de la Nueva España*, Vol. 1. Mexico City: Porrúa, 1960.

Dixon, C. W., *Smallpox*, London: J. and A. Churchill, 1962.

Dobyns, H. F., "Estimating Aboriginal American Population: an Appraisal of Techniques with a New Hemisphere Estimate," *Current Anthropology* 7 (1966), 395-415.

————————"An Outline of Andean Epidemic History to 1720," *Bulletin of the History of Medicine* 37 (1963), 493-515.

Dols, Michael W., *The Black Death in the Middle East*, Princeton: Princeton University Press, 1977.

Donkin, R. A., *Agricultural Terracing in the Aborginal New World*, Tucson, Arizona: The University of New Mexico Press for the Wenner-Gren Foundation for Anthropological Research, Inc., 1979.

Doolittle, W. E., *Canal Irrigation in Prehistoric Mexico*, Austin: University of Texas Press, 1990.

Elliott, J. H., "The Spanish Conquest and Settlement of America," in Leslie Bethell (ed.), *The Cambridge History of Latin America,* Vol. 1. Cambridge: Cambridge University Press, 1984, 149-206.

Evans, A. S., "Epidemiological Concepts and Methods," in A.S. Evans (ed.), *Viral Infections of Humans*, New York and London: Plenum Medical Book Company, 1976, 1-32.

Eversley, D. E. C., "Population, Economy, and Society," in D.V. Glass and D.E.C. Eversley (eds.), *Population in History*, Chicago: Aldine Publishing Co., 1965, 23-69.

Farrar, W. V., "Tecuitlatl; A Glimpse of Aztec Food Technology," *Nature* 211 (1966), 341-342.

Fiset, Paul, "Clinical and Laboratory Diagnosis of Rickettsial Diseases of Man," in Gueh-Djen Hsiung and Robert H. Green (eds.), *Virology and Rickettsiology*, Volume 1 Part 2, CRC Handbook Series in Clinical Laboratory Science, West Palm Beach, Fla: CRC Press, Inc., 1978.

Flannery, K. V., *The Early Mesoamerican Village*, New York: Academic Press, 1976.

Flinn, M.W., *The European Demographic System, 1500-1820*, Brighton, UK: Harvester Press, 1981.

Forrester, J. W., *Principles of Systems*, Cambridge, MA: Wright-Allen Press, Inc., 1968.

Friede, J., "De la Encomienda Indiana a la Propiedad Territorial y su Influencia sobre el Mestizaje," *Anuario Colombiano de Historia Social y de la Cultura* 4 (1969), 35-62.

——————— "Demographic Changes in the Mining Community of Muzo after the Plague of 1629," *Hispanic American Historical Review* 47 (1967), 338-343.

Frisancho, A. R., "Nutritional Influences on Human Growth and Maturation," in K. A. Bennett (ed.), *Yearbook of Physical Anthropology*, Vol. 21. Washington, DC: American Association of Physical Anthropologists, 1978, 174-191.

Frish, R. E., "Demographic Implications of the Biological Determinants of Female Fecundity," *Social Biology* 22 (1975), 17-22.

——————— "Some Further Notes on Population, Food Intake, and Natural Fertility," in H. Levidon and J. Menken (eds.), *Natural Fertility*, Liege, Belgium: Ordina Editions, no date. 137-147.

Gerhard, P., *The Southeast Frontier of New Spain*, Princeton: Princeton University Press, 1979.

——————— *A Guide to the Historical Geography of New Spain*, Cambridge: Cambridge University Press, 1972.

Gibson, Charles, *The Aztecs Under Spanish Rule*, Stanford, California: Stanford University Press, 1964.

Gluck, L. H., "On the Climate, Diseases, and Materia Medica of the Sandwich (Hawaiian) Islands," *New York Journal of Medicine* 14 (1855), 169-211.

Gonzáles, E. R., and R. Mellafe, "La Función de la Famila en la Historia Social Hispanoamericana Colonial," *Anuario del Instituto Investigaciones Históricas* 8 (1965), 57-81.

Guerra, Francisco, "Aztec Science and Technology," *History of Science* 8 (1969), 32-52.

——————— "Aztec Medicine," *Medical History* 10 (1966), 315-338.

Habakkuk, H. J., *Population Growth and Econoomic Development Since 1750*, Leicester, U.K: Leister University Press, 1971.

Harvey, D., *Explanation in Geography*, New York: St. Martin's Press, 1969.

Hassig, Ross, *Trade, Tribute, and Transportation, The Sixteenth-Century Political Economy of the Valley of Mexico*, Norman: The University of Oklahoma Press, 1985.

————— "The Famine of One Rabbit: Ecological Causes and Social Consequences of a Pre-Colombian Calamity," *Journal of Anthropological Research* 37 (1981), 171-182.

Hatcher, John, *Plague, Population and the English Economy 1348-1530*, London and Basingstoke: The Macmillan Press Ltd., 1977.

Henige, D., "On the Contact Population of Hispañola: History as Higher Mathematics," *Hispanic American Historical Review* 58 (1978), 217-237.

Hernández, M., A., Chavez, and H. Bourges. *Valor Nutritivo de los Alimentos Mexicanos: Tablas de uso Práctico*, Mexico: Publicaciones de la División de Nutrición L 12, 6a Instituto Nacional de la Nutrición, 1974.

Hindley, K., "Reviving the food of the Aztecs," *Science News* 116 (1979), 168-169.

Hirsh, A., *Handbook of Geographic and Historical Pathology*, London: New Sydenham Society, 1883.

Hirst, L. Fabian, *The Conquest of Plague*, Oxford: Clarendon Press, 1953.

Hollingsworth, Mary F., and T. H. Hollingsworth, "Plague Mortality Rates by Age and Sex in the Parish of St. Botolph's without Bishopsgate, London, 1603," *Population Studies* 25 (1971), 131-146.

Hollingsworth, T. H., *Historical Demography*, Ithaca, NY: Cornell University Press, 1969.

Hopkins, D. R., *Princes and Peasants, Smallpox in History*, Chicago: University of Chicago Press, 1983.

Hugo, G. J., "The Demographic Impact of Famine: A Review," in B. Currey and G. J. Hugo (eds.), *Famine as a Geographical Phenomena*, Boston: D. Reidel Publishing Co., 1984, 7-31.

Huss-Ashmore, R., "Fat and Fertility: Demographic Implications of Differential Fat Storage," in K. A. Bennett (ed.), *Yearbook of Physical Anthropology*, New York: Alan R. Liss, Inc., 1980, 23, 65-91.

Jaramillo Uribe, J., "La Población Indígena de Colombia en el Momento de la Conquísta y sus Transformaciones Posteriores," *Anuario Colombiano de Historia Social y de la Cultura* 1 (1964), 239-293.

Johnson, Douglas L., and Thomas M. Whitmore, *Population Reconstruction of the Egyptian Nile Valley: 4000 B.C. to Present*, Millennial Long Waves in Human Occupance Project: Technical Paper #3, Clark University, 1987.

Joralemon, D., "New World Depopulation and the Case of Disease," *Journal of Anthropological Research* 38 (1982), 108-127.

Judd, C.S. Jr., "Depopulation in Polynesia," *Bulletin of the History of Medicine* 51 (1977), 585-593.

Kane, Peny, "The Demography of Famine," *Genus* 18 (1987), 43-58.

Katz, S. H., M. L. Hediger, and L. A. Valleroy, "Traditional Maize Processing Techniques of the New World," *Science* 184 (1974), 765-773.

Kehoe, T. F., and A. B. Kehoe, "Comments on H. F. Dobyns, 'Estimating Aboriginal American Population: an Appraisal of Techniques with a New Hemisphere Estimate'," *Current Anthropology* 7 (1966), 395-415.

Keys, A., J. Brozek, A. Henschul, O. Mickelsen, and H. L. Taylor, *The Biology of Human Starvation,* Vol. 1, Minneapolis: University of Minnesota Press, 1950.

Kicza, John E., "Migration to Major Metropoles in Colonial Mexico," in David J. Robinson (ed.), *Migration in Colonial Spanish America*, Cambridge: Cambridge University Press, 1990, 193-211.

Kroeber, A.L., *Cultural and Natural Areas of North America*, University of California Publications in American Archaeology and Ethnology Vol. 38, Berkeley: University of California Press, 1939.

Kubler, George, "Population Movements in Mexico 1520-1600," *Hispanic American Historical Review* 22 (1942), 606-643.

Lang, R., "Plagues and Pestilence in Polynesia: The Nineteenth-Century Cook Islands Experience," *Bulletin of the History of Medicine* 58 (1984), 325-346.

Las Casas, B. de, *Obras Escogidas de Fray Bartolomé de las Casas*, J. Pérez de Tudela (ed.). Madrid: Ediciones Atlas, 1957-1958.

Le Roy Ladurie, Emmanuel, "Famine Amenorrhoea (Seventeenth-Twentieth Centuries)," in Robert Forster and Orest Ranum (eds.), *Biology of Man in History: Selections from the Annales Économies, Sociétés, Civilisations*, Trans. Elborg Forster and Patricia M. Ranum, Baltimore and London: The Johns Hopkins University Press, 1975, 163-178.

247

Lipschutz, A., "La Despoblación de las Indias después de la Conquísta," *América Indígena* 26 (1966), 227-247.

MacLeod, Murdo J., *Spanish Central America A Socioeconomic History, 1520-1720*, Berkley: University of California Press, 1973.

Mata, L.J., "Malnutrition-Infection Interactions in the Tropics," *The American Journal of Tropical Medicine and Hygiene* 24 (1975), 564-574.

May, J. M., "Medical Geography: Its Methods and Objectives," *Geographical Review* 40 (1950), 9-41.

McArthur, N., "The Demography of Primitive Populations," *Science* 167 (1970), 1097-1101.

McBryde, F. W., "Influenza in America During the Sixteenth Century (Guatemala: 1523, 1559-62, 1576)," *Bulletin of the History of Medicine* 8 (1940), 296-302.

McEvedy, C., and R. Jones, *Atlas of World Population History*, London: Penguin Books, 1978.

McKeown, T., "Food, Infection, and Population," in R.I. Rotberg and T. K. Rabb (eds.), *Hunger and History, The Impact of Changing Food Production and Consumption Patterns on Society*, Cambridge: Cambridge University Press, 1983, 29-49.

McNeill, William H., *Plagues and Peoples*, Garden City, NY: Anchor Books, 1976.

Meadows, D. H., "The Unavoidable A Priori," in J. Randers (ed.), *Elements of the System Dynamics Method*, Cambridge, MA: The M.I.T. Press, 1980, 23-57.

Means, P.A., *Ancient Civilizations of the Andes*, New York: Charles Scribner's Sons, 1931.

Mercer, A. J., "Smallpox and Epidemiological-Demographic Change in Europe: The Role of Vaccination," *Population Studies* 39 (1985), 287-307.

Messer, E., "The Small but Healthy Hypothesis: Historical, Political, and Ecological Influences on Nutritional Standards," *Human Ecology* 14 (1986), 57-75.

Mooney, J., *The Aboriginal Population of America North of Mexico*, Miscellaneous Collections 80, No. 7, Washington, DC: Smithsonian Institution, 1928.

Morley, D., "The Severe Measles of West Africa," *Proceedings of the Royal Society of Medicine* 57 (1964), 846-849.

Morris, Christopher, "The Plague in Britain," *The Historical Journal* 14 (1971), 205-224.

Mosley, W. H., "The Effects of Nutrition on Natural Fertility," in H. Levidon and J. Menken (ed.), *Natural Fertility*, Liege, Belgium: Ordina Editions, no date, 85-105.

Murray, J., A. Murray, M. Murray, and C. Murray, "The Biological Supression of Malaria: an Ecological and Nutritional Interrelationship of a Host and Two Parasites," *The American Journal of Clinical Nutrition* 31 (1978), 1363-1366.

National Geographic Society, *Aztec World*, (map) Washington, DC: National Geographic Society, 1980.

Neprash, J. A., "Some Problems in the Correlation of Spatially Distributed Variables," *American Statistical Association Supplement* 29 (1934), 167-168.

Newman, M. T., "Aboriginal New World Epidemiology and Medical Care, and the Impact of Old World Disease Imports," *American Journal of Physical Anthropology* 45 (1978), 667-672.

—————— "Adaptations in the Physique of American Aborigines to Nutritional Factors," *Human Biology* 32 (1960), 288-313.

Nuttels, N., "Medical Problems in Newly Contacted Groups," In *Pan American Health Organization Scientific Publication # 165, Biomedical Challenges Presented by the American Indian*, Washington, DC: Pan American Health Organization, 1968, 77-81.

Offner, Jerome A. "Household Organization in the Texcocan Heartland: The Evidence in the Codex Vergara," in H. R. Harvey and H.J. Prem (eds.), *Explorations in Ethnohistory, Indians of Central Mexico in the Sixteenth Century*, Albuquerque: University of New Mexico Press, 1984, 127-146.

—————— "Archival Reports of Poor Crop Yields in the Early Postconquest Texcocan Heartland and their Implications for Studies of Aztec Period Populations," *American Antiquity* 45 (1980), 848-856.

Ogden, P.E. "Population Geography," in R. J. Johnston (ed.), *The Dictionary of Human Geography*, Oxford: Basin Blackwell Ltd., 1981, 355-356.

Ortíz de Montellano, B., "Aztec Cannibalism: An Ecological Necessity?" *Science* 200 (1978), 611-617.

Panum, P. L., *Observations Made During the Epidemic of Measles on the Faroe Islands in the Year 1846*, New York: American Publishing Association, 1940.

Parsons, J. R., "The Role of Chinampa Agriculture in the Food Supply of Aztec Tenochtitlan," in C. E. Cleland (ed.), *Cultural Change and Continuity: Essays in Honor of James Bennett Griffin*, New York: Academic Press, 1976, 233-257.

Patterson, K. David, *Pandemic Influenza 1700-1900*, Totowa, NJ: Rowman & Littlefield, 1986.

Peart, A. F. W., and F. P. Nagler, "Measles in the Canadian Arctic, 1952," *Canadian Journal of Public Health* 45: (1954), 146-157.

Petersen, W., "A Demographers View of Prehistoric Demography," *Current Anthropology* 16 (1975), 227-245, 461-463.

——————*Population*, Third ed., New York: MacMillan Publishing, Inc., 1975.

Pollitzer, R., *Plague*, World Health Organization Monograph Series No. 22, Geneva: World Health Organization, 1954.

Posey, Darrell A., "Entomological Considerations in Southeastern Aboriginal Demography," *Ethnohistory* 23 (1976), 147-160.

Post, J. D., *Food Shortage, Climatic Variability, and Epidemic Disease in Preindustrial Europe*, Ithaca, NY: Cornell University Press, 1985.

Preston, S. H., *Mortality Patterns in National populations, With Special Reference to Recorded Cause of Death*, New York: Academic Press, 1976.

Ramenofsky, A. F., *Vectors of Death The Archaeology of European Contact*, Albuquerque: University of New Mexico Press, 1987.

Razzell, P., *The Conquest of Smallpox: The Impact of Innoculation on Smallpox Mortality in Eighteenth Century Britian*, Sussex: Caliban Books, 1977.

Ricketson, O. G. Jr., and E. Bayles, *Uaxactun Guatemala, Group E - 1926-1931. Part 1: The excavations; Part 2: The Artifacts*, Carnegie Institutions of Washington Publication No. 477, 1937.

Rivet, P., "Langues Américaines," in A. Meillet and M. Cohen (eds.), *Les Langues des Monde*, Vol. 12. Paris: Collection Linguistique, Société du Linguistique, 1924.

Robertson, W., *The History of America*, Vol. 2. London, 1777.

Robinson, A. H., "The Necessity of Weighing Values in Correlation Analysis of Areal Data," *Annals of the Association of American Geographers* 46 (1956), 233-236.

Robinson, D. J., "Introduction: Towards a Typology of Migration in Colonial Spanish America," in D.J. Robinson (ed.), *Migration in Spanish Colonial America*, Cambridge: Cambridge University Press, 1990, 1-17.

——————— "Introduction," in D. J. Robinson (ed.), *Studies in Spanish American Population History*, Boulder, CO: Westview Press, 1981, 1-23.

Rogers, S. L., "A Comparison Between Sixteenth Century Medicine in Europe and Pre-Cortesian Mexico," *Actas XLI Congresso Internacional de Americanistas* 1 (1974), 49-55.

Rosenblat, A., "The Population of Hispañola at the time of Columbus," in W.M. Denevan (ed.), *The Native Population of the Americas in 1492*, Madison, WI: University of Wisconsin Press, 1976.

——————— *La Población de América en 1492, Viejos y Nuevos Cálculos*, Mexico City: El Colegio de México, 1967.

——————— *La población y el mestizaje en America*, Vol. 1, Buenos Aires: Editorial Nova, 1954.

Rotberg, R. I., and T. K. Rabb. "The Relationship of Nutrition, Disease, and Social Conditions: A Graphical Presentation," in R. I. Rotberg and T.K. Rabb (eds.), "Hunger and History," Cambridge: Cambridge University Press, 1983, 305-308.

Russell, Josiah Cox, *British Medieval Population*. Albuquerque, NM, 1948.

Sánchez-Albornoz, N., "The Population of Colonial Spanish America," in Leslie Bethell (ed.), *The Cambridge History of Latin America, Volume II: Colonial Latin America*, Cambridge: Cambridge University Press, 1984, 3-36.

——————— *The Population of Latin America: A History*, Berkeley: University of California Press, 1974.

Sanders, W. T., "The Agricultural History of the Basin of Mexico," in E. R. Wolf (ed.), *The Valley of Mexico*, Albuquerque: The University of New Mexico Press, 1976.

251

──────── "The Population of the Central Mexican Symbiotic Region, the Basin of Mexico, and the Teotihuacán Valley in the Sixteenth Century," in W.M. Denevan (ed.), *The Native Population of the Americas in 1492*, Madison, WI: University of Wisconsin Press, 1976, 85-150.

──────── "The Population of the Teotihuacan Valley, the Basin of Mexico, and the Central Mexican Symbiotic Region in the 16th Century," In *The Natural Environment, Contemporary Occupation and 16th Century Population of the Valley*, The Teotihuacan Valley Project Final Report, Vol. 1, University Park, PA: Department of Anthropology, 1970, 385-457.

Sanders, W. T., J. R. Parsons, and R. S. Santley, *The Basin of Mexico: Ecological Processes in the Evolution of a Civilization*, New York: Academic Press, 1979.

Santley, R. S., and E. K. Rose, "Diet, Nutrition, and Population Dynamics in the Basin of Mexico," *World Archaeology* 11 (1979), 185-207.

Sapper, K., "Die Zahl und die Volkdichte der Indianischen Bevolkerung in Amerika von der Conquista und in der Gegenwart," In *Proceedings of the Twenty-first International Congress of Americanists, First part*, Leiden: E.J. Brill, 1924, 95-104.

Sauer, C. O., *The Early Spanish Main*, Berkeley: University of California Press, 1966.

──────── *Aboriginal Population of Northwestern Mexico*, Ibero-Americana 10, Berkeley: The University of California Press, 1935.

Schendel, Gordon, *Medicine in Mexico*, Austin, TX: University of Texas Press, 1968.

Scrimshaw, N. S., "Functional Consequences of Malnutrition for Human Populations: A Comment," in R. I. Rotberg and T. K. Rabb (eds.), *Hunger and History, The Impact of Changing Food Production and Consumption Patterns on Society*, Cambridge: Cambridge University Press, 1983, 211-213.

──────── "Interactions of Malnutrition and Infection: Advances in Understanding," in R. E. Olson (ed.), *Protein Calorie Malnutrition*, New York: Academic Press, 1975, 353-367.

Scrimshaw, N. S., C. E. Taylor, and J. E. Gordon, *Interactions of Nutrition and Infection*, Geneva: World Health Organization, 1968.

Seckler, D., "The 'Small But Healthy?' Hypothesis: A Reply to Critics," *Economic and Political Weekly* (1984), 1886-1888.

Shea, D. E., "A Defense of Small Population Estimates for the Colonial Andes in 1520," in W. M. Denevan (ed.), *The Native Population of the Americas in 1492*, Madison, WI: University of Wisconsin Press, 1976, 157-180.

Shrewsbury, J. F. D., *A History of Bubonic Plague in the British Isles*, Cambridge: Cambridge University Press, 1970.

Simpson, L. B., *Exploitation of Land in Central Mexico in the Sixteenth Century*, Ibero-Americana 36, Berkeley: University of California Press, 1952.

Sinnecker, H., *General Epidemiology*, Translated by N. Walker, London: Wiley, 1976.

Slack, Paul, *The Impact of Plague in Tudor and Stuart England*, London: Routledge & Kegan Paul, 1985.

Slicher van Bath, B. H., "The Calculation of the Population of New Spain, Especially for the Period before 1570," *Boletín de Estudios Lationamericanos y del Caribe* 24 (1978), 67-95.

Soustelle, J., *The Daily Life of the Aztecs on the Eve of the Spanish Conquest*, London: Weidenfield and Nicholson, 1961.

Spinden, H. J., "The Population of Ancient America," *Geographic Review* 18 (1928), 641-660.

Stearn, E., and A. E. Stearn, *The Effect of Smallpox on the Destiny of the Amerindian*, Boston: Bruce Humphries Inc., 1945.

Steward, J. H., "The Native Population of South America," in J. H. Steward (ed.), *Handbook of South American Indians*, Vol. 5, Smithsonian Institution, Bureau of American Ethnology Bulletin No. 143, Washington DC: U.S. Government Printing Office, 1949, 655-668.

Taylor, C. E., and C. DeSweemer, "Nutrition and Infection," in M. Rechcigl (ed.), *Food, Nutrition and Health, World Review of Nutrition and Dietetics*, Basel: Karger, 1973, Vol. 16, 203-225.

Thomas, E. N., and D. L. Anderson, "Additional Comments on Weighting Values in Correlation Analysis of Areal Data," *Annals of the Association of American Geographers* 55 (1965), 492-505.

Tolstoy, P., and S. K. Fish, "Surface and Subsurface Evidence for Community Size at Coapexco, Mexico," *Journal of Field Archaeology* 2 (1975), 97-104.

Tooth, J. S. H., and I. C. Lewis, "Measles Epidemic in a Primative Isolated Community," *Medical Journal of Australia* 1 (1963), 182-186.

Turner, B. L. II, "The Specialist-Synthesis Approach to the Revival of Geography: The Case of Cultural Ecology," *Annals of the Association of American Geographers* 79 (1989), 88-100.

——————— *Population Reconstruction of the Central Maya Lowlands: 1000 B.C. to Present*, Millennial Long Waves of Human Occupance Project, Technical Paper #2, Clark University, 1986.

——————— "Comparisons of Agrotechnologies in the Basin of Mexico and Central Maya lowlands: Formative to the Classic Maya Collapse," in A. G. Miller (ed.), *Highland-Lowland Interaction in Mesoamerica, Interdisciplinary Approaches*, Washington, DC: Dunbarton Oaks Research Library and Collection, 1983, 13-47.

Turner, B. L. II, and S. B. Brush, "Purpose, Classification, and Organization," in B. L. Turner II and S. B. Brush, (eds.) *Comparative Farming Systems*, New York: The Guilford Press, 1987, 3-10.

United Nations Department of Economic and Social Affairs, *The Determinants and Consequences of Population Trends*, Vol. 1, New York: The United Nations, 1973.

Veblen, T. T., "Native Population Decline in Totonicapan Guatemala," *Annals of the Association of American Geographers* 67 (1977), 484-499.

Vellard, J., "Causes Biológicas de la Desaparición de los Indios Americanos," *Boletín del Instituto Riva Agüero* 2 (1956), 77-93.

Wachtel, N., "The Indian and the Spanish Conquest," in L. Bethell (ed.), *The Cambridge History of Latin America*, Vol. 1, Cambridge: Cambridge University Press, 1984, 207-248.

Watkins, S. C., and J. Menken, "Famines in Historical Perspective," *Population and Development Review* 11 (1985), 647-675.

Watkins, S. C., and E. van der Walle, "Nutrition, Mortality, and Population Size: Malthus' Court of Last Resort," in R. T. Rotberg and T.K. Rabb (ed.), *Hunger and History, The Impact of Changing Food Production and Consumption Patterns on Society*, Cambridge: Cambridge University Press, 1983, 7-28.

Whitmore, Thomas M., and B. L. Turner II, *Population Reconstruction of the Basin of Mexico: 1150 B.C. to Present*, Millennial Longwaves of Human Occupance Project: Technical Paper #1, Clark University, 1986.

Wilken, G. C., "The Ecology of Gathering in a Mexican Farming Region," *Economic Botany* 24 (1970), 286-295.

Wisseman, Charles L. Jr., "Rickettsial Diseases," in F. H. S. Top and Paul F. Wehrle (eds.), *Communicable and Infectious Diseases*, Eighth edition, Saint Louis: The C. V. Mosby Company, 1976.

Woods, R., *Theoretical Population Geography*, Burnt Mill, UK: Longman Group Ltd., 1982.

Wrigley, E. A., and R. S. Schofield, *The Population History of England 1541-1871: A Reconstruction*, London: Edward Arnold, 1981.

Zambardino, R. A., "Mexico's Population in the Sixteenth Century: Demographic Anomaly or Mathematical Illusion?" *Journal of Interdisciplinary History* 11 (1980), 1-27.

—————— "Critique of David Henige; 'On the Contact Population of Hispanola: History as Higher Mathematics'," *Hispanic American Historical Review* 58 (1978), 700-704.

Zdrodovskii, P. F., and H. M. Golinevich, *The Rickettsial Diseases*, Trans. B. Haigt, New York: Pergamon Press, 1960.

Zelinski, W. A., *Prologue to Population Geography*, Englewood Cliffs, NJ: Prentice-Hall, 1966.

Zinsser, H., *Rats, Lice and History*, Boston: Little Brown and Company, 1934.

Index

Agave worms (Hypopta agavis), 91

Agricultural demand models 83–84
consumption demand in, 86
surplus and, 83, 92–93
total production unit (PU) demand in,
86, 100, 103–104, 105
tribute demand in, 83, 93
urban demand in, 101–102

Agricultural labor, 28, 83, 84

Agricultural productivity (*see* Maize)

Agriculture, 28, (*see also* Agricultural
demand models)
adverse environmental conditions and,
105–106, 107, 122, 199
description of in Basin of Mexico,
94–97
logic of in MEXIPOP, 98
labor tribute and, 83, 124
morbidity rate (synergy) and, 28, 82,
105, 122, 124
non-agricultural population of Basin of
Mexico, 101–102, 103, 104, 105
production (food) sub-models in
MEXIPOP
baseline assumptions of, 122–124
logic of, 83, 86, 98–108
maize tribute in, 93, 99, 105, 107,
124, 129–130, 133, 135, (*see also*
Maize)
sensitivity tests of, 129–130
surplus set-aside in MEXIPOP, 83,
92–93, 99, 108
baseline assumptions of, 122–123
sensitivity tests of, 133–136

Amaranths (Amaranthus spp.), 90, 91, 92

American trypanosomiasis, 51

American leishmaniasis, 51

Amerindian population
decline in
compared with European countries,
206–207
due to epidemics, 2, 16, 18, 25–26,
161–165, 207–210, 214

due to epidemic induced famines, 21,
25, 28, 124, 130–132, 143–144,
145–146, 149–150, 166–174, 211,
214
due to famines induced by adverse
environmental conditions, 28,
174–179, 212
due to homicide and migration, 2–3,
16–17, 21, 25–26, 212, 214
due to other causes, 2, 21, 25, 17–18,
179–180, 214
role of demographic structure, 18–19,
26, 210, 214
scale of, 202–203, 213
step-like pattern of, 160, 198, 203,
213
genetic inferiority of, 208–209, 214
historical estimates of, 2, 3, 4–5,
109–118, 120, 137, 153, 213
criticism of, 5–11, 13–16, 18–19,
115, 116, 139, 203, 213
data and evidence for, 5–11, 13–16
influence of epidemics on dates of
Hispanic counts used to create,
203–204
methodology used to create, 9, 5–11,
13–16, 18–19
in Basin of Mexico
historical estimates of, 3–5
simulation of, 191, 204
compared with historical estimates,
203, 213
Mexican, compared with best
simulation, 206
North American, 7
pre-Columbian, 14–15, 204
South American, 7
Western Hemisphere, 1–2, 6–7, 13, 204,
206, 207, 211

Armadillos (Dasypus sexcintus), 91

Aquatic insects, larvae, and eggs (Ahuauhtl
and Azayacatl), 91

Arthritides, 50

255

DATE DUE

MAR 2 8 1995			
APR 1 0 1995			
NOV 1 0 1997			
OCT 2 3 1997			
DEC 5 1999			
APR 0 1 2006			

DEMCO 38-297